K.-D. Kühn

Bone Cements

Springer

Berlin
Heidelberg
New York
Barcelona
Hong Kong
London
Milano
Paris
Singapore
Tokyo

K.-D. Kühn

Bone Cements

Up-to-Date Comparison
of Physical and Chemical Properties
of Commercial Materials

With 207 Figures, 190 in colour and 132 Tables

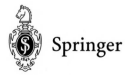 Springer

Dr. Klaus-Dieter Kühn

Heraeus Kulzer GmbH & Co. KG
Philipp-Reis-Straße 8/13,
D-61273 Wehrheim/Taunus

ISBN   3-540-67207-9 Springer-Verlag Berlin Heidelberg New York

Library of Congress Cataloging-in-Publication Data

Kühn, Klaus-Dieter:
Bone cements / Klaus-Dieter Kühn. – Berlin; Heidelberg; New York; Barcelona; Hongkong;
London; Mailand; Paris; Singapur; Tokio;
Springer, 2000
      ISBN 3-540-67207-9

Springer-Verlag is a company in the BertelmannSpringer publishing group
© Springer-Verlag Berlin Heidelberg 2000
Printed in Germany

Cover design: *design & production* GmbH, Heidelberg
Typesetting: cicero Lasersatz, Dinkelscherben
Printed on acid-free paper – SPIN: 10761226   18/3135   5 4 3 2 1 0

Foreword

Methyl methacrylate (MMA) is the basic component of bone cements. To use it, a dough is prepared from the liquid and powder by mixing right before application, which is normally done by the operating team. During its working phase the dough is then inserted into the tissue where polymerization is completed. Thus, the final implant polymethylmethacrylate (PMMA) is only created at the implantation site.

Besides methyl methacrylate, bone cements sometimes contain other methacrylates, such as butyl methacrylate. To achieve X-ray opacity, radiopacifiers (zirconium dioxide or barium sulfate) are added to the powder. Both the liquid and powder components contain additives (initiator and activator) that launch polymerization and control the setting when mixed together. Moreover, softener and emulsifiers are sometimes used. The addition of antibiotics to the powder component in order to prevent or treat infections has become especially important.

Commercial bone cements differ in composition and the course of curing. Some are designed for high and others for low viscosity. The way the user handles and applies the cement always crucially influences the quality of the implant.

This is why clear and comprehensive information about the cements should be available to show the user how all the relevant factors work together and how they depend on each other. It should also be possible to compare the different cements. Such information has not been readily available before and one can only obtain partial information by thorough study of the literature. Therefore, this book fills a definite gap and sets new standards at the same time!

The intention of the author, an excellent authority in this field, was to create a reference book on bone cements, and he succeeded. The book gives all information necessary in a clear manner. It starts with an explanation of polymerization with its associated phenomena, such as the setting characteristic, generation of heat, shrinkage or residual monomer; the relationship between molecular weight and mechanical strength is indicated, as well as the dependency of strength on the sterilization method. Then all the test methods used are presented, followed by individual chapters on all bone cements on the market. Their composition and chemical and physical properties are set forth in detail. Special emphasis is put upon the working characteristics. The packaging of the cements is described in detail and compared to the ISO 5833 requirements. All results are summarized and compared thoroughly.

Thus, this book is really a treasure for:

- the disciplines of orthopaedics, surgery, neurosurgery, cranial/facial surgery and others using bone cement,
- further examinations in the field of materials science,
- disciplines only occasionally occupied with bone cements with a need for special information (examination of allergic reactions, cases of failures of bone/joint implants).

I hope that the book is widely accepted and that it is used by people in many fields.

March, 2000   H. G. Willert

Preface

Until only a few years ago, all bone cements had to comply with the tough requirements of the German Drug Law (AMG). With the introduction of the Medical Device Law (MPG) bone cements are no longer classified as drugs but as medical devices, which facilitates the registration of new products. Unfortunately this means lowered requirements for the growing number of bone cements on the market.

Since all cements are based on the same chemical substance, methyl methacrylate, one could think that all cements are alike if further details are not taken into consideration. For the surgeon, his staff and, of course, for the patient, it is very important to make the optimal choice in order to assure the best long-term results for the patient.

For a scientifically based selection an extensive comparative examination of all cements in the market is necessary. These data were not available thus leaving the surgeon and the patient in an unsatisfactory situation. So we have performed this full comparison and compiled the results. We did not only apply tests according to the relevant standard but also developed other methods yielding worthy data about material properties of high importance for the surgeon and the patient.

Why was this work carried out in our company? We have followed the development of bone cements very closely ever since they were used, so we have gained a high competence in the field of methacrylate chemistry over some decades. Moreover, we had the unique chance to learn from Dr. W. Ege, a bone cement specialist known all over the world. It is him, a great scientist and a wonderful person, that I want to express especially my personal gratitude for helping me understand the exquisite matter of methacrylates. The cooperation of Heraeus Kulzer with the competent partners Biomet-Merck and Schering-Plough, well-tested for many years, also proved very successful.

Heraeus Kulzer GmbH & Co. KG will continue to be a center of competence in the field of bone cements.

All bone cements were tested according to ISO 5833/2. Additionally we examined the handling properties, release of antibiotic, content and release of residual monomer and the glass transition temperatures. On some products we also tested the fatigue strength to obtain indications of the long-term stability in the body.

The presented results show clearly that bone cements are not all alike.

March, 2000   K.-D. Kühn

Prefazio

Acknowledgements

I wish to express my special gratitude to Dr. Chr. Tuchscherer (department of medical R & D, Heraeus Kulzer GmbH & Co. KG, Wehrheim) for taking care of all the arduous work concerned with the making of the book, especially producing tables/charts, photographing the products and scanning the pictures as well as translating various parts of the book. Together with colleagues from the medical R & D lab, he has also carried out tests according to ISO 5833 and compiled the results. I also want to give thanks to Mrs. H. Maurer of the same department, for the carrying out of tests according to DIN standards, and for the determination of molecular weights and glass transition temperatures. Mr. H. Scheuermann and his staff (analytical lab of the QA department of Heraeus Kulzer GmbH & Co. KG) have, besides mechanical tests according to ISO done valuable analytical work, especially the determination of residual monomer and release of antibiotic. Mr. Scheuermann also made the qualitative and quantitative analysis of polymers, supported by Mr. Abraham (Röhm GmbH, Darmstadt). I also owe my gratitude to Drs. U. Soltész and Schäfer (Fraunhofer-Institut für Werkstofftechnik, Freiburg) for the fatigue tests, and to Dr. R. Specht and Mr. Kampfmann (Merck-Biomaterial GmbH, Darmstadt) for SEM and x-ray photographs. Moreover Mr. Krause (Merck-Biomaterial GmbH, Darmstadt) and Mr. P. Stearns (Schering-Plough, Kenilworth) supported our work by supplying free units of many cements. Translation work has also be done by Mrs. A. Keishold (Heraeus Kulzer GmbH & Co. KG, Wehrheim), Mrs. M. Kapahnke (Wehrheim) and Mrs. P. Kühn (Marburg/L.). Last, but not least, I would like to thank Prof. Willert (University of Hannover) for his friendly foreword.

Contents

1
Introduction and Scope

Bone cements are used for the fixation of artificial joints. The cements fill the free space between the prosthesis and the bone. The connection between the cement and the bone and between the cement and the prosthesis is only mechanical; therefore, it has been repeatedly, intensively studied ever since bone cements were introduced in hip arthroplasty. The irregularities of the bone surface and the penetration of the cement into the trabecular spongiosa are an important prerequisite for long survival of implants (Charnley, 1970). In this regard, the cement acts as an elastic zone that, because of its stiffness, cushions the forces affecting the bone.

All bone cements currently on the market are chemically based on the same basic substance: methyl methacrylate (MMA). Chemically, MMA is an ester of methacrylic acid, a substance scientists had already begun to study intensively by the beginning of the twentieth century.

In order to learn more about these interesting polymers, Professor Pechmann assigned the theme »polymerization products of acrylic acid« to his pupil Otto Röhm for his thesis more than 70 years ago in Tübingen. Based on the results of his research, Otto Röhm later founded the company Röhm and Haas. In their research laboratories, acrylates were further developed. By 1928, a large-scale technical synthesis for MMA was already established. This led to the birth of dentures using MMA. This technique was patented by Bauer (1935; patent DRP 652821) during the same year. When problems regarding the technical production had been clarified to a very large extent and the availability of the materials was thus guaranteed, scientists intensively occupied themselves with the questions of how and where to use these new substances and how to develop modifications that would lead to the unknown applications.

By 1936, the company Kulzer (1936; patent DRP 737058) had already found that a dough can be produced by mixing ground polymethylmethacrylate (PMMA) powder and a liquid monomer that hardens when benzoyl peroxide (BPO) is added and the mixture is heated to 100°C in a stone mold. The first clinical use of these PMMA mixtures was an attempt to close cranial defects in monkeys in 1938. When these experiences became known, surgeons were anxious to try these materials in plastic surgery on humans. The heat curing polymer Paladon 65 was soon used for closing cranial defects in humans by producing plates in the laboratory and later adjusting the hardened material on the spot (Kleinschmitt 1941).

When chemists discovered that the polymerization of MMA would occur by itself at room temperature if a co-initiator is added, the companies Degussa and

Kulzer (1943; patent DRP 973 590), using tertiary aromatic amines, established a protocol for the chemical production of PMMA bone cements in 1943; this process is still valid to this day. These studies must be considered to be the birth of PMMA bone cements.

At the end of World War II, many German patents in the field of methacrylates had to be forfeited to the victors because of the danger of a possible German rearmament. After that, the world-wide practical use of the studies started by Otto Röhm obviously occurred quickly. PMMA bone cements (which are still on the market today) were developed independently in several countries; these cements include CMW, Palacos R and Simplex P.

The advantageous handling properties of MMA polymer mixtures have remained the object of many research projects, in part because the cements on the market differ considerably in this respect, even though their chemical bases are identical. Kiaer (1951) first used PMMA as pure anchoring material by fixing acrylic glass caps on the femoral head after removing the cartilage (Haboush 1953; Henrichsen et al. 1953).

Studies on the use of the materials in cranial plastics were started with the large-scale technical production of the polymers (Worringer and Thomalske 1953). The fast-curing resins were then also used for filling defects of injuries of the visceral skeleton (Rau 1963).

Judet and Judet (1956) were the first to introduce an arthroplastic surgical method. Soon, however, it became apparent that the PMMA (Plexiglas) prosthesis used could not be integrated in the body (for biological and mechanical reasons). In 1958, Sir John Charnley first succeeded in anchoring femoral head prostheses in the femur with auto-polymerizing PMMA (Charnley 1960). Charnley called the material used »bone cement on acrylic basis«. His studies described a totally new surgical technique (Charnley 1970).

Essential prerequisites for the acceptance of PMMA in surgery were studies of the reaction of tissue to PMMA implants. Good biocompatibility of PMMA implants at an early date was of vital importance (Henrichsen et al. 1953; Wiltse et al. 1957). The extensive studies of Hullinger (1962) also proved the biocompatibility of hardened PMMA. For example, in extensive studies with cell cultures it was possible to show how a polyurethane (Ostamer, which was used as bone glue for treating bone fractures) led to violent tissue reactions, whereas the PMMA also studied did not cause any cytotoxic reactions (Lehmann and Jenny 1961).

At the end of the 1960s, Buchholz and the company Kulzer were the first to add an antibiotic to bone cements (Ege 1999). Based on the known diffusion process regarding the release of residual monomer, they investigated whether an active ingredient could be dissolved in the cement matrix. The addition of gentamicin sulfate in Palacos R yielded the first encouraging results. Numerous studies were started in the Endoklinik at Hamburg in Germany and resulted in the development of the brand Refobacin-Palacos R, the first antibiotic-loaded bone cement marketed, demonstrating the good cooperation of Merck and Kulzer (Buchholz and Engelbrecht 1970, Buchholz et al. 1981).

In part because of the positive results regarding its biocompatibility, both clinical interest in PMMA material and the number of bone cements on the market rose. In order to create a uniform and reproducible testing basis for PMMA bone cements, the development of a standard was begun in 1976. These attempts were started in the U.S., where standard American Society for Testing and Materials F-451-76 (Standard Specifications for Acrylic Bone Cements; 1978) was developed. On its basis, the protocol ISO 5833/1 (1979) was developed a short time later. Today, all bone cements must comply with the present standard, ISO 5833/2 (1992). While Ungethüm and Hinterberger (1978) made comparative studies of five cements, Edwards and Thomasz (1981) tested eight materials. In addition to chemical and physical properties, special features of packaging and labeling were also reported. By 1984, 15 different cements were already on the market. Scheuermann and Ege (1987) made a detailed survey of the structure and composition of the bone cements current at that time. In addition to chemical and mechanical data for the different cements, their packages (including the labels) were compared with regard to the requirements of the then-valid German drug law (AMG 1998). A short description of the sterilization methods, according to which the cements are treated, was included.

The increasing interest in bone cements and their use in orthopedic surgery led Willert and Buchhorn (1987) to arrange a symposium on bone cement in 1984. They especially wanted to gather together specialists in the field of hip arthroplasty and discuss the properties and clinical significance of the material. The difficulty in comparing the published mechanical and physical properties of PMMA bone cements was a main point of criticism.

Comparative studies of various bone cements have frequently been published. However, they often only deal with a few cement types and some special questions. Hansen and Jensen (1992) compared ten different bone cements strictly according to ISO 5833. New cements can easily be introduced into comparative studies with the so-called old pharmaceutical specialties, Simplex P or Palacos R. For example, Kindt-Larson et al. (1995) made a detailed comparison of Boneloc, a newly developed bone cement that had to be withdrawn from the market (Havelin et al. 1995b), and four other bone cements registered for the U.S. market. Usually, only some of the cements' properties are compared in such studies, and the methods used often cannot be applied to all cements. This unsatisfactory situation makes the user unsure of the relative merits of each cement, as he cannot easily compare the cements on the market. Recently, Lewis (1997) published another detailed review of the properties of six cements, mainly products on the U.S. market.

While there have been great efforts to create a basis valid for all cements by continuously revising the harmonizing standards for PMMA bone cements, the requirements for the manufacture of these sterile materials have, unfortunately, been relaxed. This is surprising; the fields of application of these cements are extremely critical, so the requirements for the manufacturing conditions for bone cements should be quite exacting. For this reason, an abundance of legal requirements has to be heeded in the manufacturing, packaging and sterilization of bone cements. These requirements are not explicitly included in standards but are recorded in general (not always uniform) regulations, such as the European Union Good Manufacturing Practices (EU-GMP) regulations, e.g., EU Guide for the Manufacture of Sterile Products (1998), etc.

The world-wide differences in the categorization of bone cements pose a big problem in the evaluation of the presentation, quality and manufacture of bone cements. In Europe, for example, bone cements were considered to be drugs (according to AMG 1998) until the end of an interim period in June 1998, and manufacturers required registration at the appropriate health authority before placing the product on the market. However, bone cements are today looked upon as medical devices according to the Medical device law (=MPG 1994). Thus, registration can be obtained much more easily via an authorized notified body, and EU-GMP regulations (1998) are no longer imperative. Recently, bone cements were also re-classified in the U.S.; in the future, they will no longer need a PMA (pre-market approval) by the Food and Drug Administration before being placed on the market. The registration of a bone cement can now be attained via a 510-K (pre-market notification process). The consequences this will have (especially on the quality of newly registered materials) remains to be seen.

Ultimately, the surgeon in the operating theater must be assured that products have been manufactured under strict statutory regulations. Relaxation of the statutory injunctions for the registration (and thus the manufacture) of bone cements would probably lead to a flood of new products on the market; this might initially be advantageous for the patient due to the ensuing competition. However, the risk that a cement not manufactured under strict safety regulations will show unsatisfactory clinical results will increase dramatically.

Although intense efforts to create constantly reproducible clinical conditions in hip arthroplasty with valid operating techniques have been made lately (Draenert et al. 1999), a variation in the quality of bone cements caused by a relaxation of statutory injunctions might jeopardize the validity of their use in the future. The handling properties of the cements are of extreme importance for the orthopedic surgeon, because they determine the planning of the operation and the final adjustments before, during and after arthroplastic implantation. Even though ISO 5833 (1992) obliges the manufacturer to print a graph of the handling properties in the manufacturer's instructions, the user often has great difficulty in reproducing the statements on these material parameters. More than 90% of customers' complaints are related to faulty handling properties of the cements. This unsatisfactory situation can be explained as due to the lack of a methodological basis for the determination of the handling properties. The chemical bases of all PMMA cements are comparable; their most evident difference, however, lies in the handling properties of the various cements. These properties are changed by even slight variations of the composition (Wixon and Lautenschlager 1998).

Manufacturers of bone cements supply hospitals with a polymer powder in primary packaging and a monomer liquid in an ampoule; this constitutes the so-called two-component system. The surgical nurse prepares both components during the sterile part of the surgery. Thus, the actual production of the cement dough is performed by nurses in the operating room. Therefore, the nurses (together with the surgeon) have enormous influence on the quality of the cement dough produced; in the end, this will considerably influence the clinical long-term result of a cemented hip, acetabulum or cemented knee.

Hence, it is especially important that the orthopedic surgeon know why and how the numerous bone cements on the market differ and what consequences this may have for the physical, mechanical and biological properties and the handling properties. Usually, the user has no idea of such connections. Unfortunately, if these cement properties and the surgeon's clinical experience are regarded in combination, the considerable differences in the quality of the various cements will only become apparent too late; **not all cements are alike!**

Considerable clinical differences are observed in the current bone cements (as determined using radiostereometric studies, a method of evaluation of micromovements; Mjöberg et al. 1990). In the Swedish Hip Arthroplasty Register (Malchau and Herberts 1996, 1998), a documentation of clinical results with an extremely large group of patients, revision risks depending on the cements used are also discussed. The authors make recommendations regarding the cementing technique and indicate the advantages of certain cements for minimizing the danger of loosening, from a clinical point of view (Havelin et al. 1995b). Furthermore, this independent study clearly shows that a cemented shaft – particularly in the hip – is far superior to a non-cemented shaft (Havelin et al. 1995a). Since cost is a consideration in medical repair measures, long-term studies and the survival of the implant have become especially important. Since a long survival time also depends on the quality of the cement, the choice of the right material is of great consequence. The cost is (at present) approximately 15,000–20,000 DM per total hip arthroplasty (Könning et al. 1997), so long-term studies and survival times are also becoming increasingly important from a political point of view.

This is why the goal of this study was to furnish the user of bone cements with a reference book enabling him to quickly and easily gain a general idea of all bone cements on the market and make a suitable choice of the cement that will produce the best clinical results. For this purpose, all bone cements currently on the market are described in the following chapters. The material properties of the different cements are compared, and advantages and disadvantages for the surgeon and patient will be indicated. Comparative tests for all PMMA bone cements on the market were carried out according to ISO 5833 (1992). Furthermore, new test methods that make possible the characterization and comparison of the cement properties that are most important to the user were introduced.

2
Test Material and Applied Methods

2.1
Material

In Table 1, all bone cements known to us are listed. Therefore, cements that at present play only a minor role, are only used in certain countries, have already been withdrawn from the market or could not be purchased in time by us despite our efforts (CMW 2000, Cemex XL) are also listed. Only the most important cements, however, will be described in detail and will be included in comparative tests.

Table 1. List of bone cement types known to the author

Bone Cements	Responsible Manufacturer	Viscosity type	on the market?
Acrybond	Richards	low	no
AKZ (Antibiotic Simplex®)	Stryker Howmedica	medium	yes
Allofix®-G	Sulzer	low	no
Biocryl 1	Bioland	medium	no
Biocryl 3	Bioland	low	no
Biolos 1	Bioland	medium	no
Biolos 3	Bioland	low	no
Boneloc®	Biomet Inc.USA	System	no
Bonemite	Mochida Pharmaceutical	low	no
C-ment® 1	E. M. C. M. B. V.	high	yes
C-ment® 3	E. M. C. M. B. V.	low	yes
Cemex® Isoplastic (HV)	Tecres	high	yes
Cemex® RX (LV)	Tecres	medium	yes
Cemex®-Genta HV	Tecres	high	yes
Cemex®-Genta LV	Tecres	medium	yes
Cemex® XL	Tecres	low	yes
Cerafix® LV	Ceraver Osteal	low	yes
Cerafixgenta®	Ceraver Osteal	low	yes
CLL 50	Chevalier Prosthetics	low	no
CMW® 1 Gentamicin	DePuy/Johnson & Johnson	high	yes
CMW® 1 radiolucent	DePuy/Johnson & Johnson	high	yes
CMW® 1 radiopaque	DePuy/Johnson & Johnson	high	yes
CMW® 2	DePuy/Johnson & Johnson	high	yes
CMW® 2 G	DePuy/Johnson & Johnson	high	yes
CMW® 2000	DePuy/Johnson & Johnson	high	yes
CMW® 2000 Gentamicin	DePuy/Johnson & Johnson	high	yes
CMW® 3	DePuy/Johnson & Johnson	low	yes
CMW® 3 Gentamicin	DePuy/Johnson & Johnson	low	yes
Copal®	Merck	high	yes
Duracem™ 3	Sulzer	low	yes

Table 1. Continued

Bone Cements	Responsible Manufacturer	Viscosity type	on the market?
Durus® H	Macmed Orthopedics	medium	yes
Durus® HA	Macmed Orthopedics	medium	no
Durus® L	Macmed Orthopedics	low	no
Durus® LA	Macmed Orthopedics	low	no
Endurance®	DePuy/Johnson & Johnson	low	yes
Genta C-ment® 1	E. M. C. M. B. V.	high	yes
Genta C-ment® 3	E. M. C. M. B. V.	low	yes
Implast	Beiersdorf	low	no
Kallokryl K	VEB Spezialchemie	low	no
Medifix 1	Bioland	medium	no
Medifix 3	Bioland	low	no
Nebacetin-Sulfix-6	Sulzer	low	no
Omniplastik	Johnson & Johnson	low	no
Osteobond®	Zimmer	low	yes
Osteopal®	Merck	low	yes
Osteopal® G	Merck	low	yes
Osteopal® HA	Merck	high	no
Osteopal® VS	Merck	high	no
Palacos® LV/E Flow	Schering Plough	low	yes
Palacos® LV/E Flow mit Gentamicin	Schering Plough	low	yes
Palacos® R	Merck/Schering Plough	high	yes
Palacos® R with Gentamicin	Schering Plough	high	yes
Palamed®	Merck	high	yes
Palamed® G	Merck	high	yes
Palavit® HV	Schering Plough	high	no
Palavit® LV	Schering Plough	low	no
Refobacin®-Palacos® R	Merck	high	yes
Scellos 3	Fii	low	no
Subiton	Prothoplast	high	yes
Subiton G	Prothoplast	high	yes
Sulfix®-6	Sulzer	low	no
Sulfix®-60	Sulzer	low	no
Surgical Simplex® P	Stryker Howmedica	medium	yes
Surgical Simplex® P with Microlok®	Stryker Howmedica	medium	yes
Zimmer® dough-type radiolucent	Zimmer	medium	no
Zimmer® dough-type radiopaque	Zimmer	low	yes
Zimmer® LVC	Zimmer	low	no

2.2
Applied Test Methods

All tests described in the following have been performed at the Quality Control lab and the R & D lab of Heraeus Kulzer, Wehrheim, Germany. Some exceptions are mentioned.

2.2.1
Description of the Cements

In addition to the chemical and physical parameters of the cements, the packaging and presentation of cements available on the market will also be described.

2.2.2
Determination of the Polymer Composition

To determine of the monomers on which the polymer is based, pyrolyze a sample of approximately 0.25 g for 5 s at 610°C. Determine the type and quantity of the monomers in the pyrolysate by high-performance liquid chromatography (HPLC) and compare them as far as possible using this method. For reflection scanning electron microscope photographs, the powders were sputtered with gold and pictures were taken using a Hitachi-S-520 camera (Kühn 1991). This was done at Merck Biomaterial GmbH, Darmstadt, Germany.

The polymer compositions have partly also been determined at Röhm GmbH, Darmstadt, Germany (method: GC-MS).

2.2.3
Determination of the Benzoyl Peroxide Content

2.2.3.1
Titration

Weigh approximately 0.5 g of the powder with analytical scales and dilute with 25 ml of chloroform in an Erlenmeyer flask. Seal the flask. After the specimen has dissolved by shaking (with the exception of the insoluble parts), add approximately 20 ml of 10% methanolic potassium iodide. Leave the Erlenmeyer flask in the dark for 20 min.

Titrate the contents of the flask with 0.01 N sodium thiosulfate solution until it is colorless. The calculation is:

percentage of benzoyl peroxide = volume of sodium thiosulfate
(in milliliters) x F x 0.121/weight of the powder (in grams),

where F is the factor of the sodium thiosulfate solution.

2.2.3.2
High-Performance Liquid Chromatography

Mix 0.25 g of the powder (the polymer) with 10 ml of methanol for 10 min, then centrifuge. Analyze the clear solution against standards (0.5%, 1.0% or 2.0% solutions of benzoyl peroxide in methanol).

2.2.4
Determination of the Content of Radiopaque Medium

In cement powders and cements that do not contain any non-volatile components except the radiopaque medium, the content of the radiopaque medium can easily be determined by incineration, as follows. Weigh a sample of the powder in a pre-annealed (approximately 1 h at 700°C in a muffle furnace), weighed crucible cooled to a constant weight.

Heat carefully in an open, not very hot muffle furnace or above a burner (beware of the danger of loss of solid substance by smoking and foaming), then anneal the crucible containing the sample for approximately 1 h at 700°C in a muffle furnace. No traces of carbon (black) should remain. Weigh after cooling to room temperature in a desiccator. The calculation is:

> content (percentage) = 100x[end weight – (weight of empty crucible/ weight of crucible with sample – weight of empty crucible)].

2.2.5
Representation of the Radiopacity

The measurements of the specimen should be 10 x 15 x 3.2 mm. Glue test specimens of the different bone cements of the same size (particularly the same thickness) onto paper. Take a radiograph of the specimens, choosing an energy with which medium blackening is attained and differences in the opacity can easily be seen (40–41 kV, 2–2,5 mAs). The radiographs were taken at Merck Biomaterial GmbH, Darmstadt, Germany.

2.2.6
Release of Residual Monomer

The measurements of the specimen should be 3 x 10 x 15 mm. Prepare the test specimen as follows. Mix the cement according to the manufacturer's instructions. When it is no longer sticky, press the dough into a mold between two foils and wait for it to harden. Saw the test specimens off the plate taken from the mold.

Place five specimens (weighed) with 5 ml of distilled water each in Head-Space Vials 1 h after preparation. Close the vials, and store them at 37°C. After various times (1, 3, 7, 14 days), check the eluate with HPLC against a methyl methacrylate (MMA) standard to determine the residual monomer content. State the results in micrograms of MMA per gram of bone cement (Ege and Scheuermann 1987).

2.2.7
Residual Monomer Content

The measurements of the specimen should be 3 x 10 x 15 mm. Prepare the test specimen as follows. Mix the cement according to the manufacturer's instructions. When it is no longer sticky, press the dough into a mold between two foils and wait for it to harden. Saw the test specimens off the plate taken from the mold.

Store the specimens in distilled water at 37°C. Weigh 0.2 g of a sample into a 22 ml vial and dilute with 5 ml of acetone after various times (0, 1, 3, 7, 14, 28 days). Agitate the tightly closed vial with a magnetic stirrer for 24 h.

Next, add 15 ml of a standard solution; the polymer should totally precipitate. Use the supernatant, a clear solution (centrifuge if necessary), for the analysis (inject 0.5 µl after calibration of the system). State the result as the percentage of MMA relative to the weighed portion of the sample (Ege and Scheuermann 1987).

2.2.8
Determination of the Gentamicin Content

Weigh a powder sample (~3 g). Mix it with 250 ml of distilled water for 30 min and filter it. Dilute 4 ml of this with the eluant until a volume of 50 ml is reached. Calibrate the HPLC system with standard gentamicin. Determine the content in the sample by post-column derivatization; use a fluorescence indicator for detection.

2.2.9
Determination of the Release of Gentamicin

The measurements of the specimen should be 3 x 10 x 15 mm. Prepare the test specimen as follows. Mix the cement according to the manufacturer's instructions. When it is no longer sticky, press the dough into a mold between two foils and wait for it to harden. Saw the test specimens off the plate taken from the mold (3.3 x 10 x 15 mm). Store two specimens each (weighed powder) in 10 ml of distilled water at 37°C. After various times, test the eluate against a gentamicin standard for its content of the antibiotic via HPLC. State the result as milligrams of gentamicin per gram of bone cement.

2.2.10
Determination of the Molecular Weight

Weigh a sample of polymethylmethacrylate (PMMA) or hardened bone cement, respectively, into a volumetric flask. Fill the flask with chloroform and dissolve the sample by shaking. Filter the solution through a glass frit and pour it into a suitable Ubbelohde viscometer. Keep the temperature of the water bath at 20°C.

Determine the flow time after approximately 15 min with at least three corresponding measurements. Determine the time for pure chloroform in the same way. The calculation is:

$$\text{reduced viscosity } (\eta) = (t_1/t_0 - 1) \times 100/c,$$

where c is the concentration (in percent) and t_0 is the time for chloroform.

The average molecular weight of the PMMA sample can be determined with a table or calibration curve (Fig. 1) by means of the η value (as described in the technical information report TC 1348 by Röhm). For copolymers with a predominant PMMA component, the PMMA calibration curve will still offer an acceptable accuracy.

2.2.11
Determination of the Monomer Composition

Determine the monomer composition (MMA, other methacrylates, dimethyl-*p*-toluidine) by gas chromatography. Determine the content of hydroquinone colorimetrically.

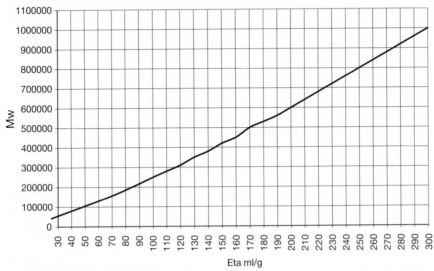

Fig. 1. Relationship between reduced viscosity (η value) and the average molecular weight of poly-methylmethacrylate

2.2.12
Determination of the Monomer Stability According to ISO 5833

Heat a sample of the liquid in a closed vessel to $60 \pm 2°C$ for 48 ± 2 h in the dark. Cool to $23°C$ for an adequate time. Determine the flow time in a viscometer at $23 \pm 0.1°C$ and compare with the flow time of an untreated sample. The flow time of the heat-treated sample should not increase by more than 10%.

2.2.13
Determination of the Bending Strength (Three-Point) According to German Industrial Standard 53435

Prepare the test specimen as follows. Mix the cement according to the manufacturer's instructions. When it is no longer sticky, press the dough into a mold between two foils and wait for it to harden. Saw the test specimens off the plate taken from the mold. Maintain the test specimens in a standard climate for at least 12 h and perform the test under the same conditions.

Place the test specimens in the supports and smoothly load to achieve deflection at a deforming rate of 150°/min. The deflection moment attained will be indicated by the maximum indicator.

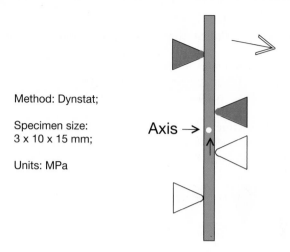

Method: Dynstat;

Specimen size:
3 x 10 x 15 mm;

Units: MPa

2.2.14
Determination of the Impact Strength According to German Industrial Standard 53435

Prepare the test specimen as follows. Mix the cement according to the manufacturer's instructions. When it is no longer sticky, press the dough into a mold between two foils and wait for it to harden. Saw the test specimens off the plate taken from the mold.

Maintain the test specimens in a standard climate for at least 12 h and perform the test under the same conditions. Use the appropriate impact direction (test specimens should absorb between 10% and 80% of the maximum impact).

Place the test specimens exactly vertically in the test device and adjust the pendulum to 90% of the height of the drop. The impact used will be indicated by the maximum indicator.

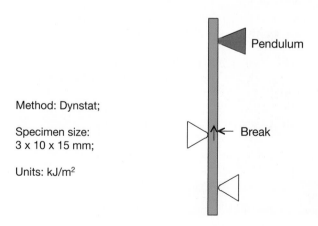

Method: Dynstat;

Specimen size:
3 x 10 x 15 mm;

Units: kJ/m²

2.2.15
Determination of Bending Strength (Four-Point) According to ISO 5833

Prepare the test specimen as follows. Mix the cement according to the manufacturer's instructions. When it is no longer sticky, press the dough into a mold between two foils and wait for it to harden. Saw the test specimens off the plate taken from the mold.

Place the test specimens in water at 37 ± 1°C for 50 ± 2 h. Measure the thickness after taking the specimens from the water, and place a strip symmetrically on the four-point bending-test rig.

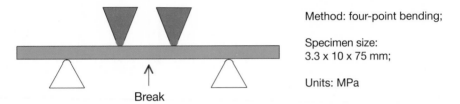

Method: four-point bending;

Specimen size:
3.3 x 10 x 75 mm;

Units: MPa

Break

Start the machine at once and increase the bending load at a cross-head speed of 5 mm/min until breakage occurs. Record the obtained bending strength.

2.2.16
Determination of Compressive Strength According to ISO 5833

Prepare the test specimen as follows. Mix the cement according to the manufacturer's instructions. Press the dough into the drill holes of a special brass mold and wait for it to harden. Saw the test specimens off the cylinders pushed from the mold. After 24 ± 2 h, precisely measure the diameter of the cement cylinder with plane-parallel ends, and place the cylinder upright in the test device.

Continue compressive loading at a cross-head speed of 20 mm/min until there is a sudden decline in strength. Use this maximum strength for calculation of the compressive strength.

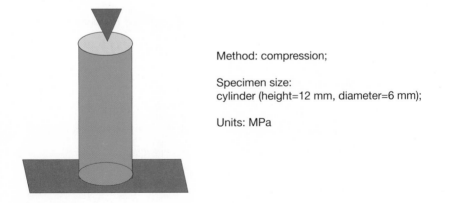

Method: compression;

Specimen size:
cylinder (height=12 mm, diameter=6 mm);

Units: MPa

2.2.17
Determination of the Bending Modulus According to ISO 5833

Prepare the test specimen as follows. Mix the cement according to the manufacturer's instructions. When it is no longer sticky, press the dough into a mold between two foils and wait for it to harden. Saw the test specimens off the plate taken from the mold.

Place the test specimens in water at 37 ± 1°C for 50 ± 2 h. Measure the thickness after taking the specimens from the water, and place a strip symmetrically on the four-point bending-test rig.

Method:
four-point bending;

Specimen size:
3.3 x 10 x 75 mm;

Units: MPa

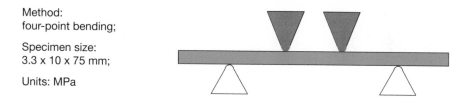

Start the machine at once and increase the bending load at a cross-head speed of 5 mm/min until breakage occurs. Calculate the bending modulus from the recorded curve (deformation versus strength) in the range between 15 N and 50 N.

2.2.18
Determination of Intrusion According to ISO 5833

Maintain the cement in a standard climate (23 ± 1°C, 50 ± 10% humidity) and perform the test under the same conditions. Mix a package according to the manufacturer's instructions and place the cement in a special Teflon mold.

One minute after the end of the sticky phase, load the plunger for 1 min with 49 N. After hardening and disassembly of the mold, measure the depth of the intrusion at the four drill holes and calculate the average value.

Method: compressive load of the dough;

Units: mm

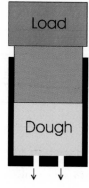

2.2.19
Determination of the Setting Temperature/Time According to ISO 5833

Mix a package of cement in an air-conditioned room (23 ± 1°C, 50 ± 10% humidity) and place it in a shallow, round Teflon mold as soon as the doughing time has been reached. Press an accurately fitting round plunger (which has drill holes to allow superfluous dough to escape) until it stops in the mold. A »cylinder of dough« with a diameter of 60 mm and a height of 6 mm will remain in the mold.

cylindrical sample of dough in teflon mould

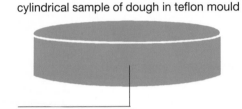

to recorder

Method: temperature/
time curve;

Quantity: one single unit;

Units: degrees
Celsius and minutes,
respectively

In its center is the soldered tip of a thermocouple; the wires are passed outside and to the measuring device via a small central drill hole in the bottom of the mold. Record the setting curve (temperature/time) and use it to determine the maximum temperature and the setting time (at the turning point; Fig. 2).

A slight increase in temperature after 2 min characterizes the filling of the mold with dough. Read the setting time (according to the standard) from the turning point of the curve in the range of the steepest ascent.

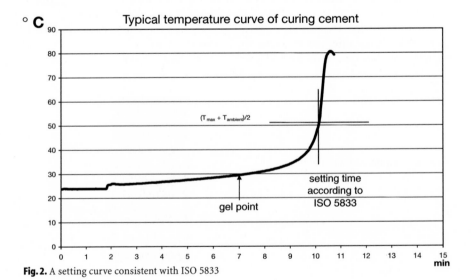

Fig. 2. A setting curve consistent with ISO 5833

2.2.20
Determination of the Doughing Time According to ISO 5833

Mix a complete package (maintained at 23 ± 1°C and 50 ± 10% humidity) and start a stopwatch when the liquid is first added to the powder. Probe the surface of the dough gently with a gloved finger (use a latex, dry, non-powdered glove). Observe whether fibers form between the dough and the glove as the finger leaves the surface.

Repeat the process at intervals of approximately 15 s at fresh points on the dough and clean parts of the glove until the gloved finger separates cleanly from the dough. Record this time as the »doughing time«.

2.2.21
Determination of the Working Properties

In a porcelain crucible, mix an original package that has been maintained in an air-conditioned room (standard climate; 23 ± 1°C and 50 ± 10% humidity; possibly 18 ± 1°C or 25 ± 1°C) for at least 12 h, as described in the manufacturer's instructions. Start a stopwatch when the liquid is first added to the powder. After thorough mixing, determine the time at which the dough is homogeneous (this marks the end of phase I).

Every 5 s, determine whether the dough still sticks to the finger (this constitutes waiting phase or phase II). The working time starts when the dough is no longer sticky (phase III). Knead the dough until it cannot be joined smoothly any longer (this marks the end of the working phase, when prosthesis can no longer be placed; it is also the start of phase IV). The setting time is the time of complete hardening, which can be recognized from the hard sound of a cement ball when knocked onto the table.

All times concerning handling properties and setting, consistent ISO 5833, are recorded in our study in minutes (Fig. 3). The examined cements are divided (according to their viscosity) as low, medium or high viscosity, using the above-mentioned method. We define these properties as follows:
– Low viscosity. Bone cements with a long-lasting liquid phase or a low-viscosity wetting phase. The material usually remains sticky for 3 min. During its working phase, the viscosity quickly increases and the dough becomes warm fast. The end of the working phase and the time of hardening are not more than 1–2 min apart.
– Medium viscosity. Bone cements with a low-viscosity wetting phase. As a rule, the material is no longer sticky after 3 min at the latest. During the working phase, the viscosity remains essentially the same and increases slowly and continuously. During that phase, the cement behaves like a high-viscosity material. Hardening occurs 1.5–2.5 min after the end of the working phase.
– High viscosity. Bone cements with only a short wetting phase; these cements quickly lose their stickiness. During the working phase, the viscosity remains unchanged and slowly increases toward the end of the phase. Generally, the working phase is especially long. Hardening occurs 1.5–2 min after the end of the working phase.

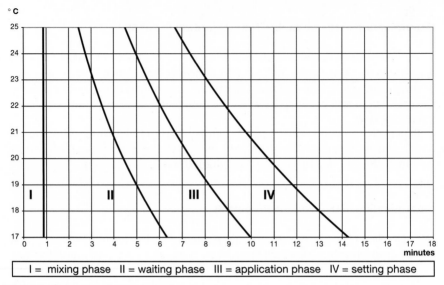

| I = mixing phase   II = waiting phase   III = application phase   IV = setting phase |

Fig. 3. Working curves of a bone cement

2.2.22
Determination of the Glass Transition Temperature

Measure the sawed bone-cement specimens in a dry state or after storage in an aqueous medium at 37°C. Accurately measure the length of the specimens, and fix them in a horizontal dilatometer (two at a time for parallel determination).

Slow heating leads to an increase in length; precisely record this as a function of temperature. At the start of softening, the length will no longer increase; eventually, it will even decrease.

Determine the glass transition temperature (T_g) from the length/temperature diagram (Fig. 4). The material starts to soften at T_g; thus, further extension does not occur despite increased heat (Ege et al. 1998a, b).

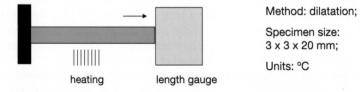

heating   length gauge

Method: dilatation;

Specimen size:
3 x 3 x 20 mm;

Units: °C

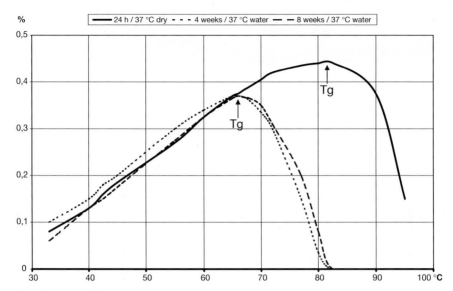

Fig. 4. Examples of dilatation/temperature curves of a bone cement

2.2.23
Determination of Fatigue Strength

The following method for determination of fatigue strength is similar to German Industrial Standard 5833.1, according to Soltesz (1994) and Soltesz et al. (1998a, 1998b). Prepare the test specimen as follows. Mix the cement according to the manufacturer's instructions. When it is no longer sticky, press the dough into a mold between two foils and wait for it to harden. Saw the test specimens off the plate taken from the mold.

Use the four-point bending test device as described in ISO 5833, with specimen sizes of 75 x 10 x 3.3 mm, a distance of 60 mm for the outer loading points and a distance of 20 mm for the inner loading points. Perform the test at 37°C in Ringer solution. Before testing, maintain the specimens under the same conditions for at least 1 month. During this time, they reach an aqueous saturation of at least 95%. Furthermore, all important continuing polymerization processes that might influence the strength should be completed by this time. Therefore, somewhat comparable initial conditions in the properties of the materials can be expected during the alternating-load measurements for a long period.

Determine the quasi-static strength of five test specimens and establish the average as reference value. Load the specimens until fracture occurs, constantly increasing the load at a rate of 90 N/min (50 MPa/min). In isolated cases where the material behaves extremely visco-elastically or plastically and fracture does not occur with a deflection of a few millimeters, increase the load to 900 N/min.

Follow the procedure described by Wöhler for measurements performed under alternating loads. Submit the specimens to a sine-shaped cyclic load of 5 Hz; this

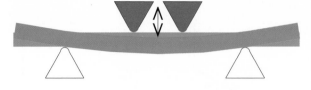

Method: oscillating load, regulated four-point bending;

Specimen size: 3.3 x 10 x 75 mm;

Frequency: 5 Hz;

Number of cycles: a maximum of one million

practically corresponds to a dynamic load (the minimum load should be 5% of the reference value, which is the quasi-static strength). Loading should continue until fracture occurs; record the number of cycles endured as the time of survival. When the maximum number of cycles (one million) without fracture is exceeded, terminate the test. Test five or six specimens, each at different load levels (but with the same maximum load). Choose these load levels at intervals of 10% of the quasi-static strength. Usually, this results in five or six load levels (between 30% and 90% of the quasi-static strength). Perform all tests under controlled loads, as physiological strain is almost exclusively controlled by force. A procedure controlled by displacement would result in under-rating the risk of failure.

Plotting the load at the time of fracture against the logarithm of the obtained number of loads (a half-logarithmic representation) results in a descending line (stress-number curve; Fig. 5). All tests of the fatigue strength of bone cements were carried out at the Fraunhofer-Institut für Werkstofftechnik institute of materials technology in Freiburg, Germany. For estimation of the fatigue strength for the tests, the annual number of double steps taken by a man was estimated to be approximately 10^6, which corresponds to approximately 2×10^6 steps annually. Ten million load alternations would correspond to survival of the implant for approximately 5–10 years.

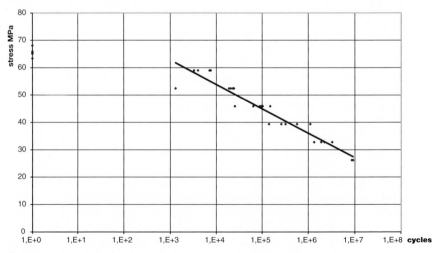

Fig. 5. Typical stress-number curve of a bone cement, according to Soltesz (1994)

3
Results and Discussion

First, several important chemical and physical aspects of the polymethylmethacrylate (PMMA) bone cements will be described to present a basis for comparative studies of the different materials. Later, all bone cements on the market at
this time are described on the basis of ISO 5833. When in this book reference is
made to ISO 5833 it always should be interpreted as standard 5833/2 of the International Organization for Standardization. Additionally, we have tested other (in
our opinion) important parameters that have been either only superficially
described in standards or not described at all but which are of vital importance
for the surgeon. All bone cements were tested according to the same method,
using the same devices and the same laboratory staff in order to guarantee un-
equivocal comparability.

3.1
PMMAs as Bone Cements

When methacrylates are used as bone cements, they must be polymerized. The
most important functional group of the molecule is the $C=C$ double bond
(Fig. 6). However, one cannot produce bone cement from monomer methyl methacrylate (MMA) alone; polymerization would take much too long, and the polymerization shrinkage would be extremely high. In addition, the heat occurring
during the polymerization of the monomer could not be controlled.

$$H_2C = C - CH_2 - O - CH_3 \qquad \text{chemical formula}$$
$$|$$
$$CH_3$$

- ester of methacrylic acid: $C - O - CH_3$ colourless liquid of intense odour
- normally stabilized by hydroquinone or derivative (radical catcher)
- polymerizable by $C = C$ double bond
- boiling point: 100 °C
- density: 0.94 g/cm^3
- molecular weight: 100 g/mol
- OSHA PEL: 100 ppm = 420 mg/m^3
- smellable already at 1 ppm

Fig. 6. Properties of methyl methacrylate

Pure MMA exhibits a shrinkage of approximately 21% during polymerization, which means 1 l of monomer only yields 800 cm³ of polymer. The polymerization temperature can increase to far above 100°C, and the monomer may even boil.

Such a high shrinkage is, of course, intolerable for use in a bone cement. For this reason, bone cements are offered as two-component systems in the marketplace. The MMA in aqueous suspension is pre-polymerized in easily cooled reaction boilers. The polymer, obtained in the form of tiny balls (1–125 μm), is easily dissolved in the monomeric MMA (Fig. 6). By using the pre-polymerized polymer powder, both the shrinkage of the sample and the temperature of the reaction can be considerably decreased.

With regard to the shrinkage, we would like to cite two results from the literature: Haas et al. (1971) found 2–5% shrinkage for Simplex P; Rimnac et al. (1986) found 3% for Palacos. Vacuum mixing (to avoid pores) leads to a slightly higher shrinkage (Davies et al. 1990). This, however, is not disadvantageous if the cement polymerizes from the prosthesis into the bone; in the crevices of the spongiosa, the re-vascularization and building of new bone will occur very fast (Draenert et al. 1999).

The polymer components of commercial bone cements usually consist of PMMA and/or copolymers. Additionally, the powder contains dibenzoyl peroxide (BPO) as an initiator for radical polymerization. The BPO can be either contained in the polymer balls or added to the polymer as a powder. Furthermore, the powder always contains a radiopaque medium and sometimes contains an antibiotic (Fig. 7).

Macroscopically, differences in the polymer composition can hardly be seen. This is quite different when watching them by scanning electron microscopy (Fig. 8). In addition to the surface structure of the polymer beads, the radiopaque medium (and sometimes the BPO) can be seen clearly. The significant differences are shown in Fig. 8 for the examples Palacos R and Simplex P. The main components in the liquid phase are MMA (Fig. 9) and, in some bone cements, other esters of acrylic acid or methacrylic acid, one or more amines (as activators for the formation of radicals), a stabilizer and, possibly, a colorant.

$$R-(CH_2-\underset{\underset{COOCH_3}{|}}{\overset{\overset{CH_3}{|}}{C}}-CH_2-\underset{\underset{COOCH_3}{|}}{\overset{\overset{CH_3}{|}}{C}}-CH_2-\underset{\underset{COOCH_3}{|}}{\overset{\overset{CH_3}{|}}{C}}-)_n-R \qquad \text{chemical formula}$$

- material marketed under many brands
- fine powder (polymer beads)
- bead diameter: 1-125 μm
- soluble in monomer
- density: 1.18 g/cm³
- molecular weight: 800.000 Da

Fig. 7. Properties of polymethylmethacrylate

Fig. 8a, b. Scanning
electron microscopy
photographs of poly-
methylmethacrylate
bone cements.
a Palacos R. *1*, polymer
bead; *2*, zirconium
dioxide.
b Simplex P. *1*, polymer
bead; *3*, barium sulfate

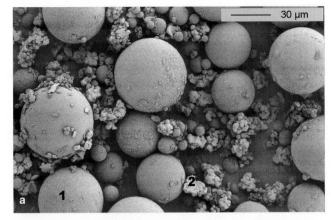

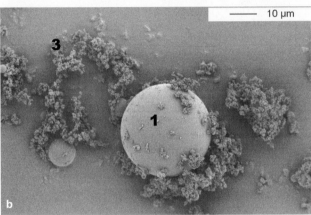

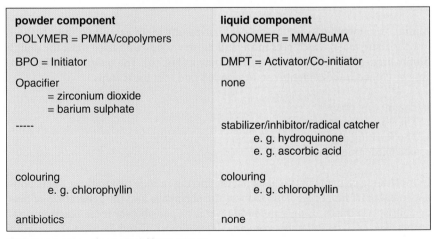

powder component	liquid component
POLYMER = PMMA/copolymers	MONOMER = MMA/BuMA
BPO = Initiator	DMPT = Activator/Co-initiator

Opacifier
     = zirconium dioxide
     = barium sulphate
	none

-----	stabilizer/inhibitor/radical catcher
	     e. g. hydroquinone
	     e. g. ascorbic acid

colouring
     e. g. chlorophyllin
	colouring
	     e. g. chlorophyllin

antibiotics	none

Fig. 9. Composition of commercial bone cements

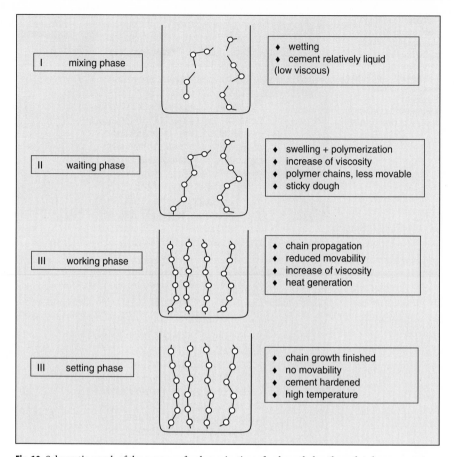

Fig. 10. Schematic graph of the process of polymerization of polymethylmethacrylate bone cements

Adding the polymer to the monomer first results in an essentially highly fluid, low-viscosity mass, which gets more and more viscous with time until the dough finally hardens completely into a solid matrix (Fig. 10). The polymerization process of PMMA bone cements can be divided into four basic steps:

1. The mixing phase
2. The waiting phase
3. The working phase
4. The hardening phase

In most bone cements on the market, the mixing ratio is two to three parts powder to one part monomer. This reduces the shrinkage and the generation of heat by at least two thirds, as only the monomer is responsible for these reaction symptoms (Fig. 11). The following cements deviate most distinctly from the original 2:1 ratio: all Cemex cements, Allofix G, Duracem 3, Cerafix (with and without gen-

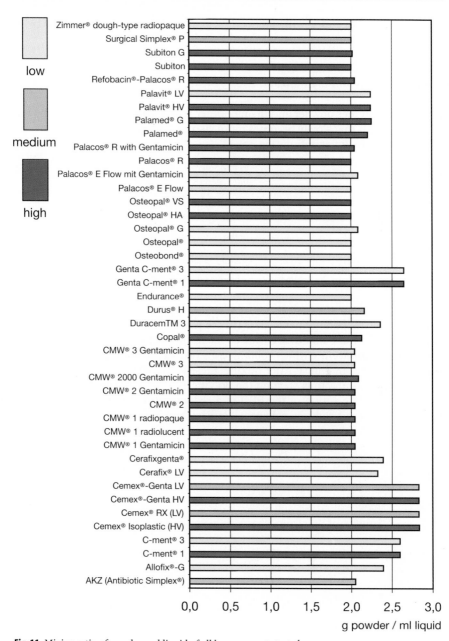

Fig. 11. Mixing ratio of powder and liquid of all bone cements tested

tamicin), C-ment 1 and 3 (with and without gentamicin), Durus H, Palamed (with and without gentamicin), Palavit LV and Palavit HV (Fig. 11).

3.1.1
Initiator System for Polymerization

Mixing the polymer powder and the monomer liquid would result in nothing but a cement dough that slowly becomes more viscous. Initiators are therefore necessary to induce polymerization (Fig. 12).

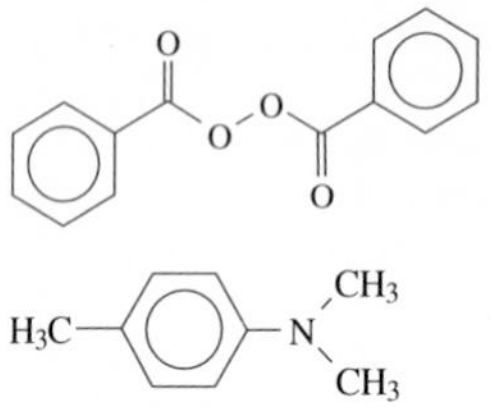

in the polymer
dibenzoyl peroxide (BPO)
– white crystals melting point: 105 °C
– thermal decomposition above
– approximately 80 °C

in the monomer
dimethyl-p-toluidine (DmpT)
– liquid boiling point: 211 °C

Fig. 12. Initiator system for the polymerization of methyl methacrylate.

In all commercial bone cements, BPO (in the powder) and *N,N*-dimethyl-*p*-toluidine, = DmpT (in the liquid) are used as the initiator system. The only exception is the cement Duracem 3, which contains 2-(4-(dimethylamino)phenyl)ethanol in the liquid instead of DmpT. After mixing, these substances can produce radicals at room temperature, thus starting the polymerization. The DmpT in the liquid causes the decomposition of the BPO in a reduction/oxidation process by electron transfer that produces a benzoyl radical and a benzoate anion (Fig. 13).

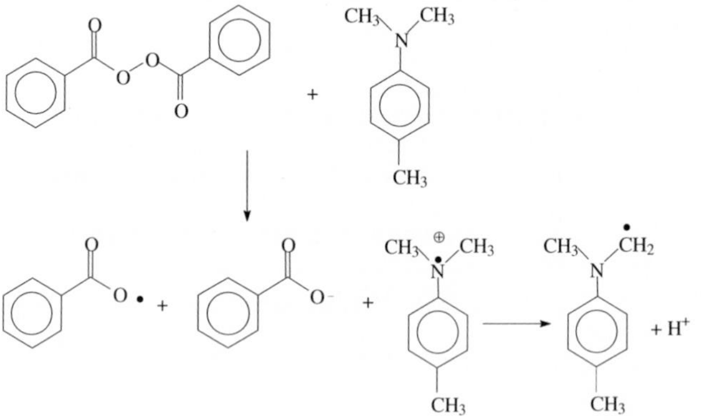

Fig. 13. Formation of radicals induced by the *N,N*-dimethyl-*p*-toluidine in polymethylmethacrylate bone cements

A radical cation is produced from the DmpT as an oxidation product; this can be rearranged into a neutral radical by proton separation. As polymerization starters, these radicals can induce an immediate formation of chains by adding themselves to the C = C double bond in the MMA (Fig. 14).

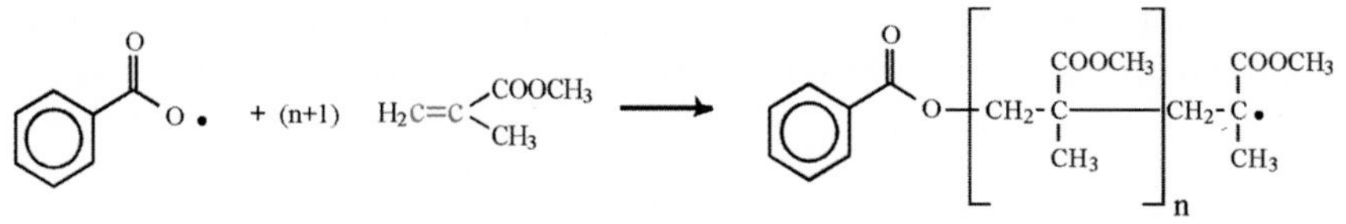

Fig. 14. Formation of chains (radical polymerization) in polymethylmethacrylate bone cementss

Due to the number of polymerization-initiating radicals, a multitude of polymer chains develop, all of which react according to the process described in Fig. 14. A great number of chains – growing with lightning speed and having molecular weights of 10^5–10^6 g/mol or more – develops (Ege 1993).

3.1.2
Polymerization Heat

With the increase of the viscosity of the dough associated with this reaction, the temperature also increases, because an energy of 52 kJ (13 kcal) is released per mole of MMA. When two reactive radical-chain ends meet, they react to form non-reactive, completed polymer chains. As a result of this termination of the reaction and the depletion of the monomer, polymerization comes to a standstill. At that moment, the polymerization temperature has usually reached its peak, and the shrinkage effect described earlier becomes obvious. Because only a few large polymer molecules develop from the multitude of monomer molecules during the progressive formation of chains, and because these molecules draw together, the material inevitably contracts.

For a long time, the short temperature peak occurring during the hardening phase of the PMMA cements was given as the main reason for loosening by heat necrosis (Huiskes 1980; Mjöberg 1986). The fact that the released energy originates from only the monomer is important; the maximum temperatures measured in vitro, in accordance with the standard, do not correspond with the actual

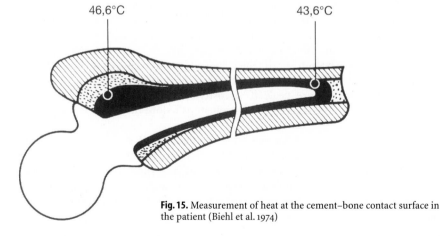

Fig. 15. Measurement of heat at the cement–bone contact surface in the patient (Biehl et al. 1974)

values in the body (Eriksson and Albrektsson 1984). Clinical tests show a considerably lower polymerization heat during the operation at the interface between bone and cement (Fig. 15); this lies significantly below the protein coagulation temperature of ~43–46°C (Biehl 1974; Labitzke and Paulus 1976; Reckling and Dillon 1977; Toksvig-Larson et al. 1991).

Reasons for this observation are the thin layer of cement (~3–5 mm) and the blood circulation and heat dissipation in the vital tissue connected with it. Moreover, further heat dissipation of the system is attained via the prosthesis.

Recently, these factors led to pre-cooling and pre-warming of the prosthesis, respectively. Some properties of the product should be taken into account. When the prosthesis is pre-cooled, the polymerization of the cement progresses toward the bone. In this case, the material shrinks at the cement–prosthesis interface, which will significantly increase the risk of early loosening. If, however, the prosthesis is significantly warmed (to over 50°C), polymerization will start from the bone and proceed toward the prosthesis. As a result of such warming, the prosthesis will lose its thermal conductive capacity, and the temperature peak during polymerization will be significantly increased. Heat-necrotic defects can easily develop at the cement–bone interface, which will lead to early loosening. The warming of the prosthesis to body temperature proved to be a practicable alternative. This avoids the formation of fissures by shrinkage at the prosthesis-cement interface; in addition, the thermal-conductivity capacity of the prosthesis is preserved to a large extent (Bishop et al. 1996).

The progress of the polymerization can best be shown in a temperature/time diagram. After the initial induction phase, during which temperature increases only slowly (sometimes hardly perceptibly), it starts to rise rather quickly with increasing viscosity of the cement dough. This rise in temperature differs among the cements. Because of the gel effect occurring during the polymerization of MMA in a substance without a solvent, the temperature rises explosively and soon reaches its maximum. This is subsequently followed by a speedy decrease in temperature, which can easily be explained as due to the polymerization behavior. The continuously increasing concentration of polymer molecules leads to an increase in viscosity, which reduces the mobility of the polymer chains and results in an inhibition of the radical-chain termination reaction (Ege 1993). The decomposition of the initiator, however, is not inhibited, which is why the radical concentration increases. The monomer, too, is still very mobile, and the growth of the radical chain is not inhibited. On the whole, this results in a drastic increase in the gross polymerization speed (the gel effect) and the consequent conversion of the monomer, which is connected with a significant increase in heat and the corresponding temperature peak. If viscosity is too high, the mobility of the monomer is also inhibited, and the reaction stops before the MMA is completely converted.

The temperature peak can only by influenced to a small extent by adding heat-conducting radiopaque media or by slightly changing the chemical composition of the liquid (for example, by the use of higher methacrylates). This will, however, result in quite different dissolution properties with the polymer – which means it will result in different working properties and, usually, a significant reduction in mechanical stability.

3.1.3
Residual Monomer

Possible heat necroses and other toxic effects of released monomers are discussed in the literature (Charnley 1970; Willert 1974; Feith 1975; Lindwer and Hooff 1975; Linder et al. 1976, Linder 1977; Lindner et al. 1976; Mjöberg 1986). Generally, radical polymerization of MMA in a substance does not proceed to completion, as the mobility of the monomer is greatly decreased by the increase in viscosity at high conversion rates. The proportion of non-converted residual monomer remaining in the polymerized bone cement is in the range of 2–6%.

Investigations of Scheuermann (1976) show that, due to a slowly progressing, continuous polymerization, the proportion of residual monomers decreases to approximately 0.5% within 2–3 weeks (Fig. 16). These in vitro tests were soon confirmed by in vivo investigations of Rudigier et al. (1981). The content of residual monomer in revision-operation materials (tested 0.5, 3 or 8 years after implantation) was always 0.5% or less (Kirschner 1978).

Ege and Scheuermann (1987) reported on the release of monomer during the hardening of cement dough. They determined values in a cement surface of 1.4–1.9 mg/cm². These results are comparable to those determined by Debrunner et al. (1976; 2 mg/cm²). In this regard, it is important that the main part of the

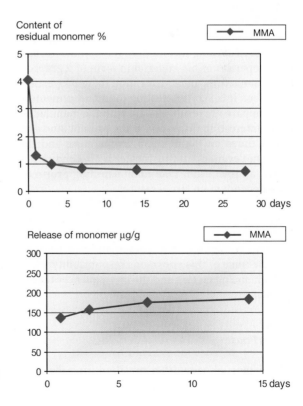

Fig. 16. Typical curves for residual monomer and released monomer versus time

eluted monomer (that is, of the 2–6% of MMA not initially converted) quickly passes into the bloodstream and (obviously) disappears just as quickly (Eggert et al. 1974, 1977; Cront et al. 1979; Wenda et al. 1985a, b).

It was discovered that the monomer is either speedily exhaled (Wenzl et al. 1973; Eggert et al. 1980) or is metabolized in the Krebs' cycle (Wenzl et al. 1973; Cront et al. 1979). Schlag et al. (1976) showed that MMA cannot be the cause of loosening or respiration and circulation reactions.

3.1.4
Handling and Viscosity

Because of the enormous importance, special attention will be directed at the description of the handling criteria of the cements. We will particularly address the important times: the point at which the surgeon obtains a homogeneous mass, the point at which the dough is no longer sticky and can be handled without syringe, and the time of complete hardening. In the description of materials, we confine ourselves to the manual mixing and application of the cements, as it would be beyond the limits of this investigation to test each cement with all mixing systems (with or without use of a vacuum) available on the market. Furthermore, we are of the opinion that the cement quality of a material manufactured according to Good Manufacturing Practices regulations will result in consistent properties of the cement. Based on this assessment, the choice of the mixing vessel should be left to the user. An essential prerequisite for judging the handling properties of bone cements is that testing take place according to a standard method. According to ISO 5833, the manufacturer is obliged to depict the handling properties of his material in form of a graph. A method, according to which the manufacturer must determine these properties, is not stated in the standard. Therefore, it is very interesting to test all cements according to the same method and compare the resulting data with the manufacturer's information.

An interesting discovery in the present study is the dependence of the determined times on the ambient temperature and the temperature of the components; not every operating theater is air-conditioned and has constant conditions during an operation. **Take note: handling properties of bone cements are extremely dependent on temperature!**

According to the ISO 5833 standard, every manufacturer is obliged to present the user with a detailed (if possible, graphic) representation of the handling properties of the cement. This is undoubtedly necessary, as the nurse in the operating theater mixes the two-component materials and thus produces the final product. Because of this enormous responsibility, we think it important to represent the influencing factors and the consequences they have for the quality of the final product.

3.1.4.1
Mixing Phase

The cements already differ greatly during the mixing phase. Some cements can be easily mixed; others can only be homogenized only with great difficulty and the utmost caution. Breusch et al. (1999) studied the cementing techniques used in total hip arthroplasty in Germany using a questionnaire and found that the mixing sequence stated in the manufacturer's instructions is only observed in two thirds of all cases. The mixing phase is by no means trivial. During this process, so many air bubbles can be mixed into the dough by overly thorough mixing that the porosity of the material can be high and the mechanical stability endangered (Jasty et al. 1990). This phenomenon was described by Charnley (1970) when bone cements were first used. The more powerfully and longer the dough is mixed, the more porous it will be!

Lee et al. (1973, 1978), Kummer (1974), Haas (1975), Müller (1975), Debrunner (1976), Connelly et al. (1978), Kusy (1978), Miller and Krause (1981), Demarest et al. (1983), Jasty et al. (1984, 1991), Lautenschlager et al. (1984), Linden (1988) and Schreurs et al. (1988) showed the influence of the porosity on the mechanical properties of bone cements. Similar studies were carried out by De Wijn et al. (1972, 1975a, 1975b) who, like Debrunner (1976), also describe the mechanism of pore formation and the mechanical properties of porous and non-porous materials. Apparently, the form of the mixing vessel and the spatula, the speed of mixing and the number of strokes have an influence on the result. Of immense importance (especially during manual mixing) is the observation that careful kneading when the dough is no longer sticky can subsequently significantly reduce porosity (Eyerer and Jin, 1986).

In addition to the described cause for the inclusion of air, it must be taken into account that air bubbles are already present in the polymer powder, and monomer bubbles, which may develop during the evaporation of the monomer while evacuating the system or later during the polymerization under high pressure, can easily appear (especially by faulty use of vacuum mixing systems; Oest et al. 1975). The formation of bubbles (caused by boiling monomer) is one of the main problems in the development of mixing systems under vacuum conditions (Draenert 1988).

The influence of vacuum mixing on the pores results in a 15–30% improvement of the bending strength of Palacos R (Lidgren et al. 1984; Wang et al. 1993, 1994, 1995). Centrifugation is another method of pore reduction (Burke et al. 1984; Rimnac et al. 1986). Davies et al. (1989), for example, found a reduction of porosity from 9.4% to 2.9% for Simplex P when centrifuged, resulting in an increase of fatigue strength.

3.1.4.2
Working Phase

The working phase is the time during which the surgeon can easily apply cement to the femur. For manual application, the cement must no longer be sticky during this phase, and the viscosity must not be too high. With regard to this parameter, the cements differ significantly. So far, no one has succeeded in comparing all cements (probably because of the lack of a determination method) in order to characterize this phase, which is eminently important in practice. We have tried to do this (as described in Sect. 2.2.21), and we state the results in the descriptions of the cements.

Evidently, the working phase of the cements changes with the use of mixing systems because, with these systems, the user need not wait until the cement is no longer sticky. However, a viscosity that is not too low during the early phase must be guaranteed. If it is not, the applied cement cannot withstand the bleeding pressure in the femur. Blood is included in the cement (Draenert 1988), and these inclusions must be looked upon as distinct weak points with a high fracture risk (Soltesz et al. 1998a, 1998b). This phenomenon is the main problem when using low-viscosity cements (compare Sect. 3.2.5.1), because these are often applied to the body at too early a point due to their short working phase (Draenert et al. 1999).

3.1.4.3
Hardening Phase

The hardening phase indicates the moment at which the surgeon can expect the cement to be completely hardened. The manufacturer can only conduct in vitro tests of this phase and can only determine the hardening times in the laboratory under defined conditions (of temperature, humidity, etc.). Although a complete package of cement is often handled in the laboratory (and, thus, a large quantity with a long diameter of a cement ball is tested), the surgeon attempts to form a cement thickness of not more than 2–5 mm under operation conditions in vivo. The hardening behavior of the cement under operating conditions (particularly under the influence of the operating-room temperature, the temperature of the components, the body temperature and the cement thickness) can significantly differ from the statements in the manufacturer's instructions. The many different factors influencing the polymerization kinetics of PMMA are probably the reason for this discrepancy.

According to Breusch et al. (1999), the moment at which the cement is applied to the femur and the acetabulum is standardized to a large extent (in approximately 88% of all cases); the mixing time of the bone cement, however, is standardized in only two thirds of all cases. In slightly more than 50% of all cases, the cement is apparently still mixed by hand and is mixed without pre-cooling of components and mixing vessels in approximately 40%.

The pre-cooling of the monomer, polymer and mixing vessels and the use of vacuum systems during mixing result in a significant reduction of the number and the volume of pores. As a consequence, a considerable improvement of the fatigue strength of bone cements has been described (Demarest et al. 1983; Keller and Lautenschlager 1983; Wixson et al. 1985, 1987; Draenert 1988; Soltesz and Ege 1993; Soltesz et al. 1998a, 1998b).

An essential prerequisite for the use of vacuum mixing systems is their correct use. Nothing is worse than an incorrect mixing technique! In the Swedish Hip Arthroplasty Register the vacuum mixing technique is recommended – but only when used correctly (Malchau and Herberts 1998). The authors report on a learning effect in the users of mixing systems; this was reflected in the fact that satisfactory clinical results were achieved only after several years of experience.

3.1.5
Molecular Weight

The molecular weight of the hardened cement matrix depends on the following parameters:

> – The molecular weights of the raw materials used in the polymer
> – The method used to sterilize the polymer powder (sterilization via irradiation results in a reduction of the molecular weight to approximately 50%)
> – The molecular weight of the monomer
> – The concentration of the initiator system or the ratio of the initiator to the activator
> – The changes in temperature during the reaction
> – The presence of regulators

For this reason, we determined the molecular weights of all bone cements on the market according to the method described in Sect. 2.2.10. The molecular weight influences the swelling properties of the cements, the mechanical strength (especially the fracture strength) and the working phases of the different materials (Lewis and Austin 1994).

The sterilization method used has a particular influence on the molecular weight. It is well known, for example, that γ sterilization of bone cements reduces the molecular weight by half, while the (much more complicated) fumigation with ethylene oxide has no influence on the molecular weight (Kim et al. 1977; Tepic and Soltesz 1996; Lewis and Mladsi 1998). Because the reduction of the molecular weight during sterilization with γ rays also changes the non-sterile primary product, significant changes in the handling properties and mechanical strength are to be expected. This phenomenon is of special importance, because most bone cements on the market are still sterilized by γ irradiation. Recently, a number of newer studies of these problems have been published. These describe the decisive influence of the sterilization method (especially on the reduction of the molecular weight) and its importance for the fatigue strength of bone cements (Tepic and Soltesz 1996; Harper et al. 1997; Lewis 1997; Lewis and Mladsi 1998). In a comparative evaluation of the fatigue strength (Sect. 3.2.5.3), we will also discuss the influence of the molecular weight (Sect. 3.2.5.2) on the results (several examples will be cited) and will give a short description of the sterilization methods used in bone cements (Sect. 3.2.5.3).

3.1.6
Mechanical Properties

Because the connection between the bone and the bone cement and between the bone cement and the prosthesis is mechanical, the cement layer has the function of an elastic buffer. The main task of the cement is to transfer the forces of the impact affecting the bone as evenly as possible. Ultimately, it is the transfer of forces that is decisive for the long-term stability of the implant. If the external stress factors are greater than the ability of the cement to transfer the force, a break will result. For this reason, it is necessary to test the mechanical properties of bone cements under standard conditions (Kusy 1978; Saha and Pal 1984, Ege 1994; Lewis 1997; Kühn et al. 1999).

For this purpose, material scientists have a number of methods at their disposal. First, there are several static tests of, e.g., tensile, compressive, bending or impact strength. These tests can be performed at different times after polymerization, or specimens can be stored in water or Ringer's solution at 37°C before testing.

The stiffness of the bone cements can be calculated (from tensile, compressive or bending tests) as the bending modulus. This is a measure of the ability of the bone cement to act as an elastic buffer between the prosthesis and the bone.

In addition to static tests, dynamic tests (i.e., a long-term alternating-load tests) are possible. These can also be conducted as tensile, compressive or bending tests. Usually, the fatigue strength is determined in a bending test, because the test device necessary for this test is comparatively simple. Such investigations, which should be made using 10^7 (or, even better, 10^8) alternating loads, take a great deal of time, as the number of load alternations should be between three and five per second (Soltesz et al. 1998a, 1998b).

In the literature a multitude of data on the mechanical properties of bone cements can be found. Unfortunately, the data determined and published by different authors can rarely be compared. Often, the reason is that necessary information regarding the preparation of specimens, their storage or the test itself is missing. Moreover, the tests are often performed according to standards suitable for metals and resins but not bone cements (Ege 1994).

To avoid this, an early attempt to define a standard applicable for all bone cements were made in the United States (American Society for Testing and Materials 451F) in 1978; this was quickly adopted as an international standard (ISO 5833) in 1979. In the first edition of this standard, the only mechanical test included was that for compressive strength. Only in the last revision was it agreed to also include tests of bending strength and bending modulus.

3.1.7
Glass Transition Temperature

On heating, resins change their state from glass-like and brittle to elastic. This physical law also applies to PMMA (and, therefore, to bone cements). Due to the distribution of the molecular weight, only a softening range (rather than an exact transition temperature) exists (Vieweg and Esser 1975).

When the glass transition temperature (T_g) is attained, Brownian motions cease; these micro-movements themselves are the reason for some changes in the materials' parameters. They influence the thermal expansion coefficient, the bending modulus and mechanical and electric absorption. T_g depends on the molecular weight, water content and, of course, the molecular structure of the monomer used.

Especially during recent years, T_g has been used for additional characterization of bone cements (Thanner et al. 1995). Some researchers postulate that the T_gs of older pharmaceutical specialties are much too high; the materials were brittle, and this was often one of the reasons for loosening of the components.

It was discovered that T_g can be adjusted to approximately 50°C by using a methacrylate with a longer alkyl side chain. Unfortunately, either only theoretical calculations on the composition were made in these studies or the few measurements were carried out on dry specimens.

The researchers unfortunately neglected the fact that bone cements are always in a humid environment at 37°C after implantation and become saturated with water after only a few weeks. A plasticizing effect develops, and T_g inevitably decreases (Table 2; Ege et al. 1998a and b, 1999).

Table 2. Glass transition temperatures of Palacos R (in degrees Celsius) after storage at 37°C

Substance in which storage occurred	1 week	2 weeks	4 weeks
Dry		86	86
Water	78	66	67
Intralipid (10%)	76	73	64

3.2
Descriptions of the Cements

In the following sections, all bone cements currently on the market are described in terms of their composition, physical and chemical properties, and presentation and packing, as described in ISO 5833 (Table 3). These descriptions should be

Table 3. Requirements of ISO 5833 (1992) for bone cements

Requirements for the liquid	
Appearance of the liquid	Free of particles and other contaminants
Stability of the liquid (48 h/60°C)	The flow time should not increase by more than 10%
Accuracy of contents	The maximum deviation should be ±5% of the volume stated on the package
Requirements for the powder	
Appearance of the powder	Free of agglomerates and extraneous material
Accuracy of the contents	The maximum deviation should be ±5% of the mass stated on the package
Requirements for the dough	
Hardening characteristics	Doughing time: a maximum of 5 min (not applicable to syringe usage)
	Setting time: 3–15 min for dough, 6.5–15 min for syringe usage
	Maximum temperature: 90°C
Intrusion	Not less than 2 mm (not applicable to syringe usage)
Requirements for the set and cured cement	
Compressive strength	A minimum of 70 MPa
Bending modulus	A minimum of 1800 MPa
Bending strength	A minimum of 50 MPa
Special requirements of ISO 5833 concerning packaging	
Components	Is the powder double packaged?
	Is the liquid double packaged?
Information on the package about the components of the powder	Qualitative / Quantitative
Information on the package about the components of the liquid	Qualitative / Quantitative
Warning concerning the monomer	Highly flammable (text or a symbol may be used)
Instruction concerning the conditions of storage	≤ 25°C, in the dark
Statement concerning the sterility	Possible statement of the kind of sterilization (a symbol may be used)
	Warning against re-use
Statement of batch number(s)	With symbol
Statement of the expiration date	With symbol
Statement concerning the manufacturer or supplier	Name and address
Number and date of the standard	If available; state if not available
Information in the accompanying documentation	Instructions for mixing and handling of the components
	Warning of the dangers to the patient
	Instructions regarding whether intended for use with a syringe or in dough state
	Statement concerning the effect of temperature on the handling properties
	Graphical representation of the effects of temperature on the handling properties

regarded as a reference for the various cements. Short summaries of the most important characteristic values are given at the end of each description. The most important parameters of the various cements are compared and discussed with reference to literature reports.

Even though manufacturers having several products on the market often use uniform packaging with different labels, every cement (including packaging) is described separately (particularly because the different cements were tested independently); the packaging of each cement is also described. Sometimes, slight differences were found in the labels; we indicate these differences. However, it is possible that a number of cements are marketed with different packaging in countries where special legal requirements apply.

Due to the situation described above, repetitions in the descriptions of the cements often occur. We are aware of this but include all the cements in order to provide a thorough reference book.

First, we describe all known antibiotic-free cements on the market, followed by comparative observations with reference to reports found in the literature. We then describe all antibiotic-loaded cements currently on the market, again followed by comparative observations with reference to literature reports.

Finally, we comparatively discuss several important parameters. These topics have not been described in any standards, but we believe them to be important for the assessment of the quality of the cements and to facilitate the user's choice of a particular cement. The comparative observations of these parameters and the methods introduced for their determination are suggested as standards and should be made obligatory in the testing of PMMA bone cements.

All tested bone cements complied with the requirements of the standards regarding intrusion (Sect. 2.2.18), stability of the monomer (Sect. 2.2.12) and doughing time (Sect. 2.2.20). Therefore, these results are not described in detail.

3.2.1
Antibiotic-Free (Plain) Cements

Table 4 shows the cements examined in our study and lists some relevant information. We tested at least three different batches of each of these cements. We contacted the distributors directly or bought the cements from clinic drug stores. Therefore, only practically marketed products were used in the study.

Before going into the details of the cements of Table 4, we want to give comparative overviews about the compositions of powders (Fig. 17) and liquids (Fig. 18) and note the differences and similarities. Moreover, the initiators (Fig. 19) and the radiopaque media (Fig. 20) will be compared.

The powder composition shows significant variation. Sometimes, we found data differing from the information given by the manufacturer.

The Cemex cements contain approximately 3% styrene, the Subiton cement contains approximately 20% n-butyl methacrylate. The C-ment cements show even two extra co-monomers besides MMA: methyl acrylate and ethyl acrylate, and Durus H contains ethylhexyl (meth)acrylate. All these were not declared on the labels (see special marking *IIIIII* for the declared PMMA in Fig. 17). The

Table 4. Plain cements

Name	Responsible Manufacturer	Viscosity type	Powder sterilization	Market
C-ment® 1	E. M. C. M. B. V.	high	beta irradiation	Central Europe, G
C-ment® 3	E. M. C. M. B. V.	low	beta irradiation	Central Europe, G
Cemex® Isoplastic (HV)	Tecres	high	ethylene oxide	South Europe, I
Cemex® RX (LV)	Tecres	medium	ethylene oxide	South Europe, I
Cerafix® LV	Ceraver Osteal	low	gamma irradiation	South Europe, F
CMW® 1 radiolucent	De Puy	high	gamma irradiation	worldwide
CMW® 1 radiopaque	DePuy	high	gamma irradiation	worldwide
CMW® 2	DePuy	high	gamma irradiation	worldwide
CMW® 3	DePuy	low	gamma irradiation	worldwide
Duracem™ 3	Sulzer	low	ethylene oxide	Central Europe, CH
Durus® H	Macmed Orthopedics	medium	gamma irradiation	South Africa
Endurance®	DePuy	low	gamma irradiation	USA
Osteobond®	Zimmer	low	gamma irradiation	USA
Osteopal®	Merck	low	ethylene oxide	worldwide
Osteopal® HA	Merck	high	ethylene oxide	F
Osteopal® VS	Merck	high	ethylene oxide	F
Palacos® LV/E Flow	Schering Plough	low	ethylene oxide	worldwide
Palacos® R	Merck/Schering Plough	high	ethylene oxide	worldwide
Palamed®	Merck	high	ethylene oxide	worldwide
Palavit® HV	Schering Plough	high	ethylene oxide	F, CH
Palavit® LV	Schering Plough	low	ethylene oxide	F, CH
Subiton	Prothoplast	high	ethylene oxide	Argentina
Surgical Simplex® P	Howmedica	medium	gamma irradiation	worldwide, USA
Zimmer® dough-type radiopaque	Zimmer	low	gamma irradiation	USA

F, France; *G*, Germany; *I*, Italy; *CH*, Switzerland

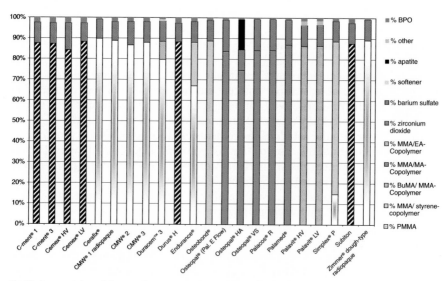

Fig. 17. Composition of the powder components of all investigated plain cements

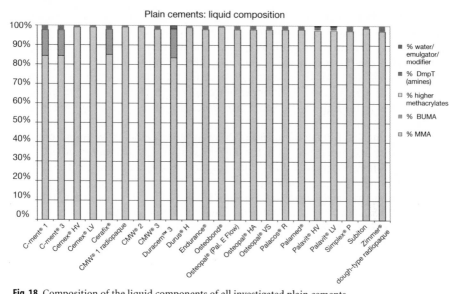

Fig. 18. Composition of the liquid components of all investigated plain cements

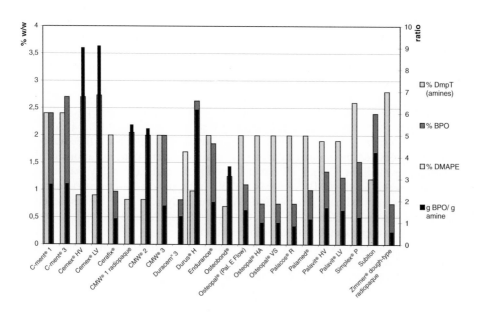

Fig. 19. Initiator/activator ratios of plain cements. DMAPE = 2-[4-(dimethylamino)phenyl]ethanol

exact percentage of co-monomer can be found by nuclear magnetic resonance. These cements contain both pure PMMA and co-polymers.

Some manufacturers offer different variants of their cements. In these cases, the variants are chemically alike. They may have a common polymer basis with different additives. This holds especially true for the cements of Heraeus-Kulzer, almost all of which have a green polymer component. Only the Palavit powders are colorless; the liquids, however, are greenish, as is typical of the Kulzer cements.

Concerning the BPO content in the different bone cements we found out that for the most examined products the BPO is within the polymer beads. This is obviously different for all Palacos-like products and Cerafix, where the BPO is admixed to the polymer separately.

Regarding the composition of the liquids, only a few brands differ from the known MMA-DmpT system. Figure 18 shows the liquid compositions in a manner similar to that used in Figure 17 for the powders.

In C-ment-1, C-ment-3, Cerafix and Duracem 3, there is a component of the liquid in addition to MMA.

The Palavit liquids contain long methacrylates and special components in order to lower the setting temperature. The exact compositions are given in the appropriate sections of this text.

The amounts of initiators (BPO and amine) differ significantly. Duracem 3 is the only cement using 2-[4-(dimethylamino)phenyl]ethanol instead of DmpT as the activator (Fig. 19).

Figure 19 shows the percentage (w/w) of the initiators in the powder and liquid, respectively. It also gives the ratio of BPO to DmpT in the mixed cement with respect to the powder/liquid mixing ratio (Fig. 11).

These data are important for the understanding of the problem of residual monomer and residual DmpT (Stea et al. 1997). In Sect. 3.2.5.5, this is discussed in detail.

Only zirconium dioxide and barium sulfate are used as radio-opacifiers (in different percentages) (Fig. 20). The lowest radio-opacifier content (~9%) is found in Cemex LV, Cerafix, CMW 1 and Durus H. Sometimes, the different variants produced by one manufacturer contain different concentrations of the radiopaque medium. Cemex LV has a low content, and Cemex HV has a high content (~13%). Of the CMW cements, CMW 3 has a 10% radio-opacifier content, CMW 2 has approximately 11.3%, and CMW has only 9.1%. The highest level is found in Osteopal, Palacos LV/E Flow, Osteopal VS and Palacos R (15%). Palamed only contains approximately 12% radio-opacifier.

Most manufacturers have an approximately 10% radio-opacifier content. In Sect. 3.2.5.4, it is shown how the different concentrations of the different radiopaque media affect the actual X-ray opacity.

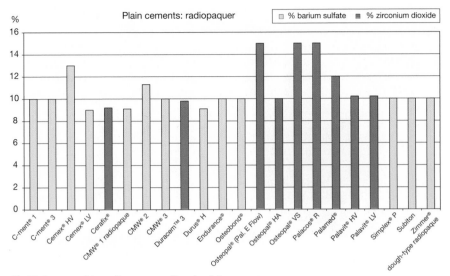

Fig. 20. Content of the radiopaque medium in plain cements

3.2.1.1
C-ment 1

The polymer powder and monomer liquid of C-ment 1 are packed in a rather small and very solid outer carton. The carton may be easily opened on the upper side. The outer carton itself is printed with the most important information (for example, the compositions of the powder and liquid). Two small, separate labels show the batch number and the expiration date. Indications regarding the registration and the distributor may also be clearly displayed.

The outside of the packing contains a polyethylene pouch that encloses a blister pack (Fig. 21). This blister pack contains the powder (in a glass bottle) and the monomer (in an ampoule). Furthermore, there is an insert and four chart stickers for patients' records. To our knowledge, this type of packing of the polymer powder (i.e., in a brown glass bottle) is otherwise used only by the company Sulzer for the cements Allofix G and Duracem 3.

The peel-off pouch consists of a Tyvek side and a transparent polyethylene side. On the cardboard side, there is a label that indicates the composition of both cement components, the expiration date and the batch number.

The peel-off pouch may be easily opened. The blister pack contained in it consists of transparent, molded polyvinyl chloride (PVC) and is sealed with unprinted Tyvek. The powder bottle and the monomer ampoule may be well visualized through the PVC. The blister pack may be easily opened. Both primary packed materials bear a batch number related to the product; this number is not identical to the number on the peel-off pouch on the outer carton. An expiration date is missing on the polymer bottle and the monomer ampoule. The brown glass

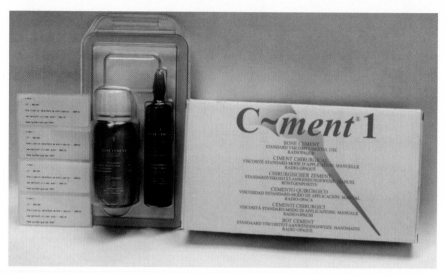

Fig. 21. The packaging of C-ment 1

bottle that contains the polymer powder is a screw-cap bottle. The lock is different from those of the powder bottles of Allofix G and Duracem 3.

A stopper made of plastic serves as a locking aid on the bottle. This bottle is printed with white letters. Instructions are given regarding sterilization by means of X-rays, and the composition, batch number and manufacturer are listed. The polymer powder contains 87.6% PMMA, 2.4% BPO and 10.0% barium sulfate (as an opacifier; Fig. 22) according to the manufacturer. However, analysis shows that the polymer also contains a low percentage of methyl acrylate and ethyl acrylate.

The ampoule is also printed like the polymer bottle. The top of the ampoule features a white dot, which shows the breaking shaft.

In addition to monomer quantity and composition, the batch number and manufacturer are given as information. The liquid consists of two different methacrylates – 84.4% MMA and 13.2% butylmethacrylate (BuMA) – in addition to 2.4% DmpT and approximately 20 ppm hydroquinone (as a stabilizer; Fig. 22).

powder		liquid
35,04 g	poly(methyl methacrylate) containing some % of methyl acrylate and ethyl acrylate	12,15 g methyl methacrylate (=12,93 ml)
		1,90 g butyl methacrylate (=2,12 ml)
		0,35 g N,N-dimethyl-p-toluidine (=0,37 ml)
0,96 g	benzoyl peroxide	20 ppm hydroquinone
4,00 g	barium sulphate	
----------		-----------
40,00 g		14,40 g (15,42 ml) = Biocryl 1
	C-ment 1	

Fig. 22. Composition of C-ment 1

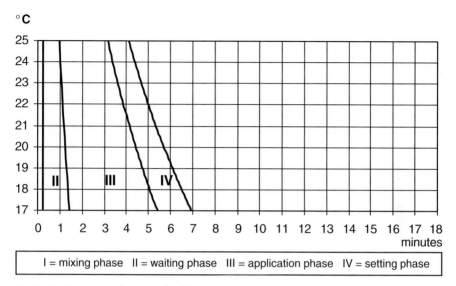

I = mixing phase   II = waiting phase   III = application phase   IV = setting phase

Fig. 23. Working curves of C-ment 1 for different ambient/component temperatures

The compositions of the powder and liquid are identical to those of Biocryl 1 (manufactured by Bioland), a bone cement that is no longer sold under this trademark. In former times, Biocryl cements could be obtained in France and other Southern European countries.

To mix the dough, the powder is put into the vessel, and the liquid is then added. The wetting occurs very quickly, although it often seems that the material is too dry at first. However, after approximately 15–20 s, the dough is rather viscous and completely homogeneous. From the beginning, the cement shows a high viscosity and may be taken out of the vessel after less than 1 min, and processing may be continued. This viscosity is so high that processing without problems is not easy. After 3 min 30 s, the dough may no longer be handled.

After 4 min, a clear warming may be noticed. After between 4 min 50 s and 5 min, the dough is completely hardened (Fig. 23).

Due to these properties, C-ment 1 has to be regarded as a high-viscosity cement. The mechanical strengths all correspond to those listed in the ISO standard (Table 5). The low impact strength and the slight deviations between the bending strengths listed in Dynstat and ISO 5833 are striking.

Table 5. Mechanical strength according to ISO 5833 and German Industrial Standard DIN 53435 for C-ment 1

| | ISO 5833 | | | DIN 53435 | |
	Bending strength (MPa)	Bending modulus (MPa)	Compressive strength (MPa)	Bending strength (MPa)	Impact strength (kJ/m²)
Limit given in the standard	>50	>1800	>70		
Actual strength	67.4	2584	89.3	70.2	3.9

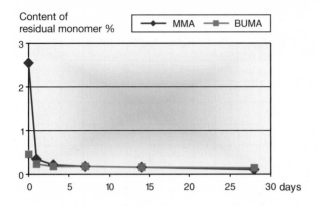

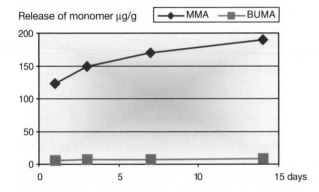

Fig. 24. Content and release of residual monomers of C-ment 1 with time

The setting time (determined according to ISO 5833 protocols) was 8 min 30 s; the polymerization temperature is given as 84.6°C. Thus, this material has a high polymerization temperature, which is unexpected, due to the favorable powder/liquid ratio (Fig. 11). The residual monomer has not been considered in the comparison (Fig. 24); both MMA and BuMA monomers are contained in the liquid.

Regarding the packing components and their labeling, it is striking that the batch number is only printed on the primary container; an expiration date is completely missing. Moreover, a notice regarding the present standard (ISO 5833; Table 6) is missing. The key characteristics of C-ment 1 are listed in Table 7.

Table 6. ISO 5833 (1992) requirements for the packaging of C-ment 1

Requirements		Com- pliance	Location of information
General	Is the powder packed in a double-layered, sealed container?	+	–
	Is the liquid packed in a double-layered, sealed container?	+	–
Information regarding the powder ingredients	Qualitative	+	PF, FS, POB, PB
	Quantitative	+	PF, FS, POB, PB
Information regarding the liquid ingredients	Qualitative	+	A, POB, FS, PB
	Quantitative	+	A, POB, FS, PB
	Warning that the package contains flammable liquid	+	PB, A, FS
	Instructions for storage ($\leq 25°C$, darkness)	+	FS, POB
	Statement of the sterility of the contents	+	A, PF, FS, PB, POB
	Warning against reusing the package	+	FS, POB, PB, PF
	Batch number(s)	+	A, PF, FS, POB
	Expiration date	+	FS, POB
	Name/address of the manufacturer/distributor	+	A, PF, POB, FS, PB
	Number and date of the standard	–	–
Information in the package insert	Detailed instructions for handling the components and preparing the cement	+	PB
	A statement drawing attention to the dangers for the patient	+	PB
	Recommendations for using the cement (syringe/dough state)	+	PB
	A statement regarding the influence of the temperature on working times	+	PB
	Graphical representation of the effects of temperature on the length of the phases of cement curing	+	PB

+, complies; –, does not comply; *A*, ampoule; *FS*, carton; *PB*, package insert; *PF*, powder bottle; *POB*, peel-off pouch

Table 7. The key characteristics of C-ment 1

High viscosity
The monomer contains BuMA
The polymer contains methyl acrylate and ethyl acrylate
Barium sulfate is the radiopaque medium
The polymer is γ irradiated
The polymer is packaged in a brown glass bottle
The polymer bottle and ampoule are in one blister
Mixing sequence: powder, then monomer
Working time: short
ISO 5833 is fulfilled
Molecular weight less than 350,000 Da
Low bending strength
Low impact strength

BuMA, butyl methacrylate

3.2.1.2
C-ment 3

The polymer powder and monomer liquid of C-ment 3 are packed in a rather small and very solid outer carton. The carton may be easily opened on the upper side. The outer carton itself is printed with the most important information (for example, the compositions of the powder and liquid). Two small, separate labels show the batch number and the expiration date. Indications regarding the registration and the distributor may also be clearly displayed.

The outside of the packing contains a polyethylene pouch that encloses a blister pack (Fig. 25). This blister pack contains the powder (in a glass bottle) and the monomer (in an ampoule). Furthermore, there is an insert and four chart stickers for patients' records. To our knowledge, this type of packing of the polymer powder (i.e., in a brown glass bottle) is otherwise only used by the company Sulzer for the cements Allofix G and Duracem 3.

The peel-off pouch consists of a Tyvek side and a transparent polyethylene side. On the paper side, there is a label that indicates the composition of both cement components, the expiration date and the batch number.

The peel-off pouch may be easily opened. The blister pack contained in it consists of transparent, molded PVC and is sealed with unprinted Tyvek. The powder bottle and the monomer ampoule may be well visualized through the PVC. The blister pack may be easily opened. Both primary packed materials bear a batch number related to the product; this number is not identical to the number on the peel-off pouch on the outer carton. An expiration date is missing on the polymer

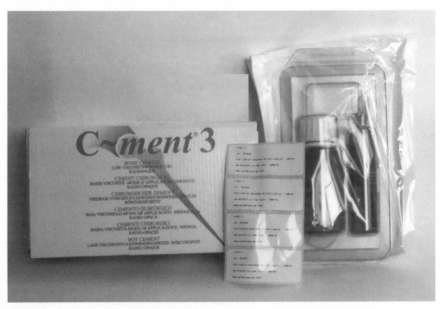

Fig. 25. The packaging of C-ment 3

bottle and the monomer ampoule. The brown glass bottle that contains the poly-mer powder is a screw-cap bottle. The lock is different from those of the powder bottles of Allofix G and Duracem 3.

A stopper made of plastic serves as a locking aid on the bottle. This bottle is printed with white letters. Instructions are given regarding sterilization by means of X-rays, and the composition, batch number and manufacturer are listed. The polymer powder contains 87.3% PMMA, 2.7% BPO and 10.0% barium sulfate (as an opacifier; Fig. 26) according to the manufacturer. However, analysis shows that the polymer also contains a low percentage of methyl acrylate and ethyl acrylate.

powder	liquid
34,92 g poly(methyl methacrylate) containing some % of methyl acrylate and ethyl acrylate 1,08 g benzoyl peroxide 4,00 g barium sulphate ------------ 40,00 g	13,85 g methyl methacrylate (=14,73 ml) 2,16 g butyl methacrylate (=2,42 ml) 0,39 g N,N-dimethyl-p-toluidine (=0,42 ml) 20 ppm hydroquinone ------------ 16,40 g (17,57 ml)
C-ment 3	

Fig. 26. Composition of C-ment 3

The ampoule is also printed like the polymer bottle. The top of the ampoule fea-tures a white dot, which shows the breaking shaft.

In addition to monomer quantity and composition, the batch number and manufacturer are given as information. The liquid consists of two different met-hacrylates – 84.4% MMA and 13.2% BuMA – in addition to 2.4% DmpT and approximately 20 ppm hydroquinone (as a stabilizer; Fig. 26).

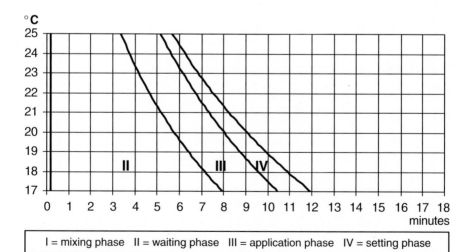

I = mixing phase   II = waiting phase   III = application phase   IV = setting phase

Fig. 27. Working curves of C-ment 3 for different ambient/component temperatures

Table 8. Mechanical strength according to ISO 5833 and German Industrial Standard DIN 53435 for C-ment 3

	ISO 5833 Bending strength (MPa)	Bending modulus (MPa)	Compressive strength (MPa)	DIN 53435 Bending strength (MPa)	Impact strength (kJ/m²)
Limit given in the standard	>50	>1800	>70		
Actual strength	68.5	2801	102.9	73.9	5.3

The compositions of the powder and liquid are identical to those of Biocryl 3 (manufactured by Bioland), a bone cement that is no longer sold under this trademark. In former times, Biocryl cements could be obtained in France and other Southern European countries.

It can be seen that the liquid monomers of C-ment 1 and C-ment 3 do not differ from each other, but different amounts of monomer have been used (14.4 g for C-ment 1 and 16.4 g for C-ment 3).

To mix the dough, the powder is put into the vessel, and the liquid is then added. The wetting occurs very quickly; after approximately 15–20 s, the dough has rather low viscosity and is completely homogeneous. The end of the sticky phase is reached at 4 min, and processing may be continued. After 6 min, the

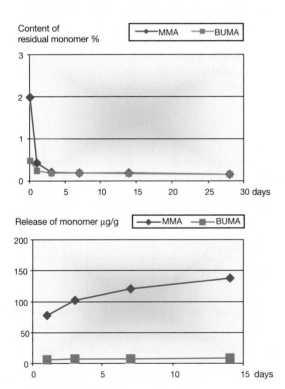

Fig. 28. Content and release of the residual monomers of C-ment 3 with time

dough may no longer be handled. The material shows a very short working phase.

After 5 min 30 s, a clear warming may be noticed. After between 6 min 40 s and 6 min 45 s, the dough is completely hardened (Fig. 27). Due to these handling properties, C-ment 3 has to be regarded as a low-viscosity cement.

The mechanical strengths all correspond to those listed in the ISO standard (Table 8). High compressive strength and low impact strength can be observed.

The hardening temperature (determined according to ISO 5833 protocols) is 80.8°C. Thus, this material has a high polymerization temperature, which is expected, due to the favorable powder/liquid ratio (Fig. 11). The setting time has a value of approximately 7 min 40 s. The residual monomer has not been considered in the comparison (Fig. 28); both MMA and BuMA monomers are contained in the liquid.

Regarding the packing components and their labeling, it is striking that the batch number is only printed on the primary container; an expiration date is completely missing. Moreover, a notice regarding the present standard (ISO 5833; Table 9) is missing. The key characteristics of C-ment 3 are listed in Table 10.

Table 9. ISO 5833 (1992) requirements for the packaging of C-ment 3

Requirements		Com-pliance	Location of information
General	Is the powder packed in a double-layered, sealed container?	+	–
	Is the liquid packed in a double-layered, sealed container?	+	-
Information regarding the powder ingredients	Qualitative	+	PF, FS, POB, PB
	Quantitative	+	PF, FS, POB, PB
Information regarding the liquid ingredients	Qualitative	+	A, POB, FS, PB
	Quantitative	+	A, POB, FS, PB
	Warning that the package contains flammable liquid	+	PB, A, FS
	Instructions for storage (≤25°C, darkness)	+	FS, POB
	Statement of the sterility of the contents	+	A, PF, FS, PB, POB
	Warning against reusing the package	+	FS, POB, PB, PF
	Batch number(s)	+	A, PF, FS, POB
	Expiration date	+	FS, POB
	Name/address of the manufacturer/distributor	+	A, PF, POB, FS, PB
	Number and date of the standard	–	–
Information in the package insert	Detailed instructions for handling the components and preparing the cement	+	PB
	A statement drawing attention to the dangers for the patient	+	PB
	Recommendations for using the cement (syringe/dough state)	+	PB
	A statement regarding the influence of the temperature on working times	+	PB
	Graphical representation of the effects of temperature on the length of the phases of cement curing	+	PB

+, complies; –, does not comply; A, ampoule; FS, carton; PB, package insert; PF, powder bottle; POB, peel-off pouch

Table 10. The key characteristics of C-ment 3

Low viscosity
The monomer contains BuMA
The polymer contains methyl acrylate and ethyl acrylate
Barium sulfate is the radiopaque medium
The polymer is γ irradiated
The polymer is packaged in a brown glass bottle
The polymer bottle and monomer ampoule are in one blister
Mixing sequence: powder, then monomer
Working time: short
ISO 5833 is fulfilled
Molecular weight less than 350,000 Da
High compressive strength
Low bending strength

BuMA, butyl methacrylate

3.2.1.3
Cemex Isoplastic (High Viscosity)

The cement components of Cemex Isoplastic (HV) are packed in a little, rectangular, navy-blue, marked outer carton. This carton is printed on all sides except the lower front side. On the back of the outer carton, the composition of the components and some storage advice are indicated. A little label on one of the front sides gives the necessary information regarding the batch number and expiration date. This label also contains all necessary EC indications.

The distributor and the manufacturer are clearly indicated. The outer carton can only be opened on one side. Inside the carton, there is an insert and a blister pack that contains the polymer pouch and the monomer ampoule (Fig. 29).

The molded PVC part is covered by printed Tyvek. This side contains all necessary product information, such as composition, batch number and expiration date. The batch number and expiration date are not directly printed but are printed on chart stickers that have been put on the Tyvek. These labels can later be used for documentation in the patients' records. On older blister packs, a large, completely printed label was used. Furthermore, a striking brown indicator strip denotes successful sterilization. A notice explaining the way in which this indicator indicates sterility is not included.

The Tyvek may be separated from the PVC lower part so that the single components may be taken out easily. First, the polymer inner pouch may be seen; it consists of a paper side and a polyester side. It is striking that the inner pouch is completely unprinted; it contains no information. A mark indicates where the pouch should be opened. The pouch may easily be opened with the help of the opening instructions. The white, slightly rose-colored polymer powder consists of 84.35% PMMA (which contains approximately 3% styrene in the form of a copolymer), 2.65% BPO and 13.0% barium sulfate (as an opacifier; Fig. 30).

The monomer ampoule lies under the inner pouch in a special space in the PVC molding foil. The brown glass ampoule is printed with white lettering. The information on the ampoule is extremely sparse; there is only the storage notice and the instructions regarding how to inject the material. The batch number and

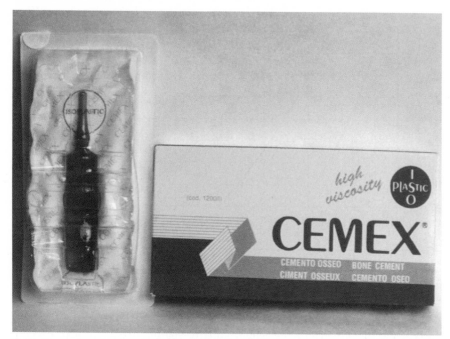

Fig. 29. The packaging of Cemex Isoplastic (High Viscosity)

expiration date are not indicated. The monomer ampoule contains the colorless monomer, which consists of 99.1% MMA, 0.9% DmpT and approximately 75 ppm hydroquinone (as a stabilizer).

It is remarkable that only one batch and one expiration date are indicated on the packing unit. Consequently, the liquid and the powder have the same batch number and the same expiration date.

To mix the dough, the liquid is first put into the mixing vessel; the powder is then added. After adding the powder, one obtains an extremely dry dough that initially may not be homogenized. The great excess of polymer powder hinders easy mixing. It gives the impression that the monomer is missing and that wetting of the polymer by the monomer will not be possible. When trying to

powder	liquid
33,72 g poly(methyl methacrylate) (with 3% styrene) 5,20 g barium sulphate 1,08 g benzoyl peroxide --------- 40,00 g	13,18 g methyl methacrylate (=14,0 ml) 0,12 g N,N-dimethyl-p-toluidine (=0,13 ml) 75 ppm hydroquinone --------- 13,30 g (14,13 ml)
Cemex Isoplastic (HV)	

Fig. 30. Composition of Cemex Isoplastic (High Viscosity)

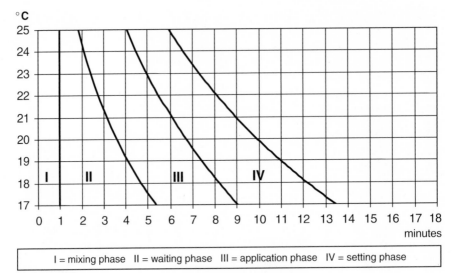

I = mixing phase   II = waiting phase   III = application phase   IV = setting phase

Fig. 31. Working curves of Cemex Isoplastic (High Viscosity) for different ambient/component temperatures

homogenize the dough with the help of a mixing spatula, one has to act especially cautiously, because the material can easily be thrown from the mixing vessel.

After approximately 50 s, one obtains a rather homogeneous dough that flows slowly together. The viscosity at the beginning is strikingly high but, at 23°C, the end of the sticky phase is only reached after 2 min 15 s. The end of the working phase occurred after 4 min 45 s in the tests we carried out; a complete hardening could be observed after 6 min 45 s (Fig. 31). The cement may be regarded as highly viscous, with a short working phase; the viscosity seems to be extremely high very early and, therefore, considerably hinders the fixation of the prosthesis.

The mechanical strengths correspond to those listed in the standard (Table 11). It is remarkable that the bending strength is at the lower limit (56.6 MPa). In contrast to the bending strength determined according to the ISO protocol, the bending strength determined according to the Dynstat protocol is very high (Fig. 29).

On the outer packaging, the manufacturer advertises a low polymerization temperature, because the component ratio of powder to liquid is 3:1. The hardening temperature (determined according to the ISO protocol) is 66.9°C.

Table 11. Mechanical strength according to ISO 5833 and German Industrial Standard DIN 53435 for Cemex Isoplastic (High Viscosity)

	ISO 5833			DIN 53435	
	Bending strength (MPa)	Bending modulus (MPa)	Compressive strength (MPa)	Bending strength (MPa)	Impact strength (kJ/m²)
Limit given in the standard	>50	>1800	>70		
Actual strength	56.6	2192	92.2	87	4.3

This demonstrates that the temperatures determined by us are essentially not lower than those of other bone cements. The setting time (determined according to the ISO protocol) is 12 min.

The residual monomer content was initially determined as 5%, although the high amount of BPO should cause a more complete reaction of the monomer (Fig. 32). It is possible that sufficient starting radicals for polymerization and chains are initially built but, due to the quick increase of viscosity, a further build-up of chains is deferred. Also, the small amount of liquid used when mixing the dough should lead to a low residual monomer content. The residual monomer release from Cemex Isoplastic (HV) is the highest among all the tested cements (more than 200 µg of monomer released per gram of cement).

The qualitative and quantitative indications regarding the components of the powder and the liquid are not printed directly on the polymer pouch or on the ampoule itself. Nevertheless, the blister pack contains all this information. Additionally, the batch number and the expiration date are not directly indicated on the primary packed polymer and monomer components. Apparently, one should avoid storing the single components separately. A graphic representation of the influence of temperature on the handling properties of the material may not be found on the insert. Furthermore, a reference to the presently valid standard (ISO 5833; Table 12) is missing on all packing units. The key characteristics of Cemex Isoplastic (HV) are listed in Table 13.

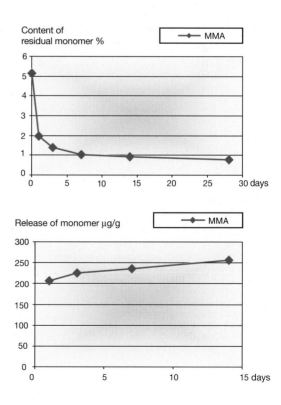

Fig. 32. Content and release of the residual monomer of Cemex Isoplastic (High Viscosity) with time

Table 12. ISO 5833 (1992) requirements for the packaging of Cemex Isoplastic (High Viscosity)

Requirements		Com-pliance	Location of information
General	Is the powder packed in a double-layered, sealed container?	+	–
	Is the liquid packed in a double-layered, sealed container?	+	–
Information regarding the powder ingredients	Qualitative	+	GB, FS, PB
	Quantitative	+	GB, FS, PB
Information regarding the liquid ingredients	Qualitative	+	GB, FS, PB
	Quantitative	+	GB, FS, PB
	Warning that the package contains flammable liquid	+	FS, PB, A, AB
	Instructions for storage (≤25°C, darkness)	+	FS, A, PB
	Statement of the sterility of the contents	+	FS, GB, PB
	Warning against reusing the package	+	FS, GB, PB
	Batch number(s)	+	FS, GB
	Expiration date	+	FS, GB
	Name/address of the manufacturer/distributor	+	GB, FS, A, PB
	Number and date of the standard	–	–
Information in the package insert	Detailed instructions for handling the components and preparing the cement	+	PB
	A statement drawing attention to the dangers for the patient	+	PB
	Recommendations for using the cement (syringe/dough state)	+	PB
	A statement regarding the influence of the temperature on working times	+	PB
	Graphical representation of the effects of temperature on the length of the phases of cement curing	+	PB

+, complies; –, does not comply; *A*, ampoule; *AB*, ampoule blister; *FS*, carton; *GB*, shared blister; *PB*, package insert

Table 13. The key characteristics of Cemex Isoplastic (High Viscosity)

High viscosity
The polymer contains styrene
Barium sulfate is the radiopaque medium
The polymer is γ irradiated
The polymer is packaged in a brown glass bottle
The polymer bottle and ampoule are in one blister
Mixing sequence: monomer, then powder
The resulting mass is very voluminous
Working time: short
ISO 5833 is fulfilled
Molecular weight less than 350,000 Da
Low bending strength
Low bending modulus

3.2.1.4
Cemex RX (Low Viscosity)

The cement components of Cemex Isoplastic (Low Viscosity; LV) are packed in a little, rectangular, red, marked outer carton. This carton is printed on all sides except the lower front side. On the back of the outer carton, the composition of the components and some storage advice are indicated. A little label on one of the front sides gives the necessary information regarding the batch number and expiration date. This label also contains all necessary CE indications.

The distributor and the manufacturer are clearly indicated. The outer carton can only be opened on one side. Inside the carton, there is an insert and a blister pack that contains the polymer pouch and the monomer ampoule (Fig. 33).

The molded PVC part is covered by printed Tyvek. This side contains all necessary product information, such as composition, batch number and expiration date. The batch number and expiration date are not directly printed but are printed on chart-stickers that have been put on the Tyvek side. These labels can later be used for documentation in the patients' records. On older blister packs, a large, completely printed label was used. Furthermore, a striking brown indicator

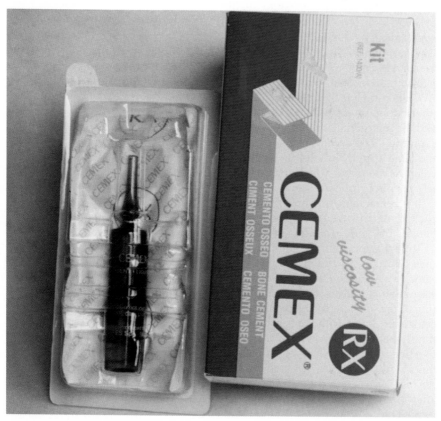

Fig. 33. The packaging of Cemex RX (Low Viscosity)

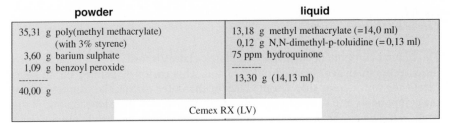

powder	liquid
35,31 g poly(methyl methacrylate) (with 3% styrene) 3,60 g barium sulphate 1,09 g benzoyl peroxide --------- 40,00 g	13,18 g methyl methacrylate (=14,0 ml) 0,12 g N,N-dimethyl-p-toluidine (=0,13 ml) 75 ppm hydroquinone --------- 13,30 g (14,13 ml)
Cemex RX (LV)	

Fig. 34. Composition of Cemex RX (Low Viscosity)

strip denotes successful sterilization. A notice explaining the way in which this indicator indicates sterility is not included.

The Tyvek foil may be separated from the PVC lower part so that the single components may be taken out easily. First, the polymer inner pouch may be seen; it consists of a paper side and a polyester side. It is striking that the inner pouch is completely unprinted; it contains no information. A mark indicates where the pouch should be opened. The pouch may easily be opened with the help of the opening instructions. The white, slightly rose-colored polymer powder consists of 88.25% PMMA (which contains approximately 3% styrene in the form of a copolymer), 2.75% BPO and 9.0% barium sulfate (as an opacifier; Fig. 34).

Obviously, both Cemex variants contain at least one styrene copolymer. Thus, the information on the package (stating that only PMMA is present) is not correct.

The monomer ampoule lies under the inner pouch in a special space in the PVC molding foil. The brown glass ampoule is printed with white lettering. The information on the ampoule is extremely sparse; there is only the storage notice and the instructions regarding how to inject the material. The batch number and expiration date are not indicated. The composition of the monomer ampoule is the same as in the case of the high-viscosity material. The ampoule contains the colorless monomer, which consists of 99.1% MMA, 0.9% DmpT and approximately 75 ppm hydroquinone (as a stabilizer).

It is remarkable that only one batch and one expiry date are indicated on the packing unit. Consequently, the liquid and the powder have the same batch number and the same expiration date.

To mix the dough, the liquid is first put into the mixing vessel; the powder is then added. After adding the powder, one obtains an extremely dry dough that initially may not be homogenized. The great excess of polymer powder hinders easy mixing. It gives the impression that the monomer is missing and that wetting of the polymer by the monomer will not be possible. When trying to homogenize the dough with the help of a mixing spatula, one has to act especially cautiously, because the material can easily be thrown from the mixing vessel.

After approximately 45–50 s, one obtains a rather homogeneous dough that flows slowly together. The viscosity at the beginning is lower than in the case of the high-viscosity version and, at 23°C, the end of the sticky phase is only reached after 3 min. The end of the working phase occurred after 5 min 45 s in the tests we carried out; a complete hardening could be observed after 8 min 15 s. The cement may be regarded as having medium viscosity, with a working phase that shows a

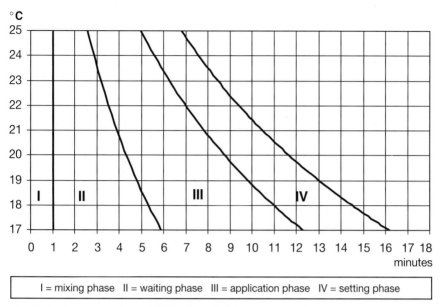

I = mixing phase   II = waiting phase   III = application phase   IV = setting phase

Fig. 35. Working curves of Cemex RX (Low Viscosity) for different ambient/component temperatures

high viscosity very early and, therefore, considerably hinders the fixation of the prosthesis. Additionally, implantation by syringes may be extremely difficult (Fig. 35).

The mechanical strengths correspond to those listed in the standard. It is remarkable that the bending strength is at the lower limit (55 MPa). In contrast to the bending strength determined according to the ISO protocol, the bending strength determined according to the Dynstat protocol (93.6 MPa) is very high (Table 14).

In the case of Cemex LV, the manufacturer advertises a low polymerization temperature on the outer packing, because the component ratio of powder to liquid is 3:1. The hardening temperature (determined according to the ISO protocol) is 71.6°C. This demonstrates that the temperatures determined by us are essentially not lower than those of other bone cements. The setting time (determined according to the ISO protocol) is 13 min 20 s.

Table 14. Mechanical strength according to ISO 5833 and German Industrial Standard DIN 53435 for Cemex RX (Low Viscosity)

	ISO 5833			DIN 53435	
	Bending strength (MPa)	Bending modulus (MPa)	Compressive strength (MPa)	Bending strength (MPa)	Impact strength (kJ/m²)
Limit given in the standard	>50	>1800	>70		
Actual strength	55	2441	92.2	93.6	5.4

The residual monomer content was initially determined as 5% (Fig. 36), although the high amount of BPO should cause a more complete monomer reaction (in comparison to the reaction occurring when DmpT is used). Therefore, there is no significant difference between the Cemex HV and Cemex LV cement. It is possible that sufficient starting radicals for polymerization and chains are initially built but, due to the quick increase of viscosity, a further build-up of chains is deferred. Also, the small amount of liquid used when mixing the dough should lead to a low residual monomer content. The residual monomer release from Cemex RX (LV) is among the highest of all the tested cements (more than 200 µg of monomer released per gram of cement; Fig. 36).

The qualitative and quantitative indications regarding the components of the powder and the liquid are not printed on the primary container. Nevertheless, the blister pack contains all this information.

The batch number and the expiration date are not directly indicated on the primary container. Apparently, one should avoid storing the single components separately.

A graphic representation of the influence of temperature on the handling properties of the material may not be found in the insert. Furthermore, a reference to the presently valid standard (ISO 5833; Table 15) is missing on all packing units. The key characteristics of Cemex RX (LV) are listed in Table 16.

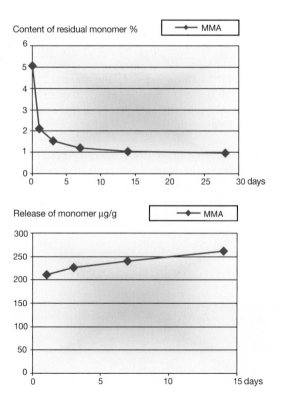

Fig. 36. Content and release of the residual monomer of Cemex RX (Low Viscosity) with time

Table 15. ISO 5833 (1992) requirements for the packaging of Cemex RX (Low Viscosity)

Requirements		Compliance	Location of information
General	Is the powder packed in a double-layered, sealed container?	+	–
	Is the liquid packed in a double-layered, sealed container?	+	–
Information regarding the powder ingredients	Qualitative	+	GB, FS, PB
	Quantitative	+	GB, FS, PB
Information regarding the liquid ingredients	Qualitative	+	GB, FS, PB
	Quantitative	+	GB, FS, PB
	Warning that the package contains flammable liquid	+	FS, PB, A, AB
	Instructions for storage (≤25°C, darkness)	+	FS, A, PB
	Statement of the sterility of the contents	+	FS, GB, PB
	Warning against reusing the package	+	FS, GB, PB
	Batch number(s)	+	FS, GB
	Expiration date	+	FS, GB
	Name/address of the manufacturer/distributor	+	GB, FS, A, PB
	Number and date of the standard	–	–
Information in the package insert	Detailed instructions for handling the components and preparing the cement	+	–
	A statement drawing attention to the dangers for the patient	+	PB
	Recommendations for using the cement (syringe/dough state)	+	PB
	A statement regarding the influence of the temperature on working times	+	PB
	Graphical representation of the effects of temperature on the length of the phases of cement curing	+	+

+, complies; –, does not comply; *A*, ampoule; *AB*, ampoule blister; *FS*, carton; *GB*, shared blister; *PB*, package insert

Table 16. The key characteristics of Cemex RX (Low Viscosity)

Medium viscosity
The polymer contains styrene
Barium sulfate is the radiopaque medium
The polymer is γ irradiated
The polymer is packaged in a brown glass bottle
The polymer bottle and ampoule are in one blister
Mixing sequence: monomer, then powder
The resulting mass is very voluminous
ISO 5833 is fulfilled
Molecular weight less than 350,000 Da
Low bending strength as defined by ISO 5833, high bending strength as defined by DIN 53435

3.2.1.5
Cerafix LV

The components of Cerafix LV are packed in a simple, rectangular, blue outer carton that may be easily opened on the front side (Fig. 37). In the outer carton,

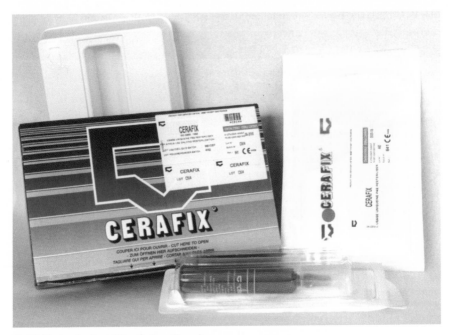

Fig. 37. The packaging of Cerafix Low Viscosity

there is a plastic tray with a space for the blister pack. On the ampoule blister pack, there is a double-packed powder pouch and the insert (in the form of a brochure) is over it. Additionally, in the outer carton is a label that can be stored with the patient's records for documentation.

The outer carton is printed on all sides. On its back, the compositions of the cement components are indicated in four different languages. The layout of the outer carton and the packaging components are consistent with the ISO packaging regulations, but the necessary information about batch number and expiration date and the »CE« characterization are only printed on a label (which was obviously attached later) on the outer carton. Moreover, it is remarkable that the typical ISO standard symbols (for example, for the batch number or the expiration date) are not used. On the additional label on the outer carton, there is a notice that the material satisfies the ISO 5833 standards for cements.

The polymer inner pouch is enclosed by a peel-off pouch that consists of an unprinted, transparent polyethylene side and a Tyvek side. On the Tyvek, there is a sterilization indicator that indicates the success of sterilization by its red color. A corresponding note appears on the label. It appears that a trilateral closed pouch (which is closed manually on its fourth side after adding the inner pouch) is used. This implies a manual filling of the pouch. The inner pouch itself bears only the brand of the product. There is an additional red sterilization indicator point. A paper label that indicates the batch and expiration date is attached. The printing on the inner pouch may be seen through the transparent polyester side of the peel-off pouch. There is no notice on the composition of the polymer

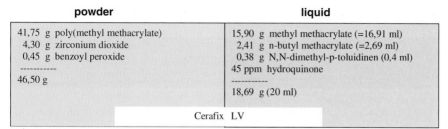

powder	liquid
41,75 g poly(methyl methacrylate) 4,30 g zirconium dioxide 0,45 g benzoyl peroxide ---------- 46,50 g	15,90 g methyl methacrylate (=16,91 ml) 2,41 g n-butyl methacrylate (=2,69 ml) 0,38 g N,N-dimethyl-p-toluidinen (0,4 ml) 45 ppm hydroquinone ---------- 18,69 g (20 ml)
Cerafix LV	

Fig. 38. Composition of Cerafix Low Viscosity

either on the peel-off ouch or on the inner pouch. Further remarks (for example, warnings) are absent. The white polymer powder consists of 89.79% PMMA, 0.96% BPO and 9.25% zirconium dioxide (as an opacifier; Fig. 38). We checked the powder for copolymers but could not find any.

The ampoule blister pack, which is in a plastic tray, contains a double-packed ampoule. Both blister packs are made of molded PVC and are covered by unprinted Tyvek. The outer blister pack contains a little label with the batch number and expiration date and a notice regarding the sterilization procedure. The function of the green stripe on the label is not clearly described. It seems to be a further sterilization indicator. On the side where it is to be opened, the second blister pack has a clearly visible green dot; in all probability, this is a sterilization indicator. The brown glass ampoule has white printing and has a plastic opening aid. Neither the packing unit nor the ampoule itself indicate the composition of the colorless liquid. This liquid contains two different methacrylates (85.1% MMA and 12.9% BuMA) and 2.0% DmpT. As a stabilizer, one can find approximately 45 ppm hydroquinone.

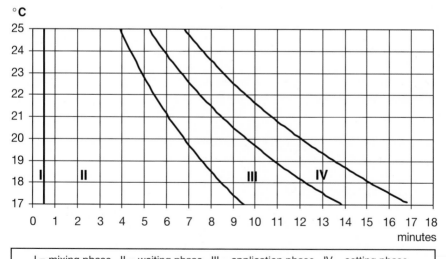

I = mixing phase   II = waiting phase   III = application phase   IV = setting phase

Fig. 39. Working curves of Cerafix Low Viscosity for different ambient/component temperatures

Table 17. Mechanical strength according to ISO 5833 and German Industrial Standard DIN 53435 for Cerafix LV

	ISO 5833 Bending strength (MPa)	Bending modulus (MPa)	Compressive strength (MPa)	DIN 53435 Bending strength (MPa)	Impact strength (kJ/m²)
Limit given in the standard	>50	>1800	>70		
Actual strength	70.6	2702	101.9	78.7	4.3

According to the instructions of the manufacturer, the powder is first put into a mixing vessel, then the liquid is added. Mixing results in a liquid, homogeneous dough in approximately 10–15 s. This dough has a slight cream-like color. The dough remains liquid and sticky for a long time. After 4 min 30 s, the dough may be taken out of the bowl; at this point, it is rather non-sticky. The sticky phase was sometimes longer than 5 min. The working phase seems to be rather short, as the viscosity of the dough increases quickly and, after 6 min 30 s, is so high that the fixation of the prosthesis may no longer be executed without risk for the patient. The complete hardening of the dough is finished after 8 min 15 s (Fig. 39).

Due to the liquid starting phase and the short working phase, manual processing is not advisable. The cement has to be regarded as a low-viscosity one (Fig. 39).

The mechanical characteristics all fulfill the standard. The high compressive strength (101.9 MPa) is striking (Table 17).

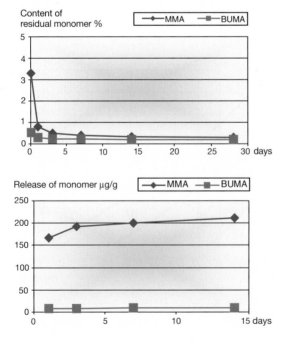

Fig. 40. Content and release of the residual monomers of Cerafix Low Viscosity with time

The setting time, determined according to the ISO protocol, was 12 min 10 s, and the polymerization temperature was clearly less than 80°C (70.4°C). The determined residual monomer content is remarkably low. However, in addition to MMA, BuMA (~13%) was used in the liquid. Comparison with other liquids exclusively containing MMA is not possible. Regarding the initiator ratio, the rather low BPO content and the comparatively high DmpT content are interesting. These conditions should have a positive influence on the completion of polymerization, resulting in a low residual monomer content (Fig. 40).

We find qualitative and quantitative indications regarding the powder and liquid constituents only on the outer carton and in the insert. Such information is, therefore, not printed on the primary vessels. The batch number and expiration date are not directly indicated on the primary vessel. Apparently, one should avoid storing the single components separately. Cerafix LV features a notice regarding the presently valid ISO 5833 standard (Table 18) on its outer carton, a notice that is missing with most other cements. The key characteristics of Cerafix LV are listed in Table 19.

Table 18. ISO 5833 (1992) requirements for the packaging of Cerafix Low Viscosity

Requirements		Compliance	Location of information
General	Is the powder packed in a double-layered, sealed container?	+	–
	Is the liquid packed in a double-layered, sealed container?	+	–
Information regarding the powder ingredients	Qualitative	+	FS, PB
	Quantitative	+	FS, PB
Information regarding the liquid ingredients	Qualitative	+	FS, PB
	Quantitative	+	FS, PB
	Warning that the package contains flammable liquid	+	FS, A
	Instructions for storage (≤25°C, darkness)	+	FS, PB
	Statement of the sterility of the contents	+	AB, IB, POB, FS, PB
	Warning against reusing the package	+	IB
	Batch number(s)	+	FS, AB, IB
	Expiration date	+	FS, AB, IB
	Name/address of the manufacturer/distributor	+	IB, FS, PB
	Number and date of the standard	+	FS
Information in the package insert	Detailed instructions for handling the components and preparing the cement	+	PB
	A statement drawing attention to the dangers for the patient	+	PB
	Recommendations for using the cement (syringe/dough state)	+	PB
	A statement regarding the influence of the temperature on working times	+	PB
	Graphical representation of the effects of temperature on the length of the phases of cement curing	+	PB

+, complies; –, does not comply; A, ampoule; AB, ampoule blister; FS, carton; IB, primary pouch; PB, package insert; POB, peel-off pouch

Table 19. The key characteristics of Cerafix Low Viscosity

Low viscosity
The monomer contains BuMA
Zirconium dioxide is the radiopaque medium
The polymer is γ irradiated
The polymer bottle and ampoule are packaged separately
Mixing sequence: powder, then monomer
Working time: short
ISO 5833 is fulfilled
Molecular weight less than 350,000 Da
High compressive strength

BuMA, butyl methacrylate

3.2.1.6
CMW 1

All the cement components of CMW 1 are packed in a rectangular outer carton that may be easily opened along its side with the help of a perforated opening aid (Fig. 41). One of the front sides of the outer carton serves as a cover under which the cement components are packed. The printing on the outer carton complies with ISO packaging regulations in every respect. The indications regarding batch number and expiration date are not printed on the front side of the carton but on the lower part. The distributor is clearly indicated.

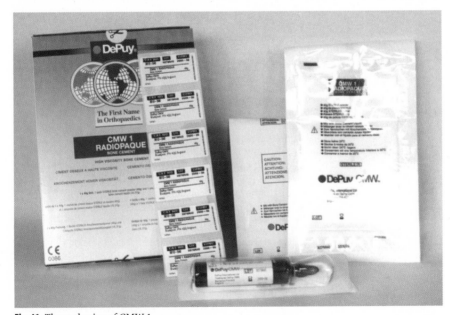

Fig. 41. The packaging of CMW 1

powder	liquid
35,54 g poly(methyl methacrylate) 0,82 g benzoyl peroxide 3,64 g barium sulphate ---------- 40,00 g	18,22 g methyl methacrylate (=19,36 ml) 0,15 g N,N-dimethyl-p-toluidine (=0,16 ml) 25 ppm hydroquinone ---------- 18,37 g (19,57 ml)
CMW 1 radiopaque	

Fig. 42. Composition of CMW 1

The outer carton contains a cardboard tray, which has a space is left for the blister pack containing the ampoule. Above and below the space is an opening that makes it easier to take out the tray. The tray has two such places on its lower part so that the unit may be used for a double pack (with two ampoule-containing blister packs).

The insert and an aluminum protective pouch (alu-pouch) that contains the polymer-containing pouch are on top of the blister-packed monomer ampoule. In the outer carton, there are also six stickers that may be attached to patients' records.

The opening of the alu-protective pouch, which has printing on both sides, should not be performed with scissors; it should be opened at the mark specially provided for opening. The alu-pouch is also printed with the batch number and the expiration date of the material. The inner surface of the alu-pouch is completely laminated with polyethylene. In the alu-pouch, there is a folded peel-off pouch, which is printed on its Tyvek side and which contains a sterilization indicator point. The pouch has a distinct sealing pattern. The inner pouch may easily

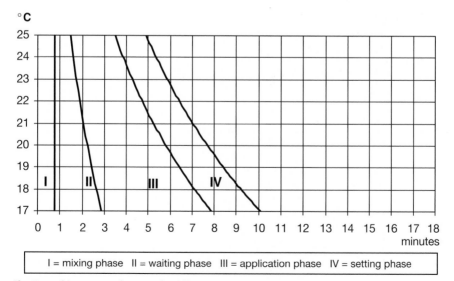

I = mixing phase   II = waiting phase   III = application phase   IV = setting phase

Fig. 43. Working curves of CMW 1 for different ambient/component temperatures

Table 20. Mechanical strength according to ISO 5833 and German Industrial Standard DIN 53435 for CMW 1

	ISO 5833 Bending strength (MPa)	Bending modulus (MPa)	Compressive strength (MPa)	DIN 53435 Bending strength (MPa)	Impact strength (kJ/m²)
Limit given in the standard	>50	>1800	>70		
Actual strength	67	2634	94.4	86.2	3.7

be distinguished through the unprinted, transparent polyethylene side, and the printing of the inner pouch can easily be read.

The polyethylene inner pouch is printed with black letters. The batch number and the expiration date are printed on the lower part, outside the seal. The polymer powder consists of 88.85% PMMA, 2.05% BPO and 9.1% barium sulfate (as an opacifier; Fig. 42).

The ampoule, which is packed in a blister pack, has the same batch number and the same expiration date as the powder. These indications are on the Tyvek side of the blister pack, which also contains all necessary warning symbols. The brown glass ampoule is in the molded, PVC part of the blister pack. A label that contains all necessary information is attached to it.

It seems that there was a change in the composition of the monomer in August 1997; earlier, the ampoules contained 0.17 g ethanol (as a plasticizer) and 0.004 g

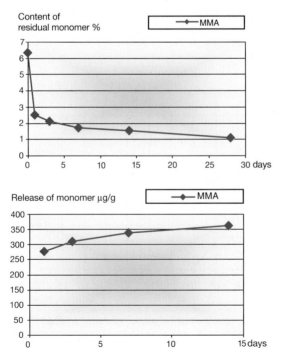

Fig. 44. Content and release of the residual monomer of CMW 1 with time

ascorbic acid (as an additional stabilizer). At the present, the colorless monomer liquid consists of 99.18% MMA and 0.82% DmpT. As a stabilizer, approximately 25 ppm hydroquinone is used.

There is no opening help included for the opening of the brown glass ampoule. The polymer pouch should be opened with the help of a scissors. The polymer powder is easily poured out of the pouch into the mixing vessel.

First, the polymer is put into the bowl for mixing. The monomer is added next. The wetting is remarkably slow. At first, it appears as though the quantity of the liquid is not sufficient. The result is a dry dough that suddenly (after 30 s) flows together and may then be described as a homogeneous mass. The sudden falling of the dough during the wetting phase is typical of all CMW cements, including Endurance.

CMW 1 reaches the end of the sticky phase after between 1 min 20 s and 1 min 30 s. The end of the working phase occurs after 4 min 15 s. At the end of the working phase, the dough becomes remarkably warm. Complete setting may be observed after 5 min 45 s (Fig. 43).

Table 21. ISO 5833 (1992) requirements for the packaging of CMW 1

Requirements		Compliance	Location of information
General	Is the powder packed in a double-layered, sealed container?	+	–
	Is the liquid packed in a double-layered, sealed container?	+	–
Information regarding the powder ingredients	Qualitative	+	PB
	Quantitative	+	PB
Information regarding the liquid ingredients	Qualitative	+	PB
	Quantitative	+	PB
	Warning that the package contains flammable liquid	+	A, AB, FS
	Instructions for storage (≤25°C, darkness)	+	IB, Alu, FS
	Statement of the sterility of the contents	+	IB, POB, A, AB, FS, Alu
	Warning against reusing the package	+	–
	Batch number(s)	+	IB, A, AB, FS, Alu
	Expiration date	+	IB, A, AB, FS, Alu
	Name/address of the manufacturer/distributor	+	IB, A, AB, FS, Alu, PB
	Number and date of the standard	–	–
Information in the package insert	Detailed instructions for handling the components and preparing the cement	+	PB
	A statement drawing attention to the dangers for the patient	+	PB
	Recommendations for using the cement (syringe/dough state)	+	PB
	A statement regarding the influence of the temperature on working times	+	PB
	Graphical representation of the effects of temperature on the length of the phases of cement curing	–	–

+, complies; –, does not comply; *A*, ampoule; *AB*, ampoule blister; *Alu*, aluminum pouch; *FS*, carton; *IB*, primary pouch; *PB*, package insert; *POB*, peel-off pouch

Table 22. The key characteristics of CMW 1

High viscosity
Barium sulfate is the radiopaque medium
The polymer is γ irradiated
The powder and ampoule are packaged separately
Mixing sequence: powder, then monomer
Working time: short
The dough is dry
ISO 5833 is fulfilled
Molecular weight less than 350,000 Da
Low impact strength

The quasi-static mechanical strength clearly corresponds to that described in the standard; therefore, the low impact strength is remarkable. Furthermore, it may be observed that the bending strengths determined according to the ISO 5833 and DIN 53435 protocols hardly differ from each other. Moreover, the compressive strength is quite high (94.4 MPa; Table 20). The setting time determined according to the ISO 5833 protocol is 8 min 10 s and the polymerization temperature is 84.3°C.

The BPO content is lower than the DmpT content, so the ratio is higher than five. The residual monomer content is higher than 6% (Fig. 44) and, therefore, is higher than in the case of CMW 3. The change in the composition of the liquid portion of CMW 1 probably leads to worse values compared with those of the low-viscosity cements.

According to the requirements of the ISO 5833 standard, the qualitative and quantitative indications regarding the ingredients of the cement components may only be found on the insert. A statement prohibiting reuse is completely missing. Furthermore, a graphic representation of the influence of temperature on the handling properties of the cement is not found in the insert. A reference to the presently valid ISO standard (Table 21) is also missing. The key characteristics of CMW 1 are listed in Table 22.

3.2.1.7
CMW 2

All the cement components of CMW 2 are packed in a rectangular outer carton that may be easily opened along its side with the help of a perforated opening aid (Fig. 45). One of the front sides of the outer carton serves as a cover under which the cement components are packed. The printing on the outer carton complies with ISO packaging regulations in every respect. The indications regarding batch number and expiration date are not printed on the front side of the carton but on the lower part. The distributor is clearly indicated.

The outer carton contains a cardboard tray, which has a space is left for the blister pack containing the ampoule. Above and below the space is an opening that makes it easier to take out the tray. The tray has two such places on its lower part so that the unit may be used for a double pack (with two ampoule-containing blister packs).

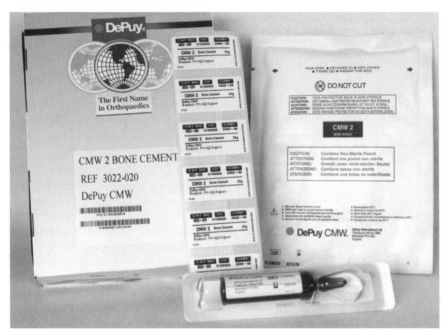

Fig. 45. The packaging of CMW 2

The insert and an alu-pouch that contains the polymer-containing pouch are on top of the blister-packed monomer ampoule. In the outer carton, there are also six stickers that may be attached to patients' records.

The opening of the alu-protective pouch, which has printing on both sides, should not be performed with scissors; it should be opened at the mark specially provided for opening. The alu-pouch is also printed with the batch number and the expiration date of the material. The inner surface of the alu-pouch is completely laminated with polyethylene. In the alu-pouch, there is a folded peel-off pouch, which is printed on its Tyvek side and which contains a sterilization indicator point. The pouch has a distinct sealing pattern. The inner pouch may easily be distinguished through the unprinted, transparent polyethylene side, and the printing of the inner pouch can easily be read.

The polyethylene inner pouch is printed with black letters. The batch number and the expiration date are printed on the lower part, outside the seal. The polymer powder consists of 86.7% PMMA, 2.0% BPO and 11.3% barium sulfate (as an opacifier; Fig. 46).

The ampoule, which is packed in a blister pack, has the same batch number and the same expiration date as the powder. These indications are on the Tyvek side of the blister pack, which also contains all necessary warning symbols. The brown glass ampoule is in the molded, PVC part of the blister pack. A label that contains all necessary information is attached to it.

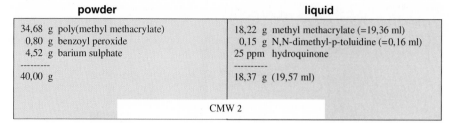

powder	liquid
34,68 g poly(methyl methacrylate) 0,80 g benzoyl peroxide 4,52 g barium sulphate --------- 40,00 g	18,22 g methyl methacrylate (=19,36 ml) 0,15 g N,N-dimethyl-p-toluidine (=0,16 ml) 25 ppm hydroquinone ---------- 18,37 g (19,57 ml)
	CMW 2

Fig. 46. Composition of CMW 2

It seems that there was a change in the composition of the monomer in August 1997; earlier, the ampoules contained 0.17 g ethanol (as a plasticizer) and 0.004 g ascorbic acid (as an additional stabilizer). At the present, the colorless monomer liquid consists of 99.18% MMA and 0.82% DmpT. As a stabilizer, approximately 25 ppm hydroquinone is used. Thus, the liquids of CMW 2 and CMW 1 show the same composition (Fig. 42).

There is no aid for the opening of the brown glass ampoule. The polymer pouch should be opened with the help of a scissors. The polymer powder is easily poured out of the pouch into the mixing vessel.

First, the polymer is put into the bowl for mixing. The monomer is added next. The wetting is extremely slow. At first, it appears as though the quantity of the liquid is not sufficient. The result is a very dry dough that suddenly (after 30–35 s) flows together and may then be described as a homogeneous mass. The sudden falling of the dough during the wetting phase is typical for CMW 2.

CMW 2 reaches the end of the sticky phase after 45–50 s, immediately after wetting. The very short working phase ends after 2 min 45 s, whereas the dough becomes remarkably warm at the end of the working phase (2 min). Complete setting may be observed after 3 min 30 s (Fig. 47).

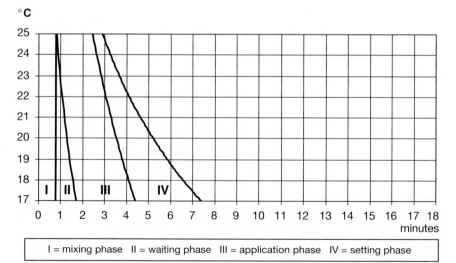

I = mixing phase   II = waiting phase   III = application phase   IV = setting phase

Fig. 47. Working curves of CMW 2 for different ambient/component temperatures

Table 23. Mechanical strength according to ISO 5833 and German Industrial Standard DIN 53435 for CMW 2

	ISO 5833 Bending strength (MPa)	Bending modulus (MPa)	Compressive strength (MPa)	DIN 53435 Bending strength (MPa)	Impact strength (kJ/m²)
Limit given in the standard	>50	>1800	>70		
Actual strength	74.3	3008	97.8	78.1	4.7

The manufacturer indicates that this high-viscosity material is not suitable for mixing under vacuum or application with syringes. Therefore, the material should not be used for total hip replacements.

The quasi-static mechanical strength clearly corresponds to that described in the standard; therefore, the low impact strength is remarkable. Furthermore, a high bending strength (determined according to the ISO 5833 protocol; 74.3 MPa) may be observed. Moreover, the compressive strength is quite high (97.8 MPa),

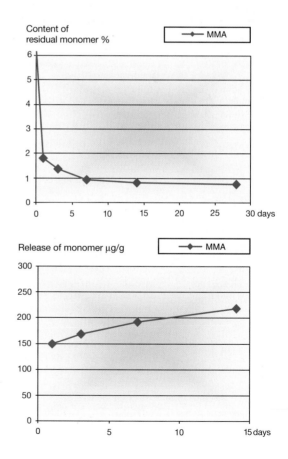

Fig. 48. Content and release of the residual monomer of CMW 2 with time

and the modulus of elasticity is 3008 MPa. This indicates a brittle material (Table 23). The setting time, determined according to the ISO 5833 protocol, is 4 min 40 s, and the polymerization temperature is 80.6°C.

The BPO content is lower than the DmpT content, so the ratio is higher than five. The residual monomer content is higher than 6% (Fig. 48) and, therefore, is higher than in the case of CMW 3 but comparable to the ratio for CMW 1. The change in the composition of the liquid portions of CMW 1 and CMW 2 probably leads to worse values compared with those of the low-viscosity cements.

According to the requirements of the ISO 5833 standard, the qualitative and quantitative indications regarding the ingredients of the cement components may only be found on the insert. A statement prohibiting reuse is completely missing. Furthermore, a graphic representation of the influence of temperature on the handling properties of the cement is not found in the insert. A reference to the presently valid ISO standard (Table 24) is also missing. The key characteristics of CMW 2 are listed in Table 25.

Table 24. ISO 5833 (1992) requirements for the packaging of CMW 2

Requirements		Com- pliance	Location of information
General	Is the powder packed in a double-layered, sealed container?	+	–
	Is the liquid packed in a double-layered, sealed container?	+	–
Information regarding the powder ingredients	Qualitative	+	PB
	Quantitative	+	PB
Information regarding the liquid ingredients	Qualitative	+	PB
	Quantitative	+	PB
	Warning that the package contains flammable liquid	+	A, AB, FS
	Instructions for storage (≤25°C, darkness)	+	IB, Alu, FS
	Statement of the sterility of the contents	+	IB, POB, A, AB, FS, Alu
	Warning against reusing the package	+	–
	Batch number(s)	+	IB, A, AB, FS, Alu
	Expiration date	+	IB, A, AB, FS, Alu
	Name/address of the manufacturer/distri-butor	+	IB, A, AB, FS, Alu, PB
	Number and date of the standard	–	–
Information in the package insert	Detailed instructions for handling the components and preparing the cement	+	PB
	A statement drawing attention to the dangers for the patient	+	PB
	Recommendations for using the cement (syringe/dough state)	+	PB
	A statement regarding the influence of the temperature on working times	+	PB
	Graphical representation of the effects of temperature on the length of the phases of cement curing	–	–

+, complies; –, does not comply; *A*, ampoule; *AB*, ampoule blister; *Alu*, aluminum pouch; *FS*, carton; *IB*, primary pouch; *PB*, package insert; *POB*, peel-off pouch

Table 25. The key characteristics of CMW 2

High viscosity
Barium sulfate is the radiopaque medium
The polymer is γ irradiated
The powder and ampoule are packaged separately
Mixing sequence: powder, then monomer
Working time: short
The dough is very dry
ISO 5833 is fulfilled
Molecular weight less than 350,000 Da
High compressive strength
High bending modulus

3.2.1.8
CMW 3

All the cement components of CMW 3 are packed in a rectangular outer carton that may be easily opened along its side with the help of a perforated opening aid (Fig. 49). One of the front sides of the outer carton serves as a cover under which the cement components are packed. The printing on the outer carton complies with ISO packaging regulations in every respect. The indications regarding batch number and expiration date are not printed on the front side of the carton but on the lower part. The distributor is clearly indicated.

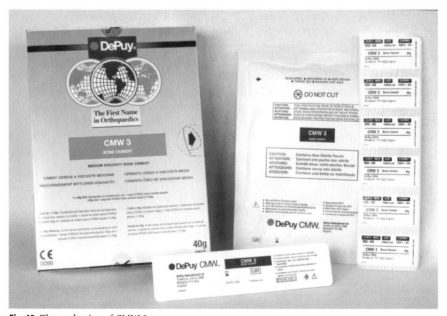

Fig. 49. The packaging of CMW 3

The outer carton contains a cardboard tray, which has a space is left for the blister pack containing the ampoule. Above and below the space is an opening that makes it easier to take out the tray. The tray has two such places on its lower part so that the unit may be used for a double pack (with two ampoule-containing blister packs).

The insert and an alu-pouch that contains the polymer-containing pouch are on top of the blister-packed monomer ampoule. In the outer carton, there are also six stickers that may be attached to patients' records.

The opening of the alu-protective pouch, which has printing on both sides, should not be performed with scissors; it should be opened at the mark specially provided for opening. The alu-pouch is also printed with the batch number and the expiration date of the material. The inner surface of the alu-pouch is completely laminated with polyethylene. In the alu-pouch, there is a folded peel-off pouch, which is printed on its Tyvek side and which contains a sterilization indicator point. The pouch has a distinct sealing pattern. The inner pouch may easily be distinguished through the unprinted, transparent polyethylene side, and the printing of the inner pouch can easily be read.

The polyethylene inner pouch is printed with black letters. The batch number and the expiration date are printed on the lower part, outside the seal. The polymer powder consists of 88.0% PMMA, 2.0% BPO and 10.0% barium sulfate (as an opacifier; Fig. 50).

The ampoule, which is packed in a blister pack, has the same batch number and the same expiration date as the powder. These indications are on the Tyvek side of the blister pack, which also contains all necessary caution notices (warning symbols). The brown glass ampoule is in the molded, PVC part of the blister pack. A label that contains all necessary information is attached to it.

It seems that there was a change in the composition of the monomer in August 1997; earlier, the ampoules contained 0.17 g ethanol (as a plasticizer) and 0.004 g ascorbic acid (as an additional stabilizer). At the present, the colorless monomer liquid consists of 97.50% MMA and 2.50% DmpT. As stabilizer, approximately 25 ppm hydroquinone is used (Fig. 50). Therefore, it obviously does not have the same liquid composition as CWM 1 or CMW 2.

There is no aid for the opening of the brown glass ampoule. The polymer pouch should be opened with the help of a scissors. The polymer powder is easily poured out of the pouch into the mixing vessel.

powder	liquid
35,20 g poly(methyl methacrylate) 0,80 g benzoyl peroxide 4,00 g barium sulphate --------- 40,00 g	17,45 g methyl methacrylate (=18,56 ml) 0,45 g N,N-dimethyl-p-toluidine (= 0,48 ml) 25 ppm hydroquinone --------- 17,90 g (19,04 ml)
CMW 3	

Fig. 50. Composition of CMW 3

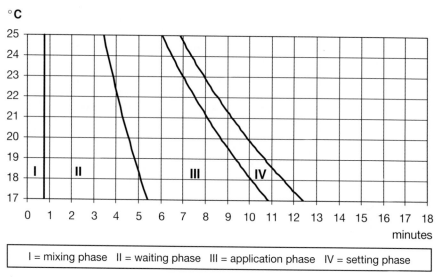

I = mixing phase   II = waiting phase   III = application phase   IV = setting phase

Fig. 51. Working curves of CMW 3 for different ambient/component temperatures

First, the polymer is put into the bowl for mixing. The monomer is added next. The wetting is slow but considerably better than in the cases of CMW 1 and CMW 2. At first, it appears as though the quantity of the liquid is not sufficient. The result is a dry dough that suddenly (after 30 s) flows together and may then be described as a liquid, homogeneous mass. In this case, the sudden falling of the dough is not as distinct as for the high-viscosity variants of the CMW cements.

CMW 3 reaches the end of the sticky phase after between 3 min 40 s and 3 min 45 s. The end of the working phase occurs after 6 min 45 s. Complete setting may be observed after 7 min 45 s (Fig. 51). Furthermore, for this low-viscosity CMW, the dough already feels warm at the end of the working phase (after approximately 6 min 45 s).

The quasi-static mechanical strength clearly corresponds to that described in the standard; therefore, the low impact strength is remarkable. Furthermore, the bending strengths determined according to the ISO 5833 and DIN 53435 protocols hardly differ from each other. Moreover, the compressive strength is quite high (96.3 MPa; Table 26).

Table 26. Mechanical strength according to ISO 5833 and German Industrial Standard DIN 53435 for CMW 3

	ISO 5833 Bending strength (MPa)	Bending modulus (MPa)	Compressive strength (MPa)	DIN 53435 Bending strength (MPa)	Impact strength (kJ/m²)
Limit given in the standard	>50	>1800	>70		
Actual strength	70.3	2764	96.3	72.4	2.9

The setting time, 9 min 55 s min, determined according to the ISO 5833 protocol, is clearly higher in the case of CMW 3 than in the cases of CMW 1 and CMW 2. The polymerization temperature, determined according to the ISO 5833 protocol, is 84.7°C.

In contrast to the both variants described before, CMW 3 has a uniform distribution of the initiators and, therefore, a ratio of a little more than one. The residual monomer content is always under 5% (Fig. 52) and, therefore, is lower than in the cases of CMW 1 and CMW 2. The change in the composition of the liquid portion of CMW 3 probably leads to better values compared with those of the high-viscosity cements.

According to the requirements of the ISO 5833 standard, the qualitative and quantitative indications regarding the ingredients of the cement components may only be found on the insert. A statement prohibiting reuse is completely missing. Furthermore, a graphic representation of the influence of temperature on the handling properties of the cement is not found in the insert. A reference to the presently valid ISO standard (Table 27) is also missing. The key characteristics of CMW 3 are listed in Table 28.

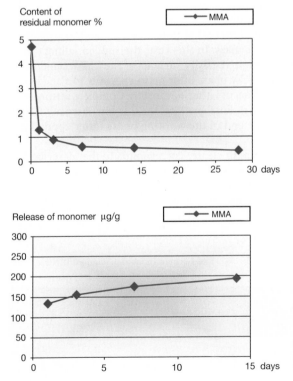

Fig. 52. Content and release of the residual monomer of CMW 3 with time

Table 27. ISO 5833 (1992) requirements for the packaging of CMW 3

Requirements		Com-pliance	Location of information
General	Is the powder packed in a double-layered, sealed container?	+	–
	Is the liquid packed in a double-layered, sealed container?	+	–
Information regarding the powder ingredients	Qualitative	+	PB
	Quantitative	+	PB
Information regarding the liquid ingredients	Qualitative	+	PB
	Quantitative	+	PB
	Warning that the package contains flammable liquid	+	A, AB, FS
	Instructions for storage (≤25°C, darkness)	+	IB, Alu, FS
	Statement of the sterility of the contents	+	IB, POB, A, AB, FS, Alu
	Warning against reusing the package	+	–
	Batch number(s)	+	IB, A, AB, FS, Alu
	Expiration date	+	IB, A, AB, FS, Alu
	Name/address of the manufacturer/distributor	+	IB, A, AB, FS, Alu, PB
	Number and date of the standard	–	–
Information in the package insert	Detailed instructions for handling the components and preparing the cement	+	PB
	A statement drawing attention to the dangers for the patient	+	PB
	Recommendations for using the cement (syringe/dough state)	+	PB
	A statement regarding the influence of the temperature on working times	+	PB
	Graphical representation of the effects of temperature on the length of the phases of cement curing	–	–

+, complies; –, does not comply; *A*, ampoule; *AB*, ampoule blister; *Alu*, aluminum pouch; *FS*, carton; *IB*, primary pouch; *PB*, package insert; *POB*, peel-off pouch

Table 28. The key characteristics of CMW 3

Low viscosity
Barium sulfate is the radiopaque medium
The polymer is γ irradiated
The powder and ampoule are packaged separately
Mixing sequence: powder, then monomer
Working time: long
The dough is dry
ISO 5833 is fulfilled
Molecular weight less than 350,000 Da
Low impact strength

3.2.1.9
Duracem 3

The polymer (powder) and monomer (liquid) of Duracem 3 are packed in a small outer carton (Fig. 53). This carton may be easily opened on the upper side before a transparent label has been removed or cut through.

The outer carton itself is printed with the most important information. On one narrow side, a white label that contains information regarding the batch numbers, expiration date, institution for registration and distributor is attached.

The outer carton contains a polyethylene pouch that encloses a blister pack. This blister pack contains the powder in a glass bottle and a monomer ampoule. Furthermore, one can find the insert and three chart stickers for patients' records. The packing of the polymer powder in a brown glass ampoule is characteristic of all cements of Sulzer Medica.

The transparent, unprinted polyethylene pouch can easily be opened. The blister pack consists of transparent PVC and is closed with printed Tyvek. This pack has no indications concerning batch number and expiration date. This information may be easily read through the PVC, as both of the brown glass bottles have a printed label.

The blister pack can easily be opened by means of a paper flap. Inside the blister, there is a packed formaldehyde tablet (which obviously guarantees the steri-

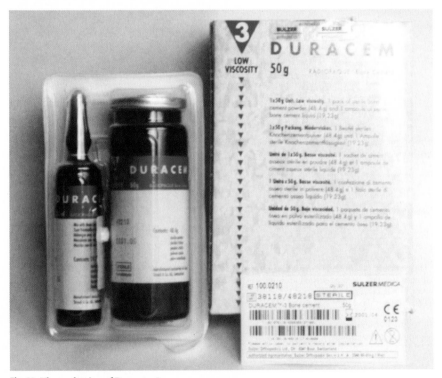

Fig. 53. The packaging of Duracem 3

powder	liquid
38,55 g poly(methyl methacrylate) 4,28 g poly(butyl methacrylate, methyl methacrylate) 4,76 g zirconium dioxide 0,40 g benzoyl peroxide 0,40 g di-cyclo-hexyl phthalate ----------- 48,39 g	16,06 g methyl methacrylate (=17,09 ml) 2,83 g butyl methacrylate (=3,16 ml) 0,31 g 2-[4-(dimethylamino)phenyl]ethanole 0,54 mg hydroquinone ---------- 19,22 g (20,55 ml)

Duracem 3

Fig. 54. Composition of Duracem 3

lity of the blister contents). A notice giving an explanation of the purpose of the tablet is missing. The user could believe that this is to be added to the cement components before mixing.

The polymer powder is packed in a brown glass bottle. It bears a label that indicates the batch number, expiration date and sterilization procedure. Consequently, the powder is sterilized by means of formaldehyde. It seems that only the surface of the brown glass bottle is sterilized by the formaldehyde tablet packed in the blister. The opening of the brown glass bottle is somewhat problematic. Often, the metal ring could not be completely removed, which sometimes led to injury of the medical staff.

The white polymer powder contains 79.7% PMMA, 8.84% poly(BuMA/MMA), 0.83% BPO, 0.83% dicyclohexylphthalate (as a plasticizer) and 9.8% zirconium dioxide (as an opacifier; Fig. 54). A printed paper label that contains all necessary information is also attached to the liquid ampoule. A notice concerning the sterile filtration of the monomer liquid is printed. The liquid consists of two diffe-

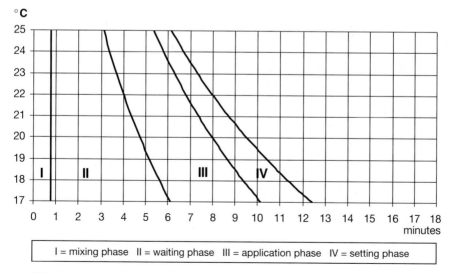

I = mixing phase   II = waiting phase   III = application phase   IV = setting phase

Fig. 55. Working curves of Duracem 3 for different ambient/component temperatures

Table 29. Mechanical strength according to ISO 5833 and German Industrial Standard DIN 53435 for Duracem 3

	ISO 5833 Bending strength (MPa)	Bending modulus (MPa)	Compressive strength (MPa)	DIN 53435 Bending strength (MPa)	Impact strength (kJ/m²)
Limit given in the standard	>50	>1800	>70		
Actual strength	70.7	2653	87.1	80	2.3

rent methacrylates (83.56% MMA and 14.78% BuMA), 1.66% 2-(4-(dimethyla-mino)phenyl)ethanol (DMAPE) and approximately 0.27 mg hydroquinone (as a stabilizer). The interesting thing concerning this composition is the use of DMAPE instead of DmpT.

Before mixing the dough, the liquid is put into the mixing vessel; the voluminous powder is then added. The wetting is very slow. It initially appears as though the quantity of liquid is not sufficient. After approximately 25–30 s, a liquid dough that is completely homogeneous arises. The end of the sticky phase occurs after 3 min 30 s (Fig. 55). The dough may then be taken out of the bowl. The end of the working phase occurs after 6 min 15 s. However, the dough is already very warm after between 5 min 45 s and 6 min. Hardening takes place after 7 min.

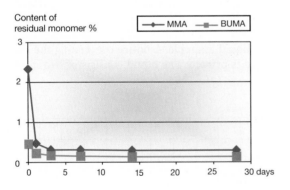

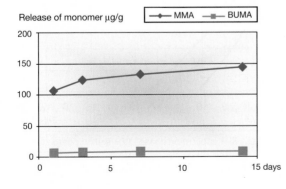

Fig. 56. Content and release of the residual monomers of Duracem 3 with time

Table 30. ISO 5833 (1992) requirements for the packaging of Duracem 3

Requirements		Com-pliance	Location of information
General	Is the powder packed in a double-layered, sealed container?	+	–
	Is the liquid packed in a double-layered, sealed container?	+	–
Information regarding the powder ingredients	Qualitative	+	PB
	Quantitative	+	PB
Information regarding the liquid ingredients	Qualitative	+	PB
	Quantitative	+	PB
	Warning that the package contains flammable liquid	+	A
	Instructions for storage (≤25°C, darkness)	+	PB, FS
	Statement of the sterility of the contents	+	PF, A, GB, FS, PB
	Warning against reusing the package	+	PB, FS
	Batch number(s)	+	A, PF, FS
	Expiration date	+	A, PF, FS
	Name/address of the manufacturer/distributor	+	A, PF, FS, PB
	Number and date of the standard	–	–
Information in the package insert	Detailed instructions for handling the components and preparing the cement	+	PB
	A statement drawing attention to the dangers for the patient	+	PB
	Recommendations for using the cement (syringe/dough state)	+	PB
	A statement regarding the influence of the temperature on working times	+	PB
	Graphical representation of the effects of temperature on the length of the phases of cement curing	+	PB

+, complies; –, does not comply; A, ampoule; FS, carton; GB, shared blister; PB, package insert; PF, powder bottle

The manufacturer recommends only syringe application in the use of Duracem 3, whereas the working criteria indicated in the insert refer only to hand application. However, there should be no important change of the handling properties in cases of application by syringe.

Due to the above-mentioned properties, Duracem 3 has to be regarded as a low-viscosity bone cement. The manufacturer points out that the material is only suitable for application by syringe.

The mechanical data correspond to the standards. The low impact strength of 2.3 kJ/m^2 (Table 29) is striking. The setting time determined according to the ISO 5833 protocol is 9 min 20 s, and the polymerization temperature is 77.5°C.

The residual monomer content (Fig. 56) is similar to that for Cerafix LV. The liquid also contains BuMA (~15%). The ratio of initiators is also comparable (a bit more than one), although Duracem 3 contains less BPO and DMAPE. A comparison with cements containing a pure MMA liquid is not possible.

Only the insert features qualitative and quantitative indications concerning the ingredients of the polymer and monomer. A notice regarding the valid ISO

Table 31. The key characteristics of Duracem 3

Low viscosity
The monomer contains BuMA and DMAPE
The polymer contains a BuMA copolymer and dicyclohexylphthalate
Zirconium dioxide is the radiopaque medium
The (very voluminous) polymer is γ irradiated
The polymer is in a brown glass bottle
The polymer bottle and monomer ampoule are in one blister
Mixing sequence: monomer, then powder
Working time: short
ISO 5833 is fulfilled
Molecular weight less than 350,000 Da
Low impact strength

BuMA, butyl methacrylate; *DMAPE*, 2-(4-(dimethylamino)phenyl)ethanol

standard (5833; Table 30) is missing. The key characteristics of Duracem 3 are listed in Table 31.

3.2.1.10
Durus H

The components of Durus H are packed in a rectangular, flat outer carton (Fig. 57). The outer carton is printed and contains all the important notices, such as the composition, batch number, expiration date and manufacturer. Furthermore, there is information regarding the manufacturing date of the components; the material obviously expires 28 months after it is manufactured. The information referring to the batch is printed on a narrow, elongated label and is subsequently attached to the outer carton. After removing a little label, the outer car-

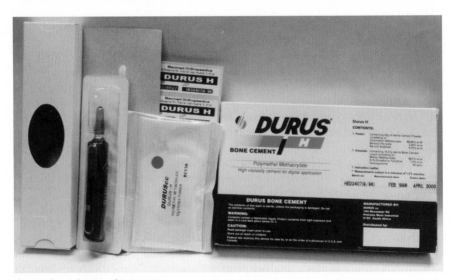

Fig. 57. The packaging of Durus H

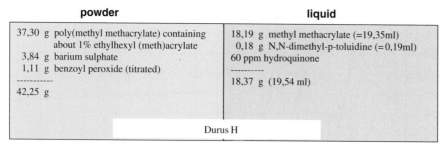

powder	liquid
37,30 g poly(methyl methacrylate) containing about 1% ethylhexyl (meth)acrylate 3,84 g barium sulphate 1,11 g benzoyl peroxide (titrated) ---------- 42,25 g	18,19 g methyl methacrylate (=19,35ml) 0,18 g N,N-dimethyl-p-toluidine (=0,19ml) 60 ppm hydroquinone ---------- 18,37 g (19,54 ml)

Durus H

Fig. 58. Composition of Durus H

ton may easily be opened. The cardboard tray inside may be taken out by means of a little flap. This tray consists of a flat sphere that contains the powder pouch, the insert and three stickers for patients' documentation, and a separate sphere that contains the blister-packed monomer ampoule.

The powder pouch is enclosed by a polyethylene/paper pouch with two indicator arrows on the upper sphere. The left one turns from red to brown in case of sufficient humidity; the right turns from light blue to yellow when penetrated by ethylene oxide. Both indicator arrows of our sample packages tested had not changed. This was not troubling because, on the insert, γ irradiation is indicated as the sterilization process for the powder pouch. The use of such a pouch may easily lead to irritation. Under extreme conditions, the user could doubt the sterility of the powder. The peel-off pouch (which may be easily opened) contains the polyethylene inner pouch, which is labeled but does not mention the batch number or expiration date. There is a red indicator dot above the label, probably meant as sterilization indicator for the γ irradiation of the powder. The polymer powder consists of two different PMMAs (90.9% altogether), 1.94% BPO and 9.1% barium sulfate (as an opacifier; Fig. 58) according to the manufacturer. However, analysis shows that the polymer also contains approximately 1% of ethylhexyl (meth)acrylate.

The blister pack of the monomer ampoule consists of molded PVC covered by medical paper. A little label is attached to the paper side; it does not show any indications regarding the batch number or expiration date, nor does the powder pouch. There is also an indicator stripe (which obviously indicates the sterility). It consists of an Indox-EO stripe that changes from yellow to red when it comes into contact with ethylene oxide. These indicator stripes had clearly turned from yellow to red. The blister pack may be opened by means of a special flap.

The brown glass ampoule is directly printed. A label with the letter »H« (for Durus H) was placed over the letter »L« (for Durus L) on some tested ampoules (Durus L, according to the manufacturer, is no longer on the market). Accordingly, the same liquid was used for both cements (Durus H and Durus L). There is a special mark on which the batch number should be printed; however, it has not been used, so a notice regarding the batch number is missing. The liquid consists of 99.02% MMA, 0.98% DmpT and approximately 60 ppm hydroquinone (as a stabilizer).

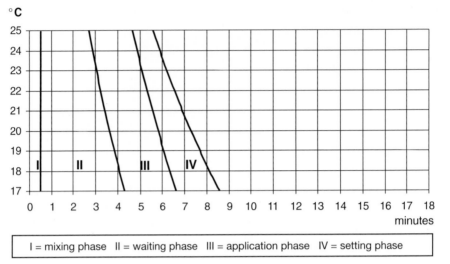

°C

| I = mixing phase   II = waiting phase   III = application phase   IV = setting phase |

Fig. 59. Working curves of Durus H for different ambient/component temperatures

According to the indications of the manufacturer, the powder component should be put into the mixing vessel, and the liquid should be added to manufacture the cement. After 10–15 s, a liquid, homogeneous dough already arises. The end of the sticky phase occurs after between 2 min 45 s and 3 min. The end of the working phase occurs after between approximately 4 min 45 s and 5 min. By this time, the dough is already very warm. Hardening of the cement may be observed after between 5 min 30 s and 6 min (Fig. 59).

Due to the working properties, Durus H has to be regarded as a medium-viscosity cement. Regarding the determined mechanical strengths (Table 32), a slight deviation of the three-point-bending strength in contrast to the bending strength as determined according to the ISO 5833 protocol is striking. The compressive strength is more than 100 MPa – rather high, as is the determined E modulus. The combination of a high E modulus and high compressive strength suggests that Durus H is a relatively brittle material.

The setting time (determined according to the ISO 5833 protocol) is 6 min 40 s. The polymerization temperature according to ISO 5833 is 81.9°C. The resi-

Table 32. Mechanical strength according to ISO 5833 and German Industrial Standard DIN 53435 for Durus H

	ISO 5833			DIN 53435	
	Bending strength (MPa)	Bending modulus (MPa)	Compressive strength (MPa)	Bending strength (MPa)	Impact strength (kJ/m²)
Limit given in the standard	>50	>1800	>70		
Actual strength	78.7	3087	100.2	78.2	4.93

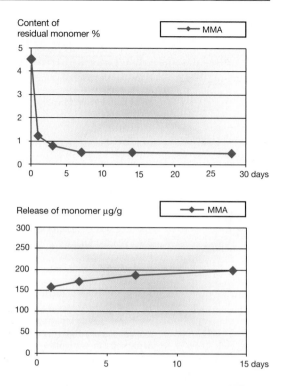

Fig. 60. Content and release of the residual monomer of Durus H with time

dual monomer content is under 5% after the preparation of the specimen (Fig. 60). The BPO content in the powder is rather high (more than 2.5%), whereas the liquid contains approximately 1% DmpT. The ratio of BPO/DmpT, therefore, is very high.

The qualitative and quantitative indications regarding the powder and liquid constituents are not printed on the primary container. Such information is only given on the outer carton and in the insert.

Batch numbers and the expiration date are not directly indicated on the primary container; they are only on the outer packing unit. Apparently, one should avoid storing the single components separately. A notice prohibiting re-use is missing. We could not find a graphic representation of the influence of temperature on the working properties of the material in the insert. A notice regarding ISO 5833 (Table 33) is also missing on all packing units. The key characteristics of Durus H are listed in Table 34.

Table 33. ISO 5833 (1992) requirements for the packaging of Durus H

Requirements		Com-pliance	Location of information
General	Is the powder packed in a double-layered, sealed container?	+	–
	Is the liquid packed in a double-layered, sealed container?	+	–
Information regarding the powder ingredients	Qualitative	+	FS, PB
	Quantitative	+	FS, PB
Information regarding the liquid ingredients	Qualitative	+	FS, PB
	Quantitative	+	FS, PB
	Warning that the package contains flammable liquid	+	A, FS, PB
	Instructions for storage (≤25°C, darkness)	+	A, PB
	Statement of the sterility of the contents	+	IB, A, AB, FS
	Warning against reusing the package	+	–
	Batch number(s)	+	FS
	Expiration date	+	FS
	Name/address of the manufacturer/distributor	+	FS, PB
	Number and date of the standard	–	–
Information in the package insert	Detailed instructions for handling the components and preparing the cement	+	PB
	A statement drawing attention to the dangers for the patient	+	PB
	Recommendations for using the cement (syringe/dough state)	+	PB
	A statement regarding the influence of the temperature on working times	+	PB
	Graphical representation of the effects of temperature on the length of the phases of cement curing	–	–

+, complies; –, does not comply; *A*, ampoule; *AB*, ampoule blister; *FS*, carton; *IB*, primary pouch; *PB*, package insert

Table 34. The key characteristics of Durus H

Medium viscosity
Barium sulfate is the radiopaque medium
The polymer is γ irradiated
The polymer contains ethylhexyl (meth)acrylate
The powder and ampoule are packed separately
Mixing sequence: power, then monomer
Working time: short
ISO 5833 is fulfilled
Molecular weight less than 350,000 Da
High compressive strength
High bending modulus

3.2.1.11
Endurance

The layout of Endurance is remarkably different from that of all other DePuy cements. In all probability, this is due to the fact that Endurance is used on the US

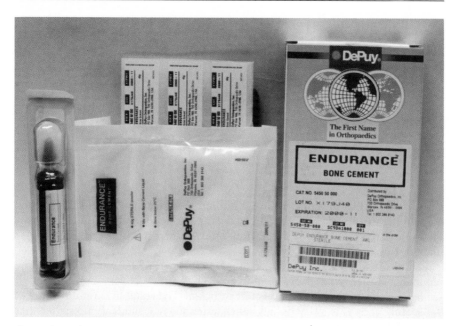

Fig. 61. The packaging of Endurance

market and, therefore, has to meet corresponding requirements. The components of Endurance are packed in a little rectangular outer carton (Fig. 61). The printed parts of the outer carton contain all the necessary information. The distributor is clearly indicated. The batch number and the expiration date are printed on an additional label that is attached to the outer carton.

The outer carton may be opened on the upper and lower, narrow side. Inside the outer carton, a tray for the ampoule blister pack is fixed. In the larger area, in addition to the tray, there is a double-packed inner pouch that contains the polymer. This packing is similar to that of Simplex P, the leader of the US market.

The outer peel-off pouch consists of an unprinted polyethylene side and a sparsely printed Tyvek side. All that is printed on this side is a notice stating the place at which the peel-off pouch may be opened and a sterilization indicator, the operation of which is not described. Furthermore, there is a warning not to use the pouch if it is damaged or opened. The peel-off pouch may be easily opened. One may read the printing of the inner pouch through the unprinted, transparent polyethylene side of the peel-off pouch. Information concerning the sterilization process, storage, batch number and expiration date is included. The white polymer powder consists of 67.05% PMMA, 21.1% MMA–styrene copolymer, 1.85% BPO and 10.0% barium sulfate (as an opacifier; Fig. 62).

The blister pack inside the separate tray of the outer carton consists of molded PVC covered with medical paper. The paper of the blister pack is printed with all the necessary information. The brown glass ampoule contains the colorless monomer liquid, which mainly consists of MMA (98.0%). It also contains 2.0% DmpT and 0.002 g hydroquinone (as a stabilizer).

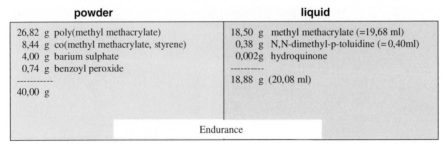

powder	liquid
26,82 g poly(methyl methacrylate) 8,44 g co(methyl methacrylate, styrene) 4,00 g barium sulphate 0,74 g benzoyl peroxide ----------- 40,00 g	18,50 g methyl methacrylate (=19,68 ml) 0,38 g N,N-dimethyl-p-toluidine (=0,40ml) 0,002g hydroquinone ---------- 18,88 g (20,08 ml)

Endurance

Fig. 62. Composition of Endurance

It is striking is that the composition is not indicated on any packing. It is located only on the insert. Furthermore, the powder component and the monomer bear the same batch number and expiration date. An expiration date of 3 years after manufacture is indicated on the insert.

Before mixing the dough, the polymer is placed in the mixing vessel. The monomer is then poured on the polymer. The wetting is very slow. At first, it seems as if the quantity of liquid is not sufficient. The result of careful moving of the spatula at 23°C is a dry dough which, after 30–35 s, suddenly flows together and may then be described as a homogeneous mass. The end of the sticky phase of Endurance is reached after approximately 3 min. The end of the working phase occurs after between 6 min and 6 min 30 s. The viscosity of the working phase is comparatively high after a short time, so the working time is only 3 min. By that time, the mass of dough is already relatively warm. Complete hardening may be observed after 8 min 15 s (Fig. 63). Due to the properties described above, Endurance has to be regarded as a low-viscosity cement.

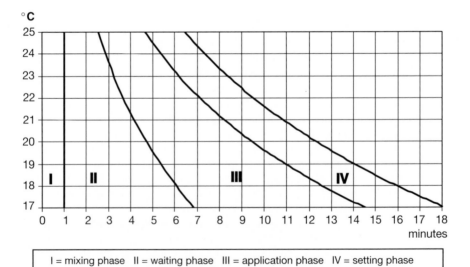

I = mixing phase   II = waiting phase   III = application phase   IV = setting phase

Fig. 63. Working curves of Endurance for different ambient/component temperatures

Table 35. Mechanical strength according to ISO 5833 and German Industrial Standard DIN 53435 for Endurance

	ISO 5833 Bending strength (MPa)	Bending modulus (MPa)	Compressive strength (MPa)	DIN 53435 Bending strength (MPa)	Impact strength (kJ/m²)
Limit given in the standard	>50	>1800	>70		
Actual strength	76.1	2896	94	76	3.2

There is a slight difference between the bending strength determined according to the protocol Dynstat protocol and that determined according to the ISO 5833 protocol (Table 35). Furthermore, the impact strength is comparatively low.

The setting time (determined according to the ISO 5833 protocol) is 13 min 25s, and the polymerization temperature is 78.5°C. The residual monomer content is approximately 6% after preparing the specimens (Fig. 64). The residual monomer release is rather high. The amounts of BPO and DmpT are nearly the same; the ratio of the initiators is a bit more than two.

Although the cement is only sold in the USA, it is nevertheless striking that indications regarding the ingredients of the single components in qualitative and

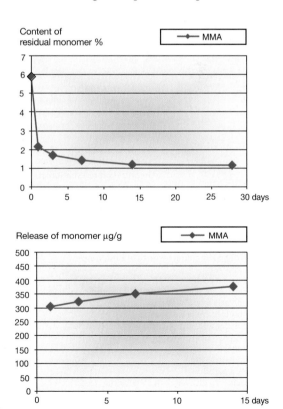

Fig. 64. Content and release of the residual monomer of Endurance with time

quantitative form are only indicated on the outer packing unit and on the outer carton. A reference to the presently valid ISO standard 5833 (Table 36) is also missing, though the symbols and notices of the ISO standard are used. The key characteristics of Endurance are listed in Table 37.

Table 36. ISO 5833 (1992) requirements for the packaging of Endurance

Requirements		Compliance	Location of information
General	Is the powder packed in a double-layered, sealed container?	+	–
	Is the liquid packed in a double-layered, sealed container?	+	–
Information regarding the powder ingredients	Qualitative	+	FS, PB
	Quantitative	+	FS, PB
Information regarding the liquid ingredients	Qualitative	+	FS, PB
	Quantitative	+	FS, PB
	Warning that the package contains flammable liquid	+	A, AB, FS, PB
	Instructions for storage (≤25°C, darkness)	+	IB, FS, PB
	Statement of the sterility of the contents	+	IB, A, AB, FS, PB
	Warning against reusing the package	+	FS
	Batch number(s)	+	IB, A, FS, AB
	Expiration date	+	IB, A, FS, AB
	Name/address of the manufacturer/ distributor	+	IB, A, FS, AB, PB
	Number and date of the standard	–	–
Information in the package insert	Detailed instructions for handling the components and preparing the cement	+	PB
	A statement drawing attention to the dangers for the patient	+	PB
	Recommendations for using the cement (syringe/dough state)	+	PB
	A statement regarding the influence of the temperature on working times	+	PB
	Graphical representation of the effects of temperature on the length of the phases of cement curing	+	PB

+, complies; –, does not comply; A, ampoule; AB, ampoule blister; FS, carton; IB, primary pouch; PB, package insert

Table 37. The key characteristics of Endurance

Low viscosity
Barium sulfate is the radiopaque medium
The polymer is γ irradiated
The polymer contains styrene
The powder and ampoule are packed separately
Mixing sequence: power, then monomer
A dry mass is produced
Working time: long
ISO 5833 is fulfilled
Molecular weight less than 350,000 Da
Low impact strength

3.2.1.12
Osteobond

The cement components of Osteobond are packed in an elongated, large, rectangular outer carton that can easily be opened on the upper, narrow side (Fig. 65). The printing on the outer carton complies with ISO packaging regulations. Nevertheless, on a label attached to a side of the outer carton, there are indications concerning the batch number of the polymer components but no indications regarding the liquid. The expiration date on the additional label is even indicated in both the usual EC manner of writing and in normal written form. In addition to the label that bears the expiration date of the material, there is an additional small, shiny label that bears all the necessary information for EC characterization. This is the only advice regarding the EC characterization of the material, because all other packing components inside the outer carton do not have such information. The name of the distributor is clearly visible.

The outer carton features two compartments; there is a greater compartment, in which the liquid ampoule is located, and a smaller one, in which the polymer pouch is located. Moreover, there is an insert and four information labels on one sheet; these may easily be pulled off and used for patients' records.

The inner pouch (which contains the polymer powder) is enclosed by a peel-off pouch. This pouch consists of a printed Tyvek side and an unprinted polyethylene side. The peel-off pouch may be easily opened without tearing the paper. The polyethylene pouch inside the peel-off pouch is placed with its printed side under the unprinted polyethylene side of the peel-off pouch so that the printing may be read through the peel-off pouch. The batch number and expira-

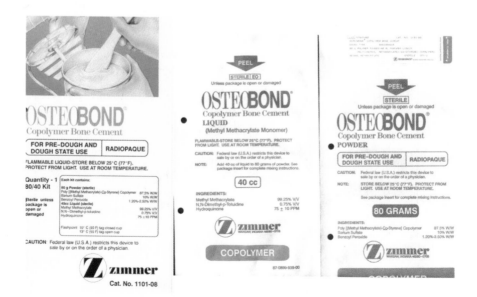

Fig. 65. The packaging of Osteobond

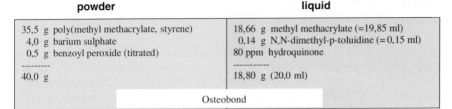

powder	liquid
35,5 g poly(methyl methacrylate, styrene)	18,66 g methyl methacrylate (=19,85 ml)
4,0 g barium sulphate	0,14 g N,N-dimethyl-p-toluidine (=0,15 ml)
0,5 g benzoyl peroxide (titrated)	80 ppm hydroquinone
---------	-----------
40,0 g	18,80 g (20,0 ml)
Osteobond	

Fig. 66. Composition of Osteobond

tion date of the polymer are printed on the peel-off pouch but not on the inner pouch itself. The inner pouch can only be opened with a scissors. The polymer powder consists of a styrene copolymer (88.75%), 1.25% BPO and 10.0% barium sulfate (as an opacifier; Fig. 66).

The monomer ampoule is packed in the same way as the polymer powder. The brown glass ampoule is enclosed by a peel-off pouch. This pouch consists of a printed Tyvek side and an unprinted polyethylene side. The peel-off pouch may be easily opened without tearing the paper. The inner pouch consists of a Tyvek side and a polyethylene side and contains the ampoule; like the peel-off pouch, it is printed on its paper side. The indicated information is identical to that on the peel-off pouch. The batch number and expiration date of the liquid are indicated on both packing units on the paper side. The inner pouch is packed in the peel-off pouch in such a way that one can clearly recognize the ampoule through the unprinted polyethylene side. The inner pouch is slightly attached to the peel-off pouch, so drawing out the inner pouch can be difficult.

The ampoule itself is printed with a white color and has an opening aid. The monomer liquid of Osteobond mainly consists of MMA (99.25%), DmpT (0.75%) and 80 ppm hydroquinone (as a stabilizer).

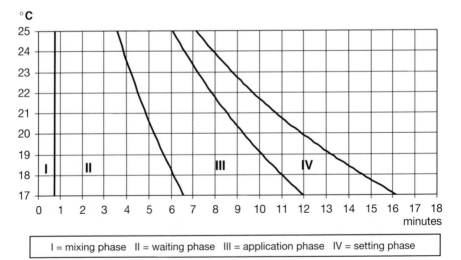

I = mixing phase   II = waiting phase   III = application phase   IV = setting phase

Fig. 67. Working curves of Osteobond for different ambient/component temperatures

Table 38. Mechanical strength according to ISO 5833 and German Industrial Standard DIN 53435 for Osteobond

	ISO 5833			DIN 53435	
	Bending strength (MPa)	Bending modulus (MPa)	Compressive strength (MPa)	Bending strength (MPa)	Impact strength (kJ/m²)
Limit given in the standard	>50	>1800	>70		
Actual strength	73.7	2828	104.6	80.1	3.5

There is an opening aid on the brown glass ampoule; the polymer pouch should be opened with a scissors. The polymer powder can easily be poured out of the pouch into the mixing vessel.

To mix the dough, the powder component is put into the mixing vessel. Due to the large volume of the powder, one should use a comparatively large vessel. After adding the liquid, it does not initially appear that the powder is wetted by the monomer. After approximately 20 s, a rather liquid, homogeneous dough appears; it reaches the end of the sticky phase after 4 min.

The working phase ends after 7 min. During the working phase, the viscosity of the dough is relatively high, so even application by syringe seems to be problematic. The hardening of the dough is finished after 8 min 15 s (Fig. 67).

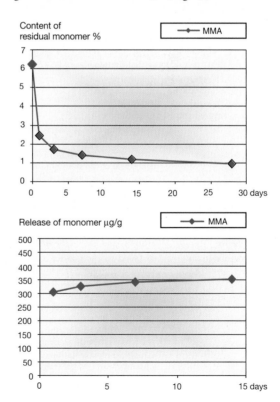

Fig. 68. Content and release of the residual monomer of Osteobond with time

The working properties of the cements show the typical low-viscosity characteristics. Despite the usual syringe application, the determined handling properties should be valid (though the material has been tested for possible hand application).

The mechanical data completely fulfill the standards (Table 38). The compressive strength (determined according to the ISO 5833 protocol) is 104.6 MPa; this is rather high. The determined bending modulus is near 3000 MPa. Osteobond seems to be a comparatively brittle material.

The setting time (determined according to the ISO 5833 protocol) is 10 min 15 s, and the polymerization temperature is well over 80°C. The determined value was 83.9°C.

The residual monomer content (more than 6%) is quite high (Fig. 68). Although the content of BPO and DmpT is comparatively low, the ratio of the initiators is a little less than four. The percentage BPO content is also higher than the DmpT content. The residual monomer release is also quite high.

Information regarding the ingredients of the single components (in qualitative and quantitative form) is only indicated on the outer packing unit and in the insert. Advice regarding the presently valid standard ISO 5833 (Table 39) is also mis-

Table 39. ISO 5833 (1992) requirements for the packaging of Osteobond

Requirements		Compliance	Location of information
General	Is the powder packed in a double-layered, sealed container?	+	–
	Is the liquid packed in a double-layered, sealed container?	+	–
Information regarding the powder ingredients	Qualitative	+	POB, PB
	Quantitative	+	POB, PB
Information regarding the liquid ingredients	Qualitative	+	POB, PB
	Quantitative	+	POB, PB
	Warning that the package contains flammable liquid	+	FS, PB
	Instructions for storage (≤25°C, darkness)	+	FS, POB, PB
	Statement of the sterility of the contents	+	FS, POB, PB
	Warning against reusing the package	+	PB
	Batch number(s)	+	FS, POB
	Expiration date	+	FS, POB
	Name/address of the manufacturer/ distributor	+	IB, POB, FS, A, PB
	Number and date of the standard	–	–
Information in the package insert	Detailed instructions for handling the components and preparing the cement	+	PB
	A statement drawing attention to the dangers for the patient	+	PB
	Recommendations for using the cement (syringe/dough state)	+	PB
	A statement regarding the influence of the temperature on working times	+	PB
	Graphical representation of the effects of temperature on the length of the phases of cement curing	–	–

+, complies; –, does not comply; A, ampoule; FS, carton; IB, primary pouch; PB, package insert; POB, peel-off pouch

Table 40. The key characteristics of Osteobond

Low viscosity
Barium sulfate is the radiopaque medium
The (very voluminous) polymer is γ irradiated
The polymer contains styrene
The powder and ampoule are packed separately
Mixing sequence: power, then monomer
Working time: long
ISO 5833 is fulfilled
Molecular weight less than 350,000 Da
High compressive strength
Low impact strength

sing, although the symbols and indicators of the ISO standard are used. Furthermore, it is striking that the insert provides no graphic description of the influence of temperature on the working properties of the cement. The key characteristics of Osteobond are listed in Table 40.

3.2.1.13
Osteopal and Palacos LV (E Flow)

Osteopal and Palacos LV (E Flow) are sold by different distributors under different trade names, but the material in each is exactly the same. All the cement components of Osteopal or Palacos LV are packed in a rectangular outer carton that may be easily opened at the upper, narrow side (Fig. 69). The printing on the outer cartons complies with ISO packaging regulations in every respect. Information regarding the batch number and expiration date is not printed on the front side of the cartons but on one of the two unprinted, small sides. The names of the distributor and manufacturer may easily be seen.

The outer cartons contain a cardboard tray in which two spaces are left for secure packaging of both ampoule-containing blister packs; in case of single versions of the bone cements, only one blister packed ampoule is located there. Usually, the insert, four to six chart-stickers and an alu-pouch that contains two inner pouches with polymer powder are placed on the two monomer ampoules, which are located in the spaces of the cardboard tray. Each of the two folded, double-packed inner pouches within the alu-pouch contains sterile pouches in which the polymer powder is located.

The paper side of the inner pouch for the polymer has printing featuring important information regarding handling and storage. Furthermore, the batch number and the expiration date are located clearly on the printed front side, as prescribed by standard protocols. The back of the inner pouch is made of polyester and is, therefore, transparent.

The green, pigmented polymer powder (the color of which is characteristic for such products and is well-known) is clearly visible. The polymer powder is sterilized by ethylene oxide. The composition of the polymer powder is 83.5% MMA–methyl acrylate copolymer, 1.5% BPO and (as an opacifier) 15.0% zirconium dioxide (Fig. 70).

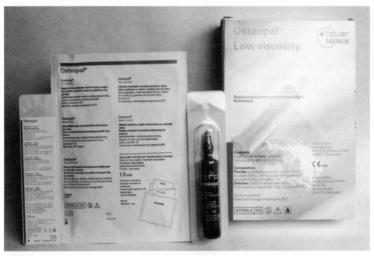

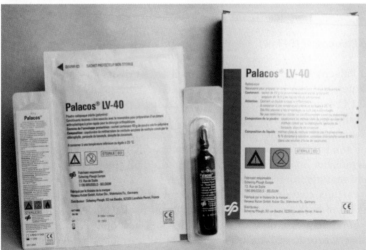

Fig. 69. The packaging of Osteopal and Palacos LV (E Flow)

These cements have a low BPO content and a high DmpT content. The ratio of the initiators is much less than two.

The sterile inner pouch is enclosed by an unprinted peel-off pouch that, like the inner pouch, consists of a paper side and a polyethylene side. As the transparent polyethylene side encloses the printed paper side of the inner pouch, the printing of the inner pouch may be clearly read through the outer pouch. On the outer pouch, a sterile label (which was obviously put on the pouch after successful sterilization) is located. Usually, two folded, peel-off pouches are packed in an alu-pouch, which also has printing on one side. The print contains all necessary instructions, including the batch number and expiration date.

powder	liquid
33,40 g poly(methyl acrylate, methyl methacrylate) 6,00 g zirconium dioxide 0,60 g benzoyl peroxide 1 mg chlorophyllin ---------- 40,00 g	18,40 g methyl methacrylate (=19,57 ml) 0,38 g N,N-dimethyl-p-toluidine (=0,43 ml) 0,4 mg chlorophyllin ---------- 18,78 g (20 ml)
Osteopal/Palacos E Flow/Palacos LV	

Fig. 70. Composition of Osteopal and Palacos LV

The two ampoules in the cardboard tray are protected not only by the blister pack but by the alu-pouch located above it. The blister pack itself consists of transparent, molded PVC and a paper cover. A printed ampoule label is attached to the paper cover; this label contains all necessary information (especially the batch number and the expiration date of the liquid monomer). A brown glass ampoule contains the sterile, filtrated green monomer, which is typical for Osteopal/Palacos LV. Each ampoule has a translucent label. The blister pack is also sterilized by ethylene oxide. The monomer consists of 98.0% MMA, 2.0% DmpT and approximately 60 ppm hydroquinone.

No opening aid is installed for the opening of the brown glass ampoule; the polymer pouch should be opened with the help of a scissors. The polymer powder may easily be poured out of the pouch into the mixing vessel.

Before mixing the cement components of Osteopal/Palacos LV, one must first pour all the liquid into the bowl. The polymer powder is then added to the monomer, and the clock is started. In a few seconds, a very liquid, low-viscosity, homo-

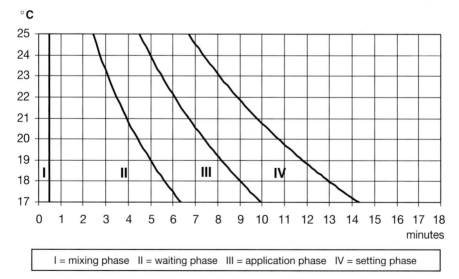

I = mixing phase   II = waiting phase   III = application phase   IV = setting phase

Fig. 71. Working curves of Osteopal/Palacos LV for different ambient/component temperatures

Table 41. Mechanical strength according to ISO 5833 and German Industrial Standard DIN 53435 for Osteopal/Palacos LV

	ISO 5833 Bending strength (MPa)	Bending modulus (MPa)	Compressive strength (MPa)	DIN 53435 Bending strength (MPa)	Impact strength (kJ/m²)
Limit given in the standard	>50	>1800	>70		
Actual strength	73.7	2828	104.6	81.9	4.4

geneous dough is easily produced. The viscosity of the dough increases very slowly, depending on the temperature of the components with respect to the temperature of the operating room. For example, the dough may be taken out of the mixing vessel in a non-sticky state after approximately 3 min if the components and the room are kept at 23°C. The working phase of Osteopal/Palacos LV varies from 2 min to 3 min and usually ends approximately 5–6 min after mixing starts. The cement hardens after approximately 7–8 min. Therefore, Osteopal and Palacos LV are characterized as low-viscosity PMMA bone cements (Fig. 71).

Osteopal and Palacos LV exist in different layouts in the marketplace. In the USA, only a single dose version that contains four chart labels is sold. Furthermore, there are specific layouts for certain countries (for example, France), and there are polyglot versions that may be used in many different countries. Mecha-

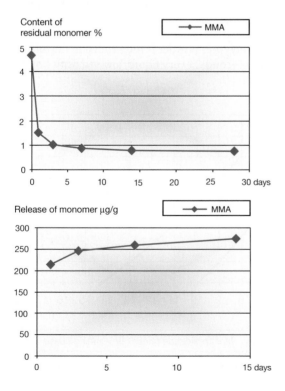

Fig. 72. Content and release of the residual monomer of Osteopal/Palacos LV with time

Table 42. ISO 5833 (1992) requirements for the packaging of Palacos LV (E Flow)/Osteopal

Requirements		Com-pliance	Location of information
General	Is the powder packed in a double-layered, sealed container?	+	–
	Is the liquid packed in a double-layered, sealed container?	+	–
Information regarding the powder ingredients	Qualitative	+	IB, Alu, FS, PB
	Quantitative	+	IB, Alu, FS, PB
Information regarding the liquid ingredients	Qualitative	+	A, AB, PB
	Quantitative	+	AB, PB
	Warning that the package contains flammable liquid	+	A, AB, FS, PB
	Instructions for storage (≤25°C, darkness)	+	IB, Alu, FS, AB, PB
	Statement of the sterility of the contents	+	IB, Alu, FS, AB, PB
	Warning against reusing the package	+	IB, Alu, FS, AB, PB
	Batch number(s)	+	IB, Alu, FS, A, PB
	Expiration date	+	IB, Alu, FS, AB
	Name/address of the manufacturer/distributor	+	IB, Alu, FS, A, AB, PB
	Number and date of the standard	–	–
Information in the package insert	Detailed instructions for handling the components and preparing the cement	+	PB
	A statement drawing attention to the dangers for the patient	+	PB
	Recommendations for using the cement (syringe/dough state)	+	PB
	A statement regarding the influence of the temperature on working times	+	PB
	Graphical representation of the effects of temperature on the length of the phases of cement curing	+	PB

+, complies; –, does not comply; *A*, ampoule; *AB*, ampoule blister; *Alu*, aluminum pouch; *FS*, carton; *IB*, primary pouch; *PB*, package insert

Table 43. The key characteristics of Palacos LV (E Flow)/Osteopal

Low viscosity
Zirconium dioxide is the radiopaque medium
The powder contains MMA/MA copolymer
The polymer is ethylene oxide sterilized
The powder and ampoule are packed separately
Mixing sequence: monomer, then powder
Working time: long
ISO 5833 is fulfilled
Molecular weight greater than 350,000 Da
Very high fatigue strength
High compressive strength
High bending strength

MMA/MA, methyl methacrylate–methyl acrylate

nical testing yielded good results. The bending strength determined according to ISO 5833 protocols is remarkably high (73.7 MPa), as is the bending strength determined according to DIN 53435 protocols (81.9 MPa; Table 41).

The hardening temperature (determined according to ISO 5833 protocols) is
83.9°C. The setting time is 10 min 15 s. For Osteopal and Palacos LV, the change in
monomer content and the monomer release rate are shown graphically in Fig. 72.
A notice regarding the presently valid ISO standard (Table 42) is missing on
packages of this type of bone cement. The key characteristics of Osteopal and
Palacos LV (E Flow) are listed in Table 43.

3.2.1.14
Osteopal HA

Osteopal HA is sold only in France today; therefore, only a French presentation
can be found. All the cement components of Osteopal HA are packed in a rectangular outer carton that may be easily opened at the upper, narrow side (Fig. 73).
The printing on the outer cartons complies in every respect with ISO packaging
regulations. Information regarding the batch number and expiration date is not
printed on the front side of the cartons but on one of the two unprinted, small
sides. The names of the distributor and manufacturer may easily be seen.

The outer cartons contain a cardboard tray in which two spaces are left for
secure packaging of both ampoule-containing blister packs; in case of single versions of the bone cements, only one blister-packed ampoule is located there.
Usually, the insert and an alu-pouch that contains two inner pouches with polymer powder are put on the two monomer ampoules, which are located in the spa-

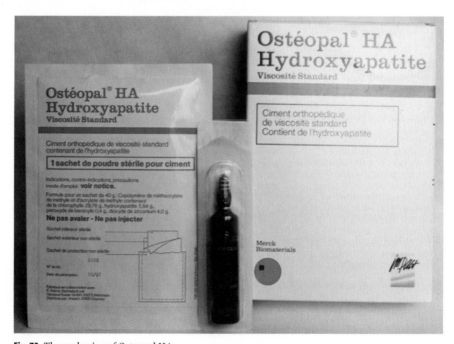

Fig. 73. The packaging of Osteopal HA

ces of the cardboard tray. Each of the two folded, double-packed inner pouches within the alu-pouch contains sterile pouches in which the polymer powder is located.

The paper side of the inner pouch for the polymer has printing featuring important information regarding handling and storage. Furthermore, the batch number and the expiration date are located clearly on the printed front side, as prescribed by standard protocols. The back of the inner pouch is made of polyester and is, therefore, transparent.

The green, pigmented polymer powder (the color of which is characteristic for such products and is well-known) is clearly visible, but a slight difference from all other green powders can be observed. Obviously, the gray hydroxyapatite within the powder leads to that slight change in the color. The polymer powder is sterilized by ethylene oxide. The composition of the polymer powder is 74.4% MMA–methylacrylate copolymer, 14.6% hydroxyapatite, 1.0% BPO and (as an opacifier) 10.0% zirconium dioxide (Fig. 74).

The sterile inner pouch is enclosed by an unprinted peel-off pouch that, like the inner pouch, consists of a paper side and a polyethylene side. As the transparent polyethylene side encloses the printed paper side of the inner pouch, the printing of the inner pouch may be clearly read through the outer pouch. On the outer pouch, a sterile label (which was obviously put on the pouch after successful sterilization) is located. Usually, two folded peel-off pouches are packed in an alu-pouch, which also has printing on one side. The print contains all necessary instructions, including the batch number and expiration date.

The two ampoules in the cardboard tray are protected not only by the blister pack but by the alu-pouch located above it. The blister pack itself consists of transparent, molded PVC and a paper cover. A printed ampoule label is attached to the paper cover; this label contains all necessary information (especially the batch number and the expiration date of the liquid monomer). A brown glass ampoule contains the sterile, filtrated green monomer, which is typical for Osteopal HA. Each ampoule has a translucent label. The blister pack is also sterilized by ethylene oxide. The monomer consists of 98.0% MMA, 2.0% DmpT, 0.4 mg chlorophyll and approximately 60 ppm hydroquinone.

No opening aid is installed for the opening of the brown glass ampoule; the polymer pouch should be opened with the help of a scissors. The polymer powder may easily be poured out of the pouch into the mixing vessel.

powder	liquid
29,76 g poly(methyl acrylate, methyl methacrylate)	18,40 g methyl methacrylate (=19,57 ml)
5,84 g hydroxyapatite	0,38 g N,N-dimethyl-p-toluidine (=0,43 ml)
4,00 g zirconium dioxide	0,4 mg chlorophyllin
0,40 g benzoyl peroxide	---------
---------	18,78 g (20 ml)
40,00 g	
	Osteopal HA

Fig. 74. Composition of Osteopal HA

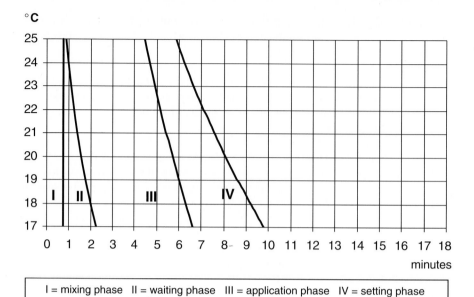

| I = mixing phase | II = waiting phase | III = application phase | IV = setting phase |

Fig. 75. Working curves of Osteopal HA for different ambient/component temperatures

Before mixing the cement components of Osteopal HA, one must first pour all the liquid into the bowl. The polymer powder is then added to the monomer and the clock is started. In 10–15 s, a homogeneous dough is easily produced. The viscosity of the dough increases very quickly. The wetting is slightly different from that of other high-viscosity materials (like Palacos R) because of the additional amount of hydroxyapatite within the polymer. The dough is gray-green in color. The dough may be taken out of the mixing vessel in a non-sticky state after approximately 1 min if the components and the room are kept at 23°C. The working phase of Osteopal HA varies from 3 min 30 s to 4 min. The cement hardens after approximately 6–7 min. Therefore, Osteopal HA is characterized as a high-viscosity, Palacos-like PMMA bone cement (Fig. 75).

Mechanical testing yielded good results, especially for the bending strength (as determined according to ISO 5833 protocols) and the impact strength (as determined according to DIN 53435 protocols; Table 44) even though the polymer powder consists of 14.6% hydroxyapatite. The hardening temperature (determined according to ISO 5833 protocols) is 68°C. The setting time is 11 min 10 s.

Table 44. Mechanical strength according to ISO 5833 and German Industrial Standard DIN 53435 for Osteopal HA

	ISO 5833 Bending strength (MPa)	Bending modulus (MPa)	Compressive strength (MPa)	DIN 53435 Bending strength (MPa)	Impact strength (kJ/m^2)
Limit given in the standard	>50	>1800	>70		
Actual strength	69.7	2849	78.4	68.9	6

For Osteopal HA, the change in monomer content and the monomer release rate are shown graphically in Figure 76. Details of the ISO standard are given in Table 45, and the key characteristics of Osteopal HA are listed in Table 46.

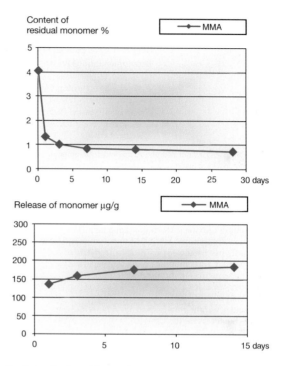

Fig. 76. Content and release of the residual monomer of Osteopal HA with time

Table 45. ISO 5833 (1992) requirements for the packaging of Osteopal HA

Requirements		Com-pliance	Location of information
General	Is the powder packed in a double-layered, sealed container?	+	–
	Is the liquid packed in a double-layered, sealed container?	+	–
Information regarding the powder ingredients	Qualitative	+	IB, Alu, FS, PB
	Quantitative	+	IB, Alu, FS, PB
Information regarding the liquid ingredients	Qualitative	+	AB, A, PB
	Quantitative	+	AB, PB
	Warning that the package contains flammable liquid	+	A, AB, FS, PB
	Instructions for storage (≤25°C, darkness)	+	IB, Alu, FS, AB, PB
	Statement of the sterility of the contents	+	IB, Alu, FS, AB, PB
	Warning against reusing the package	+	IB, Alu, FS, AB, PB
	Batch number(s)	+	IB, Alu, FS, AB
	Expiration date	+	IB, Alu, FS, A, AB, PB
	Name/address of the manufacturer/distributor	+	IB, A, FS, AB, PB
	Number and date of the standard	–	–

Table 45. Continued

Requirements		Com-pliance	Location of information
Information in the package insert	Detailed instructions for handling the components and preparing the cement	+	PB
	A statement drawing attention to the dangers for the patient	+	PB
	Recommendations for using the cement (syringe/dough state)	+	PB
	A statement regarding the influence of the temperature on working times	+	PB
	Graphical representation of the effects of temperature on the length of the phases of cement curing	+	PB

+, complies; −, does not comply; *A*, ampoule; *AB*, ampoule blister; *Alu*, aluminum pouch; *FS*, carton; *IB*, primary pouch; *PB*, package insert

Table 46. The key characteristics of Osteopal HA

High viscosity
Zirconium dioxide is the radiopaque medium
The powder contains MMA/MA copolymer and hydroxyapatite
The polymer is ethylene oxide sterilized
The powder and ampoule are packed separately
Mixing sequence: monomer, then powder
Working time: long
ISO 5833 is fulfilled
Molecular weight greater than 350,000 Da
High impact strength

MMA/MA, methyl methacrylate–methyl acrylate

3.2.1.15
Osteopal VS

Osteopal VS is sold only in France today; therefore, only a French translation can be found. All the cement components of Osteopal VS are packed in a rectangular outer carton that may be easily opened at the upper, narrow side (Fig. 77). The printing on the outer cartons complies in every respect with ISO packaging regulations. Information regarding the batch number and expiration date is not printed on the front side of the cartons but on one of the two unprinted, small sides. The names of the distributor and manufacturer may easily be seen.

The outer cartons contain a cardboard tray in which two spaces are left for secure packaging for both ampoule-containing blister packs; in case of single versions of the bone cements, only one blister-packed ampoule is located there. Usually, the insert and an alu-pouch that contains two inner pouches with polymer powder are put on the two monomer ampoules, which are located in the spaces of the cardboard tray. Each of the two folded, double-packed inner pouches within the alu-pouch contains sterile pouches in which the polymer powder is located.

The paper side of the inner pouch for the polymer has printing featuring important information regarding handling and storage. Furthermore, the batch

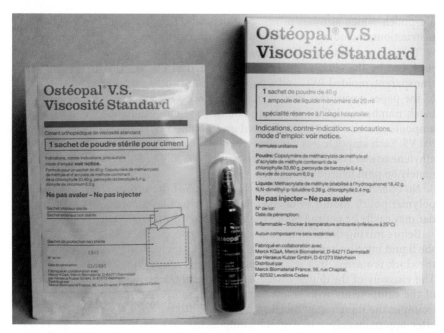

Fig. 77. The packaging of Osteopal VS

number and the expiration date are located clearly on the printed front side, as prescribed by standard protocols. The back of the inner pouch is made of polyester and is, therefore, transparent.

The green, pigmented polymer powder (the color of which is characteristic for such products and is well-known) is clearly visible. The polymer powder is sterilized by ethylene oxide. The composition of the polymer powder is 84.4% MMA–methylacrylate copolymer, 1.0% BPO and (as an opacifier) 15.0% zirconium dioxide (Fig. 78).

The sterile inner pouch is enclosed by an unprinted peel-off pouch that, like the inner pouch, consists of a paper side and a polyethylene side. As the transparent polyethylene side encloses the printed paper side of the inner pouch, the printing of the inner pouch may be clearly read through the outer pouch. On the outer pouch, a sterile label (which was obviously put on the pouch after successful sterilization) is located. Usually, two folded peel-off pouches are packed in an

powder	liquid
33,6 g poly(methyl acrylate, methyl methacrylate)	18,40 g methyl methacrylate (=19,57 ml)
	0,38 g N,N-dimethyl-p-toluidine (=0,43 ml)
6,0 g zirconium dioxide	0,4 mg chlorophyllin
0,4 g benzoyl peroxide	---------
---------	18,78 g (20 ml)
40,0 g	
Osteopal VS	

Fig. 78. Composition of Osteopal VS

alu-pouch, which also has printing on one side. The print contains all necessary instructions, including the batch number and expiration date.

The two ampoules in the cardboard tray are protected not only by the blister pack but by the alu-pouch located above it. The blister pack itself consists of transparent, molded PVC and a paper cover. A printed ampoule label is attached to the paper cover; this label contains all necessary information (especially the batch number and the expiration date of the liquid monomer). A brown glass ampoule contains the sterile, filtrated green monomer, which is typical for Osteopal VS. Each ampoule has a translucent label. The blister pack is also sterilized by ethylene oxide. The monomer consists of 98.0% MMA, 2.0% DmpT and approximately 60 ppm hydroquinone (Fig. 78).

No opening aid is installed for the opening of the brown glass ampoule; the polymer pouch should be opened with the help of a scissors. The polymer powder may easily be poured out of the pouch into the mixing vessel.

Before mixing the cement components of Osteopal VS, one must first pour all the liquid into the bowl. The polymer powder is then added to the monomer and the clock is started. In a few seconds, a homogeneous dough is easily produced. The viscosity of the dough increases very quickly, depending on the temperature of the components with respect to the temperature of the operating room. For example, the dough may be taken out of the mixing vessel in a non-sticky state after approximately 1 min if the components and the room are kept at 23°C (Fig. 79). The working phase of Osteopal VS varies from 3 min 30 s to 4 min and usually ends between approximately 4 min 30 s and 5 min after mixing starts. The cement hardens after approximately 6–7 min. Therefore, Osteopal VS is characterized as a high-viscosity, Palacos-like PMMA bone cement.

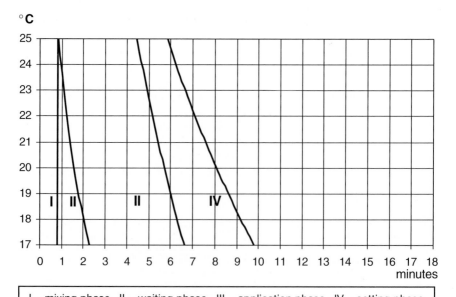

I = mixing phase   II = waiting phase   III = application phase   IV = setting phase

Fig. 79. Working curves of Osteopal VS for different ambient/component temperatures

Table 47. Mechanical strength according to ISO 5833 and German Industrial Standard DIN 53435 for Osteopal VS

	ISO 5833 Bending strength (MPa)	Bending modulus (MPa)	Compressive strength (MPa)	DIN 53435 Bending strength (MPa)	Impact strength (kJ/m²)
Limit given in the standard	>50	>1800	>70		
Actual strength	72.6	2827	76.9	87.8	7.2

The handling properties of Osteopal VS are the same as for Palacos R. Unlike all other cements, the surface of Osteopal VS is rough, not smooth (because of the granules). This facilitates the adhesion of new bone cells.

Mechanical testing yielded good results. The bending strength determined according to ISO 5833 protocols is remarkably high (73.7 MPa), as is the bending strength determined according to DIN 53435 protocols (87.8 MPa) and the impact strength (7.2 kJ/m²; Table 47). The hardening temperature (determined according to ISO 5833 protocols) is 69°C. The setting time is 9 min 30 s.

The residual monomer content of the specimens is less than 5% after setting (Fig. 80). The BPO content of these cements is clearly lower than the portion of DmpT. The ratio of initiator to activator is distinctly less than one. In contrast to the low- and medium-viscosity cements produced by this manufacturer, the high-viscosity cements show a low BPO content. The residual monomer content is not significantly lower than those of low- and medium-viscosity cement types.

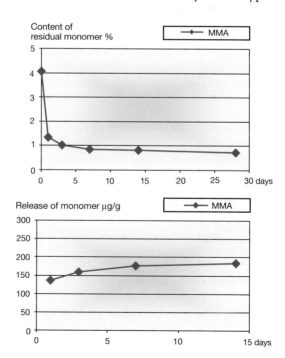

Fig. 80. Content and release of the residual monomer of Osteopal VS with time

Table 48. ISO 5833 (1992) requirements for the packaging of Osteopal VS

Requirements		Com-pliance	Location of information
General	Is the powder packed in a double-layered, sealed container?	+	–
	Is the liquid packed in a double-layered, sealed container?	+	–
Information regarding the powder ingredients	Qualitative	+	IB, Alu, FS, PB
	Quantitative	+	IB, Alu, FS, PB
Information regarding the liquid ingredients	Qualitative	+	AB, A, PB
	Quantitative	+	AB, PB
	Warning that the package contains flammable liquid	+	A, AB, FS, PB
	Instructions for storage (≤25°C, darkness)	+	IB, Alu, FS, AB, PB
	Statement of the sterility of the contents	+	IB, Alu, FS, AB, PB
	Warning against reusing the package	+	IB, Alu, FS, AB, PB
	Batch number(s)	+	IB, Alu, FS, AB
	Expiration date	+	IB, Alu, FS, A, AB, PB
	Name/address of the manufacturer/distributor	+	IB, A, FS, AB, PB
	Number and date of the standard	-	–
Information in the package insert	Detailed instructions for handling the components and preparing the cement	+	PB
	A statement drawing attention to the dangers for the patient	+	PB
	Recommendations for using the cement (syringe/dough state)	+	PB
	A statement regarding the influence of the temperature on working times	+	PB
	Graphical representation of the effects of temperature on the length of the phases of cement curing	+	PB

+, complies; –, does not comply; *A*, ampoule; *AB*, ampoule blister; *Alu*, aluminum pouch; *FS*, carton; *IB*, primary pouch; *PB*, package insert

Table 49. The key characteristics of Osteopal VS

High viscosity
Zirconium dioxide is the radiopaque medium
The powder contains MMA/MA copolymer
The polymer is ethylene oxide sterilized
The powder and ampoule are packed separately
Mixing sequence: monomer, then powder
Working time: long
ISO 5833 is fulfilled
Molecular weight greater than 350,000 Da
High impact strength
High bending strength

MMA/MA, methyl methacrylate–methyl acrylate

The same applies to the residual monomer release. A notice regarding the presently valid ISO standard (Table 48) is missing on packages of this type of bone cement. The key characteristics of Osteopal VS are listed in Table 49.

3.2.1.16
Palacos R

Palacos R bone cement is sold by different distributors under the same trade name. The material is exactly the same.

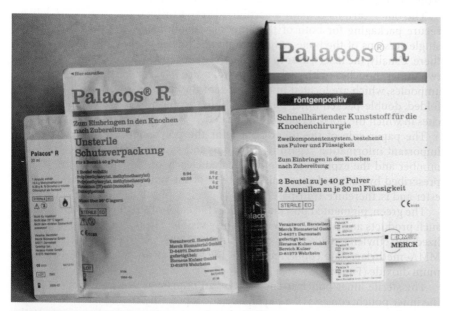

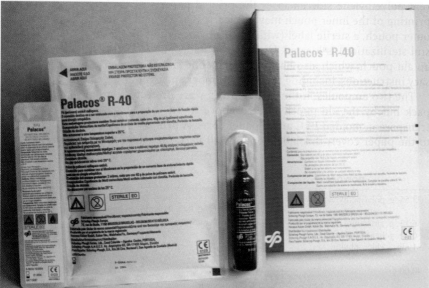

Fig. 81. The packaging of Palacos R

All the cement components of Palacos R are packed in a rectangular outer carton that may be easily opened at the upper, narrow side (Fig. 81). The printing on the outer cartons complies in every respect with ISO packaging regulations. Information regarding the batch number and expiration date is not printed on the front side of the cartons but on one of the two unprinted, small sides. The names of the distributor and manufacturer may easily be seen.

The outer cartons contain a cardboard tray in which two spaces are left for secure packaging for both of the ampoule-containing blister packs; in case of single versions of the bone cements, only one blister-packed ampoule is located there. Usually, the insert, four to six chart-stickers and an alu-pouch that contains two inner pouches with polymer powder are placed on the two monomer ampoules, which are located in the spaces of the cardboard tray. Each of the two folded, double-packed inner pouches within the alu-pouch contains sterile pouches in which the polymer powder is located.

The paper side of the inner pouch for the polymer has printing featuring important information regarding handling and storage. Furthermore, the batch number and the expiration date are located clearly on the printed front side, as prescribed by standard protocols. The back of the inner pouch is made of polyester and is, therefore, transparent.

The green, pigmented polymer powder (the color of which is characteristic for such products and is well-known) is clearly visible. The polymer powder is sterilized by ethylene oxide. The composition of the polymer powder is 84.5% MMA–methylacrylate copolymer, 0.5% BPO and (as an opacifier) 15.0% zirconium dioxide (Fig. 82).

The sterile inner pouch is enclosed by an unprinted peel-off pouch that, like the inner pouch, consists of a paper side and a polyethylene side. As the transparent polyethylene side encloses the printed paper side of the inner pouch, the printing of the inner pouch may be clearly read through the outer pouch. On the outer pouch, a sterile label (which was obviously put on the pouch after successful sterilization) is located. Usually, two folded, peel-off pouches are packed in an alu-pouch, which also has printing on one side. The print contains all necessary instructions, including the batch number and expiration date.

The two ampoules in the cardboard tray are protected not only by the blister pack but by the alu-pouch located above it. The blister pack itself consists of transparent, molded PVC and a paper cover. A printed ampoule label is attached to the paper cover; this label contains all necessary information (especially the

powder	liquid
33,55 g poly(methyl acrylate, methyl methacrylate)	18,40 g methyl methacrylate (=19,57 ml)
6,13 g zirconium dioxide	0,38 g N,N-dimethyl-p-toluidine (=0,43 ml)
0,32 g benzoyl peroxide	0,4 mg chlorophyllin
1 mg chlorophyllin	---------
---------	18,78 g (20 ml)
40,00 g	

Palacos R

Fig. 82. Composition of Palacos R

batch number and the expiration date of the liquid monomer). A brown glass ampoule contains the sterile, filtrated green monomer, which is typical for Palacos R. Each ampoule has a translucent label. The blister pack is also sterilized by ethylene oxide. The monomer consists of 98.0% MMA, 2.0% DmpT and approximately 60 ppm hydroquinone.

No opening aid is installed for the opening of the brown glass ampoule; the polymer pouch should be opened with the help of a scissors. The polymer powder may easily be poured out of the pouch into the mixing vessel.

Before mixing the cement components of Palacos R, one must first pour all the liquid into the bowl. The polymer powder is then added to the monomer and the clock is started. In a few seconds, a homogeneous dough is easily produced. The viscosity of the dough increases very quickly, depending on the temperature of the components with respect to the temperature of the operating room. For example, the dough may be taken out of the mixing vessel in a non-sticky state after approximately 1 min if the components and the room are kept at 23°C. The working phase of Palacos R varies from 3.5 min to 4 min and usually ends between approximately 4 min 30 s and 5 min after mixing starts. The cement hardens after approximately 6–7 min. Therefore, Palacos R is characterized as a high-viscosity PMMA bone cement (Fig. 83). One has to take into consideration that chilled Palacos R has completely different working characteristics.

Palacos R exists in different layouts in the marketplace. In the USA, only a single dose version that contains four chart labels is sold. Furthermore, there are specific layouts for certain countries (for example, Germany), and there are polyglot versions that may be used in many different countries.

Mechanical testing yielded good results. The bending strength determined according to ISO 5833 protocols is remarkably high (72.2 MPa), as is the bending

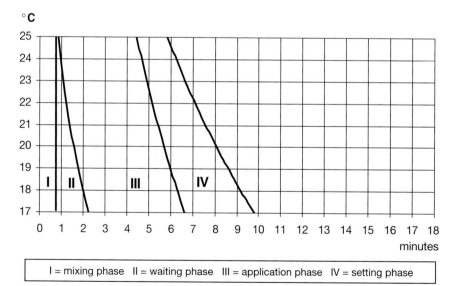

I = mixing phase   II = waiting phase   III = application phase   IV = setting phase

Fig. 83. Working curves of Palacos R for different ambient/component temperatures

Table 50. Mechanical strength according to ISO 5833 and German Industrial Standard DIN 53435 for Palacos R

	ISO 5833 Bending strength (MPa)	Bending modulus (MPa)	Compressive strength (MPa)	DIN 53435 Bending strength (MPa)	Impact strength (kJ/m^2)
Limit given in the standard	>50	>1800	>70		
Actual strength	72.2	2628	79.6	87.4	7.5

strength determined according to DIN 53435 protocols (87.4 MPa) and the impact strength (7.5 kJ/m^2; Table 50). The hardening temperature (determined according to ISO 5833 protocols) is 69°C. The setting time is 9 min 30 s.

The residual monomer content of the specimens is below 5% after setting (Fig. 84). The BPO content of these cements is clearly lower than the portion of DmpT. The ratio of initiator to activator is distinctly less than one. In contrast to the low- and medium-viscosity cements produced by this manufacturer, the high-viscosity cements show a low BPO content. The residual monomer content is not significantly lower than those of low- and medium-viscosity cement types. The same applies to the residual monomer release.

The ratio of initiators is the same for all Palacos R, Osteopal and Palamed products. A notice regarding the presently valid ISO standard (Table 51) is missing on packages of this type of bone cement. The key characteristics of Palacos R are listed in Table 52.

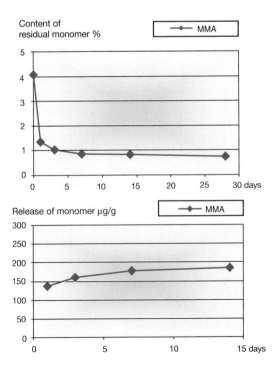

Fig. 84. Content and release of the residual monomer of Palacos R with time

Table 51. ISO 5833 (1992) requirements for the packaging of Palacos R

Requirements		Com-pliance	Location of information
General	Is the powder packed in a double-layered, sealed container?	+	–
	Is the liquid packed in a double-layered, sealed container?	+	–
Information regarding the powder ingredients	Qualitative	+	IB, Alu, FS, PB
	Quantitative	+	IB, Alu, FS, PB
Information regarding the liquid ingredients	Qualitative	+	A, AB, PB
	Quantitative	+	AB, PB
	Warning that the package contains flammable liquid	+	A, AB, FS, PB
	Instructions for storage (≤25°C, darkness)	+	IB, Alu, FS, AB, PB
	Statement of the sterility of the contents	+	IB, Alu, FS, AB, PB
	Warning against reusing the package	+	IB, Alu, FS, AB, PB
	Batch number(s)	+	IB, Alu, FS, A, PB
	Expiration date	+	IB, Alu, FS, AB
	Name/address of the manufacturer/ distributor	+	IB, Alu, FS, A, AB, PB
	Number and date of the standard	–	–
Information in the package insert	Detailed instructions for handling the components and preparing the cement	+	PB
	A statement drawing attention to the dangers for the patient	+	PB
	Recommendations for using the cement (syringe/dough state)	+	PB
	A statement regarding the influence of the temperature on working times	+	PB
	Graphical representation of the effects of temperature on the length of the phases of cement curing	+	PB

+, complies; –, does not comply; *A*, ampoule; *AB*, ampoule blister; *Alu*, aluminum pouch; *FS*, carton; *IB*, primary pouch; *PB*, package insert

Table 52. The key characteristics of Palacos R

High viscosity
Zirconium dioxide is the radiopaque medium
The powder contains MMA/MA copolymers
The polymer is ethylene oxide sterilized
The powder and ampoule are packed separately
Mixing sequence: monomer, then powder
Working time: long
ISO 5833 is fulfilled
Molecular weight greater than 350,000 Da
High fatigue strength
High impact strength
High bending strength

MMA/MA, methyl methacrylate–methyl acrylate

3.2.1.17
Palamed

All the cement components of Palamed are packed in a rectangular outer carton that may be easily opened at the upper, narrow side (Fig. 85). The printing on the outer cartons complies in every respect with ISO packaging regulations. Information regarding the batch number and expiration date is not printed on the front side of the cartons but on one of the two unprinted, small sides. The names of the distributor and manufacturer may easily be seen.

The outer cartons contain a cardboard tray in which two spaces are left for secure packaging for both of the ampoule-containing blister packs; in case of single versions of the bone cements, only one blister-packed ampoule is located there. Usually, a multilingual brochure, four to six chart stickers and an alu-pouch that contains two inner pouches with polymer powder are placed on the two monomer ampoules, which are located in the spaces of the cardboard tray. Each of the two folded, double-packed inner pouches within the alu-pouch contains sterile pouches in which the polymer powder is located.

The paper side of the inner pouch for the polymer has printing featuring important information regarding handling and storage. Furthermore, the batch number and the expiration date are located clearly on the printed front side, as prescribed by standard protocols. The back of the inner pouch is made of poly-ester and is, therefore, transparent.

The green, pigmented polymer powder (the color of which is characteristic for Palacos R-like products and is well-known) is clearly visible. The polymer powder is sterilized by ethylene oxide. The composition of the polymer powder is

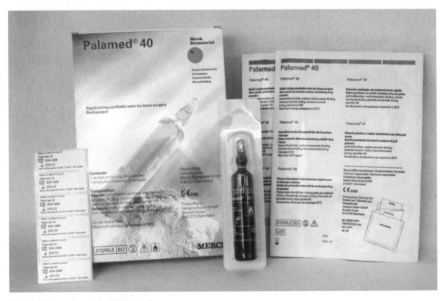

Fig. 85. The packaging of Palamed

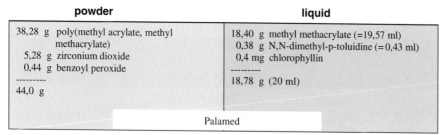

powder	liquid
38,28 g poly(methyl acrylate, methyl methacrylate) 5,28 g zirconium dioxide 0,44 g benzoyl peroxide --------- 44,0 g	18,40 g methyl methacrylate (=19,57 ml) 0,38 g N,N-dimethyl-p-toluidine (=0,43 ml) 0,4 mg chlorophyllin --------- 18,78 g (20 ml)
Palamed	

Fig. 86. Composition of Palamed

87% MMA–methyacrylate copolymer, 1.0% BPO and (as an opacifier) 12.0% zir-conium dioxide (Fig. 86).

The sterile inner pouch is enclosed by an unprinted peel-off pouch that, like the inner pouch, consists of a paper side and a polyethylene side. As the transparent polyethylene side encloses the printed paper side of the inner pouch, the printing of the inner pouch may be clearly read through the outer pouch. On the outer pouch, a sterile label (which was obviously put on the pouch after successful sterilization) is located. Usually, two folded, peel-off pouches are packed in an alu-pouch, which also has printing on one side. The print contains all necessary instructions, including the batch number and expiration date.

The two ampoules in the cardboard tray are protected not only by the blister pack but by the alu-pouch located above it. The blister pack itself consists of transparent, molded PVC and a paper cover. A printed ampoule label is attached to the paper cover; this label contains all necessary information (especially the batch number and the expiration date of the liquid monomer). A brown glass ampoule contains the sterile, filtrated green monomer, which has the same com-

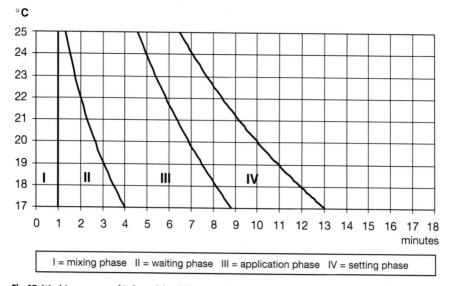

| I = mixing phase   II = waiting phase   III = application phase   IV = setting phase |

Fig. 87. Working curves of Palamed for different ambient/component temperatures

Table 53. Mechanical strength according to ISO 5833 and German Industrial Standard DIN 53435 for Palamed

	ISO 5833 Bending strength (MPa)	Bending modulus (MPa)	Compressive strength (MPa)	DIN 53435 Bending strength (MPa)	Impact strength (kJ/m^2)
Limit given in the standard	>50	>1800	>70		
Actual strength	69.4	2581	93.5	90.8	5.2

position as Palacos R. Each ampoule has a translucent label. The blister pack is also sterilized by ethylene oxide. Therefore, the monomer of Palamed consists of 98.0% MMA, 2.0% DmpT and approximately 60 ppm hydroquinone (Fig. 86).

No opening aid is installed for the opening of the brown glass ampoule; the polymer pouch should be opened with the help of a scissors. The polymer powder may easily be poured out of the pouch into the mixing vessel.

Before mixing the cement components of Palamed, one must first pour all the liquid into the bowl. The polymer powder is then added to the monomer and the clock is started. In a few seconds, a liquid, low-viscosity, homogeneous dough is easily produced. The viscosity of the dough increases slowly, depending on the temperature of the components with respect to the temperature of the operating

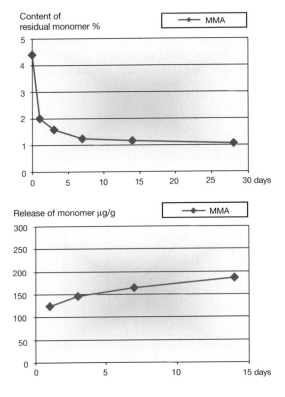

Fig. 88. Content and release of the residual monomer of Palamed with time

room. For example, the dough may be taken out of the mixing vessel in a non-sticky state after between approximately 1 min 30 s and 1 min 40 s if the components and the room are kept at 23°C (Fig. 87). The working phase of Palamed varies from 3 min 30 s to 4 min and usually ends between approximately 5 min and 5 min 30 s after mixing starts. Therefore, the working phases of Palamed and Palacos R are comparable. The cement hardens after approximately 6–8 min. So Palamed is characterized as a high-viscosity PMMA bone cement with a liquid, low-viscosity wetting phase.

Mechanical testing yielded good results. The bending strength determined according to ISO 5833 protocols is remarkably high (69.4 MPa), as is the bending strength determined according to DIN 53435 protocols (90.8 MPa; Table 53). The hardening temperature (determined according to ISO 5833 protocols) is 69.5°C. The setting time is 11 min 5 s.

The residual monomer content of the specimens is below 5% after setting (Fig. 88). The BPO content of these cements is clearly lower than the portion of DmpT. The ratio of initiator to activator is approximately one. In contrast to the

Table 54. ISO 5833 (1992) requirements for the packaging of Palamed

Requirements		Com-pliance	Location of information
General	Is the powder packed in a double-layered, sealed container?	+	–
	Is the liquid packed in a double-layered, sealed container?	+	–
Information regarding the powder ingredients	Qualitative	+	IB, Alu, FS, PB
	Quantitative	+	IB, Alu, FS, PB
Information regarding the liquid ingredients	Qualitative	+	A, AB, PB
	Quantitative	+	AB, PB
	Warning that the package contains flammable liquid	+	A, AB, FS, PB
	Instructions for storage (≤25°C, darkness)	+	IB, Alu, FS, AB, PB
	Statement of the sterility of the contents	+	IB, Alu, FS, AB, PB
	Warning against reusing the package	+	IB, Alu, FS, AB, PB
	Batch number(s)	+	IB, Alu, FS, A, PB
	Expiration date	+	IB, Alu, FS, AB
	Name/address of the manufacturer/distributor	+	IB, Alu, FS, A, AB, PB
	Number and date of the standard	–	–
Information in the package insert	Detailed instructions for handling the components and preparing the cement	+	PB
	A statement drawing attention to the dangers for the patient	+	PB
	Recommendations for using the cement (syringe/dough state)	+	PB
	A statement regarding the influence of the temperature on working times	+	PB
	Graphical representation of the effects of temperature on the length of the phases of cement curing	+	PB

+, complies; –, does not comply; *A*, ampoule; *AB*, ampoule blister; *Alu*, aluminum pouch; *FS*, carton; *IB*, primary pouch; *PB*, package insert

Table 55. The key characteristics of Palamed

High viscosity
Zirconium dioxide is the radiopaque medium
The powder contains MMA/MA copolymers
The polymer is ethylene oxide sterilized
The powder and ampoule are packed separately
Mixing sequence: monomer, then powder
Working time: long
ISO 5833 is fulfilled
Molecular weight greater than 350,000 Da
High fatigue strength
High impact strength
High bending strength

MMA/MA, methyl methacrylate–methyl acrylate

high-viscosity cements produced by this manufacturer, the medium-viscosity cement shows a higher BPO content but a lower BPO content than the low-viscosity materials. The residual monomer content is comparable to those of the high-viscosity and low-viscosity cement types. The same applies to the residual monomer release. A notice regarding the presently valid ISO standard (Table 54) is missing on packages of this type of bone cement. The key characteristics of Palamed are listed in Table 55.

3.2.1.18
Palavit HV

Palavit HV is no longer sold in France and Switzerland. Only a multilingual presentation can be found.

All the cement components of Palavit HV are packed in a rectangular outer carton that may be easily opened at the upper, narrow side (Fig. 89). The printing on the outer cartons complies in every respect with ISO packaging regulations. Information regarding the batch number and expiration date is not printed on the front side of the cartons but on one of the two unprinted, small sides. The names of the distributor and manufacturer may easily be seen.

The outer cartons contain a cardboard tray in which two spaces are left for secure packaging for both of the ampoule-containing blister packs; in case of single versions of the bone cements, only one blister-packed ampoule is located there. Usually, the insert and an alu-pouch that contains two inner pouches with polymer powder are placed on the two monomer ampoules, which are located in the spaces of the cardboard tray. Each of the two folded, double-packed inner pouches within the alu-pouch contains sterile pouches in which the polymer powder is located.

The paper side of the inner pouch for the polymer has printing featuring important information regarding handling and storage. Furthermore, the batch number and the expiration date are located clearly on the printed front side, as prescribed by standard protocols. The back of the inner pouch is made of polyester and is, therefore, transparent.

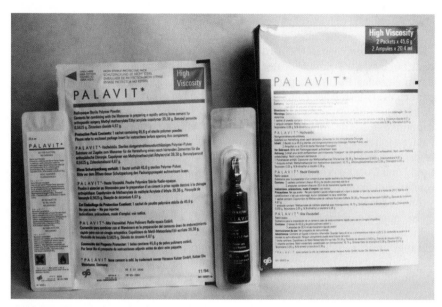

Fig. 89. The packaging of Palavit HV

The white polymer powder is clearly visible and is sterilized by ethylene oxide. The composition of the polymer powder is 86.4% MMA–ethyl acrylate copolymer, 1.2% BPO, 2.2% calcium carbonate and (as an opacifier) 10.2% zirconium dioxide (Fig. 90).

The sterile inner pouch is enclosed by an unprinted peel-off pouch that, like the inner pouch, consists of a paper side and a polyethylene side. As the transparent polyethylene side encloses the printed paper side of the inner pouch, the printing of the inner pouch may be clearly read through the outer pouch. On the outer pouch, a sterile label (which was obviously put on the pouch after successful sterilization) is located. Usually, two folded, peel-off pouches are packed in

powder	liquid
39,38 g poly(ethyl acrylate, methyl methacrylate)	18,75 g methyl methacrylate (=19,95 ml)
4,67 g zirconium dioxide	0,08 g ethylene glycole dimethacrylate (= 0,08 ml)
0,56 g benzoyl peroxide	0,36 g N,N-dimethyl-p-toluidine (=0,38 ml)
0,99 g calcium carbonate	0,05 g terpinolene
----------	0,015g chlorophyllin
45,60 g	----------
	19,26 g (20,4 ml)

Palavit HV

Fig. 90. Composition of Palavit HV

an alu-pouch, which also has printing on one side. The print contains all necessary instructions, including the batch number and expiration date.

The two ampoules in the cardboard tray are protected not only by the blister pack but by the alu-pouch located above it. The blister pack itself consists of transparent, molded PVC and a paper cover. A printed ampoule label is attached to the paper cover; this label contains all necessary information (especially the batch number and the expiration date of the liquid monomer). A brown glass ampoule contains the sterile, filtrated green monomer, which has the same composition as Palacos R liquid monomer. Each ampoule has a translucent label. The blister pack is also sterilized by ethylene oxide. The Palavit monomer consists of 97.35% MMA, 1.9% DmpT, 0.42% ethylene glycol dimethacrylate, 0.26% terpinolene, 0.015 g chlorophyll and approximately 60 ppm hydroquinone (Fig. 90). Therefore, the composition of the monomers of Palavit HV and Palavit LV are the same.

No opening aid is installed for the opening of the brown glass ampoule; the polymer pouch should be opened with the help of a scissors. The polymer powder may easily be poured out of the pouch into the mixing vessel.

Before mixing the cement components of Palavit HV, one must first pour all the liquid into the bowl. The polymer powder is then added to the monomer and the clock is started. In a few seconds, a homogeneous dough is easily produced. The viscosity of the dough increases very quickly, depending on the temperature of the components with respect to the temperature of the operating room. For example, the dough may be taken out of the mixing vessel in a non-sticky state after approximately 1 min if the components and the room are kept at 23°C (Fig. 91). The working phase of Palavit HV varies from 3.5 min to 4 min and usually ends between approximately 4 min 30 s and 5 min after mixing starts. The cement hardens after approximately 6–7 min. Therefore, Palavit HV is characterized as a high-viscosity PMMA bone cement.

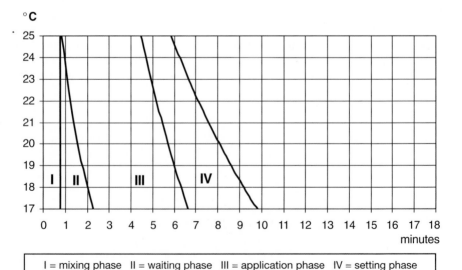

| I = mixing phase   II = waiting phase   III = application phase   IV = setting phase |

Fig. 91. Working curves of Palavit HV for different ambient/component temperatures

Table 56. Mechanical strength according to ISO 5833 and German Industrial Standard DIN 53435 for Palavit HV

	ISO 5833 Bending strength (MPa)	Bending modulus (MPa)	Compressive strength (MPa)	DIN 53435 Bending strength (MPa)	Impact strength (kJ/m²)
Limit given in the standard	>50	>1800	>70		
Actual strength	68.6	2668	98.4	74.9	6

Mechanical testing results fulfill the ISO 5833 and DIN 53435 requirements (Table 56). The impact strength is remarkably high (6 kJ/m²).

The hardening temperature (determined according to ISO 5833 protocols) had a very low value of 54°C because of the terpinolene in the liquid. The setting time is 8 min 20 s.

Table 57. ISO 5833 (1992) requirements for the packaging of Palavit HV

Requirements		Compliance	Location of information
General	Is the powder packed in a double-layered, sealed container?	+	–
	Is the liquid packed in a double-layered, sealed container?	+	–
Information regarding the powder ingredients	Qualitative	+	IB, Alu, FS, PB
	Quantitative	+	IB, Alu, FS, PB
Information regarding the liquid ingredients	Qualitative	+	A, AB, PB
	Quantitative	+	AB, PB
	Warning that the package contains flammable liquid	+	A, AB, FS
	Instructions for storage (≤25°C, darkness)	+	FS
	Statement of the sterility of the contents	+	IB, Alu, FS, AB, PB
	Warning against reusing the package	–	–
	Batch number(s)	+	IB, Alu, FS, A, AB
	Expiration date	+	IB, Alu, FS, AB
	Name/address of the manufacturer/ distributor	+	IB, Alu, FS, A, AB, PB
	Number and date of the standard	–	–
Information in the package insert	Detailed instructions for handling the components and preparing the cement	+	PB
	A statement drawing attention to the dangers for the patient	+	PB
	Recommendations for using the cement (syringe/dough state)	+	PB
	A statement regarding the influence of the temperature on working times	+	PB
	Graphical representation of the effects of temperature on the length of the phases of cement curing	+	PB

+, complies; –, does not comply; *A*, ampoule; *AB*, ampoule blister; *Alu*, aluminum pouch; *FS*, carton; *IB*, primary pouch; *PB*, package insert

Table 58. The key characteristics of Palavit HV

High viscosity
Zirconium dioxide is the radiopaque medium
The powder contains a MA/EA copolymer
The liquid contains a cross-linking agent and a radical catcher
The polymer is ethylene oxide sterilized
The powder and ampoule are packed separately
Mixing sequence: monomer, then powder
Working time: long
ISO 5833 is fulfilled
Molecular weight greater than 350,000 Da
High impact strength

MA/EA, methyl acrylate–ethyl acrylate

Because the material is no longer marketed, no tests have been done on the residual monomer content after setting. A new material based on the composition of Palavit will be introduced in the market. A notice regarding the presently valid ISO standard is missing on packages of this type of bone cement (Table 57). The key characteristics of Palavit HV are listed in Table 58.

3.2.1.19
Palavit LV

Palavit LV is no longer sold in France and Switzerland. Only a multilingual presentation can be found.

All the cement components of Palavit LV are packed in a rectangular outer carton that may be easily opened at the upper, narrow side (Fig. 92). The printing on the outer cartons complies in every respect with ISO packaging regulations. Information regarding the batch number and expiration date is not printed on the front side of the cartons but on one of the two unprinted, small sides. The names of the distributor and manufacturer may easily be seen.

The outer cartons contain a cardboard tray in which two spaces are left for secure packaging for both of the ampoule-containing blister packs; in case of single versions of the bone cements, only one blister-packed ampoule is located there. Usually, the insert and an alu-pouch that contains two inner pouches with polymer powder are placed on the two monomer ampoules, which are located in the spaces of the cardboard tray. Each of the two folded, double-packed inner pouches within the alu-pouch contains the sterile pouches in which the polymer powder is located.

The paper side of the inner pouch for the polymer has printing featuring important information regarding handling and storage. Furthermore, the batch number and the expiration date are located clearly on the printed front side, as prescribed by standard protocols. The back of the inner pouch is made of polyester and is, therefore, transparent.

The white polymer powder is clearly visible and is sterilized by ethylene oxide. The composition of the polymer powder is 86.4% MMA–ethyl acrylate copoly-

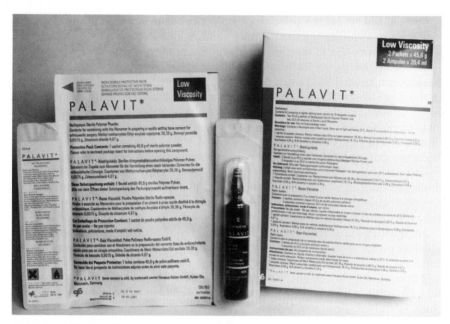

Fig. 92. The packaging of Palavit LV

mer, 1.3% BPO, 2.1% calcium carbonate and (as an opacifier) 10.2% zirconium dioxide (Fig. 93).

The sterile inner pouch is enclosed by an unprinted peel-off pouch that, like the inner pouch, consists of a paper side and a polyethylene side. As the transparent polyethylene side encloses the printed paper side of the inner pouch, the printing of the inner pouch may be clearly read through the outer pouch. On the outer pouch, a sterile label (which was obviously put on the pouch after successful sterilization) is located. Usually, two folded, peel-off pouches are packed in an

powder	liquid
39,38 g poly(ethyl acrylate, methyl methacrylate)	18,75 g methyl methacrylate (=19,95 ml)
4,67 g zirconium dioxide	0,08 g ethylene glycole dimethacrylate (= 0,08 ml)
0,61 g benzoyl peroxide	0,36 g N,N-dimethyl-p-toluidine (=0,38 ml)
0,94 g calcium carbonate	0,05 g terpinolene
----------	0,015g chlorophyllin
45,60 g	----------
	19,26 g (20,4 ml)
Palavit LV	

Fig. 93. Composition of Palavit LV

alu-pouch, which also has printing on one side. The print contains all necessary instructions, including the batch number and expiration date.

The two ampoules in the cardboard tray are protected not only by the blister pack but by the alu-pouch located above it. The blister pack itself consists of transparent, molded PVC and a paper cover. A printed ampoule label is attached to the paper cover; this label contains all necessary information (especially the batch number and the expiration date of the liquid monomer). A Palavit brown glass ampoule contains the sterile, filtrated green monomer, but with a composition completely different from that of Palacos R liquid monomer. Each ampoule has a translucent label. The blister pack is also sterilized by ethylene oxide. The Palavit monomer consists of 97.35% MMA, 1.9% DmpT, 0.42% ethylene glycol dimethacrylate, 0.26% terpinolene, 0.015 g chlorophyll and approximately 60 ppm hydroquinone (Fig. 94). Therefore, the composition of the monomers of Palavit HV and Palavit LV are the same.

No opening aid is installed for the opening of the brown glass ampoule; the polymer pouch should be opened with the help of a scissors. The polymer powder may easily be poured out of the pouch into the mixing vessel.

Before mixing the cement components of Palavit LV, one must first pour all the liquid into the bowl. The polymer powder is then added to the monomer and the clock is started. In a few seconds, a very liquid, low-viscosity, homogeneous dough is easily produced. The viscosity of the dough increases very slowly, depending on the temperature of the components with respect to the temperature of the operating room. For example, the dough may be taken out of the mixing vessel in a non-sticky state after between approximately 2 min 30 s and 3 min if the components and the room are kept at 23°C. The working phase of

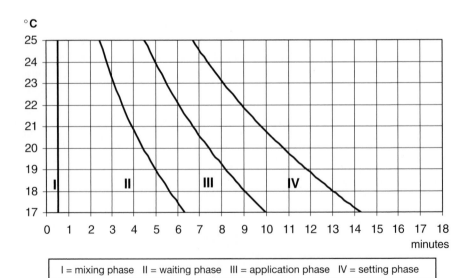

I = mixing phase   II = waiting phase   III = application phase   IV = setting phase

Fig. 94. Working curves of Palavit LV for different ambient/component temperatures

Table 59. Mechanical strength according to ISO 5833 and German Industrial Standard DIN 53435 for Palavit LV

	ISO 5833 Bending strength (MPa)	Bending modulus (MPa)	Compressive strength (MPa)	DIN 53435 Bending strength (MPa)	Impact strength (kJ/m^2)
Limit given in the standard	>50	>1800	>70		
Actual strength	69.1	2768	112.9	78.4	5.2

Palavit LV varies from 3 min to 5 min 30 s. The cement hardens after approximately 6–8 min. Therefore, Palavit LV is characterized as a low-viscosity PMMA bone cement.

Mechanical testing results fulfill the ISO 5833 and DIN 53435 requirements. The compressive strength is remarkable high (112.9 MPa; Table 59).

Table 60. ISO 5833 (1992) requirements for the packaging of Palavit LV

Requirements		Compliance	Location of information
General	Is the powder packed in a double-layered, sealed container?	+	–
	Is the liquid packed in a double-layered, sealed container?	+	–
Information regarding the powder ingredients	Qualitative	+	IB, Alu, FS, PB
	Quantitative	+	IB, Alu, FS, PB
Information regarding the liquid ingredients	Qualitative	+	A, AB, PB
	Quantitative	+	AB, PB
	Warning that the package contains flammable liquid	+	A, AB, FS
	Instructions for storage (≤25°C, darkness)	+	FS
	Statement of the sterility of the contents	+	IB, Alu, FS, AB, PB
	Warning against reusing the package	–	–
	Batch number(s)	+	IB, Alu, FS, A, AB
	Expiration date	+	IB, Alu, FS, AB
	Name/address of the manufacturer/distributor	+	IB, Alu, FS, A, AB, PB
	Number and date of the standard	–	–
Information in the package insert	Detailed instructions for handling the components and preparing the cement	+	PB
	A statement drawing attention to the dangers for the patient	+	PB
	Recommendations for using the cement (syringe/dough state)	+	PB
	A statement regarding the influence of the temperature on working times	+	PB
	Graphical representation of the effects of temperature on the length of the phases of cement curing	+	PB

+, complies; –, does not comply; *A*, ampoule; *AB*, ampoule blister; *Alu*, aluminum pouch; *FS*, carton; *IB*, primary pouch; *PB*, package insert

Table 61. The key characteristics of Palavit LV

Low viscosity
Zirconium dioxide is the radiopaque medium
The powder contains a MA/EA copolymer
The liquid contains a cross-linking agent and a radical catcher
The polymer is ethylene oxide sterilized
The powder and ampoule are packed separately
Mixing sequence: monomer, then powder
Working time: long
ISO 5833 is fulfilled
Molecular weight greater than 350,000 Da
High compressive strength

MA/EA, methyl acrylate–ethyl acrylate

The hardening temperature (determined according to ISO 5833 protocols) had a very low value of 52°C because of the terpinolene in the liquid. The setting time is 9 min 50 s.

Because the material is no longer marketed, no tests have been done on the residual monomer content after setting. A new material based on the composition of Palavit will be introduced in the market. A notice regarding the presently valid ISO standard is missing on packages of this type of bone cement (Table 60). The key characteristics of Palavit LV are listed in Table 61.

3.2.1.20
Surgical Simplex P and Surgical Simplex P with Microlok

The components of Surgical Simplex P with Microlok are packaged in a simple flat carton to be opened at the side via a marked flap (Fig. 95). Surgical Simplex P, however, is opened via its upper flap. The printed front sides contain all the rele-

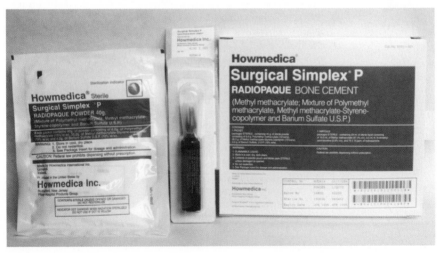

Fig. 95. The packaging of Surgical Simplex P

vant information. An additional label features the batch number, sterilization date and expiration date of the polymer and monomer and an extra control number. Moreover, there are two bar codes on the label. The carton is not printed directly. The information given conforms to the ISO packaging regulations. The back side of the carton of Surgical Simplex P with Microlok has additional information normally presented in the package insert (contraindications, warnings and precautions). The name of the manufacturer is also given.

The outer carton of Surgical Simplex P with Microlok contains a cardboard tray with a flap by which the tray can be drawn out of the carton. Sometimes this tray fits very tightly in the outer carton, thus hindering withdrawal. In the front part of the tray, the space for the ampoule is punched out. The ampoule should be taken out first. The polymer pouch, visible through a square window in the tray and protected from both sides, can then easily be taken out.

The outer cartons of Surgical Simplex P don't contain such a tray. An additional partition in the carton keeps the blistered ampoule away from the double-packaged polymer pouch. There are also four chart labels for the patients' documentation, allowing tracing via the control number. The rest of the packaging is the same for both Surgical Simplex P and Surgical Simplex P with Microlok.

The polyethylene peel-off pouch of the polymer, which has printing on one side, is opened via a Tyvek flap. The inner pouch can then easily be taken out. The polyethylene peel-off pouch gives instructions for use of the contents. There is an adhesive, dark-red indicator point; however, on the package of Surgical Simplex P with Microlok, no clear explanation is given that this means sterility, unlike the case for Surgical Simplex P. The Tyvek opening flap on the transparent back side of the peel-off pouch extends half the length of the pouch. The information on the inner pouch (batch number, sterilization number and expiration date) can easily be read through the transparent polyethylene foil. This information is not on the printed part of the peel-off pouch. Differences between Simplex P and Simplex P with Microlok could only be found as to the packaging!

The polymer powder of Surgical Simplex P consists of 15.0% PMMA, 75.0% MMA–styrene copolymer, 1.5% BPO and 10.0% barium sulfate (as an opacifier). The content of BPO is not given on the package, though it is obviously part of the polymer (Fig. 96).

The ampoule blister consists of molded PVC and Tyvek. The printed Tyvek part has all necessary the information, such as the batch number, expiration date

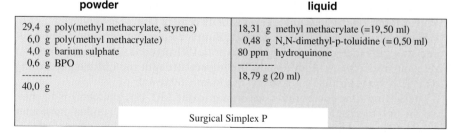

powder	liquid
29,4 g poly(methyl methacrylate, styrene) 6,0 g poly(methyl methacrylate) 4,0 g barium sulphate 0,6 g BPO -------- 40,0 g	18,31 g methyl methacrylate (=19,50 ml) 0,48 g N,N-dimethyl-p-toluidine (=0,50 ml) 80 ppm hydroquinone ----------- 18,79 g (20 ml)
Surgical Simplex P	

Fig. 96. Composition of Surgical Simplex P

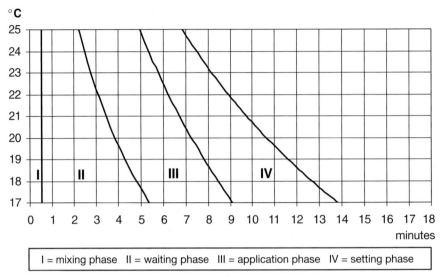

Fig. 97. Working curves of Surgical Simplex P for different ambient/component temperatures

and sterilization number. Unlike the powder pouch, there is a warning not to use the ampoule if the four indicator points appear blue. The colorless liquid consists of 97.4% MMA, 2.6% DmpT and 80 ppm hydroquinone (Fig. 96).

The ampoule has an opening aid; the polymer pouch should be opened with scissors. Due to the very bulky nature of the powder, it cannot be poured out easily.

Because of its high volume, the powder must be put into a large bowl. The monomer liquid is then added, and the stopwatch is started. At first, it appears that the amount of liquid not will be sufficient to wet all the powder. Thus, stirring has to be done very carefully. After 15–20 s, the powder breaks down abruptly, and total wetting is achieved. The relatively low viscosity then allows easy homogenization of the dough. At 23°C (room and components), the dough can be taken out of the mixing vessel after 2 min 45 s without causing it to stick to the gloves. The working time of Surgical Simplex P is between 3 min and 6 min. The viscosity, however, is already quite high after between 4 min and 4 min 30 s, thus preventing further handling. Hardening occurs after between 7 min 45 s and 8 min. Surgical Simplex P must be judged a medium-viscosity cement (Fig. 97).

The mechanical properties of Surgical Simplex P are not very good. The bending strengths (determined according to both ISO 5833 and DIN 53435 protocols) are comparatively low. Additionally, the impact strength (determined according to the DIN 53435 protocol) is also low (3.9 kJ/m²; Table 62).

The setting time (determined according to the ISO 5833 protocol) is 10 min, and the polymerization temperature is 89.7°C. The content of residual monomer immediately after hardening is slightly above 5%. The DmpT content (>2.5%) is one of the highest among all the cements (together with Zimmer dough-type

Table 62. Mechanical strength according to ISO 5833 and German Industrial Standard DIN 53435 for Surgical Simplex P

	ISO 5833 Bending strength (MPa)	Bending modulus (MPa)	Compressive strength (MPa)	DIN 53435 Bending strength (MPa)	Impact strength (kJ/m²)
Limit given in the standard	>50	>1800	>70		
Actual strength	67.1	2643	80.1	70.5	3.9

cement). The BPO percentage is only 1.5%, resulting in a favorable ratio of the initiators (1.5).

Information regarding the compositions of the powder and liquid are only given on the carton and in the package insert. The ampoule blister features the batch number and expiration date; the inner polymer pouch has none of these data. The symbols of the applicable product standard are used; the number of the standard, however, is not given (Table 63). A graphic representation of the temperature dependence of the working time is also not presented (Fig. 98). The key characteristics of Surgical Simplex P are listed in Table 64.

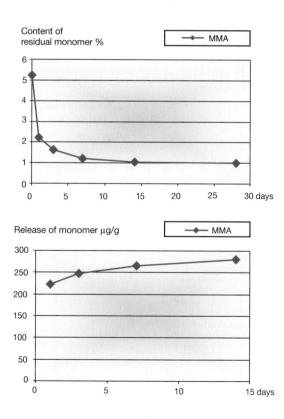

Fig. 98. Content and release of the residual monomer of Surgical Simplex P with time

Table 63. ISO 5833 (1992) requirements for the packaging of Surgical Simplex P

Requirements		Com-pliance	Location of information
General	Is the powder packed in a double-layered, sealed container?	+	–
	Is the liquid packed in a double-layered, sealed container?	+	–
Information regarding the powder ingredients	Qualitative	+	FS, PB
	Quantitative	+	FS, PB
Information regarding the liquid ingredients	Qualitative	+	FS, PB
	Quantitative	+	FS, PB
	Warning that the package contains flammable liquid	+	A, AB, FS
	Instructions for storage (≤25°C, darkness)	+	A, FS, IB, PB
	Statement of the sterility of the contents	+	A, AB, POB, FS, PB
	Warning against reusing the package	+	AB
	Batch number(s)	+	FS, AB
	Expiration date	+	FS, AB
	Name/address of the manufacturer/distributor	+	AB, POB, FS, PB
	Number and date of the standard	–	–
Information in the package insert	Detailed instructions for handling the components and preparing the cement	+	PB
	A statement drawing attention to the dangers for the patient	+	PB
	Recommendations for using the cement (syringe/dough state)	+	PB
	A statement regarding the influence of the temperature on working times	+	PB
	Graphical representation of the effects of temperature on the length of the phases of cement curing	–	–

+, complies; –, does not comply; *A*, ampoule; *AB*, ampoule blister; *FS*, carton; *IB*, primary pouch; *PB*, package insert; *POB*, peel-off pouch

Table 64. The key characteristics of Surgical Simplex P

Medium viscosity
Barium sulfate is the radiopaque medium
The powder contains a styrene copolymer
The polymer is γ irradiated
The powder and ampoule are packed separately
Mixing sequence: powder, then monomer
Working time: long
The viscosity is relatively high
ISO 5833 is fulfilled
Molecular weight less than 350,000 Da
Low impact strength

3.2.1.21
Surgical Subiton RO

The cement components of Surgical Subiton RO are packed in a flat, rectangular outer carton that may easily be opened on the upper, narrow side (Fig. 99). The printing on the blue-colored outer carton conforms to the valid ISO packaging regulations. Instructions concerning batch number and expiration date are printed on an additional attached label, not on the outer packing. A notice regarding the distributor may be clearly seen. The packing has an EC character, though the material is nearly exclusively sold in Argentina. A further notice on the outer packing indicates that the material fulfills ISO standard 5833 for bone cements.

In the outer carton, there is only a blister pack containing the polymer powder pouch and the monomer ampoule. The sterilization of the different components is obviously performed simultaneously inside this blister pack. An alu-pouch is not present. The molded PVC is designed in such a way that two ampoule blisters could be packed into it. In the middle of the blister pack is the doubly packed inner pouch. The printing on the inner pouch may be clearly read through the transparent PVC, but the back of the ampoule label cannot be identified on this package.

The back of the blister pack is made of medical paper on which some general information is indicated. A notice concerning the expiration date and the batch number is missing. The paper side cannot be easily separated from the PVC; usually, the paper becomes torn.

The doubly packed inner pouch slightly sticks to the laminated inner side of the paper of the outer blister. The paper that encloses the PVC molded blister

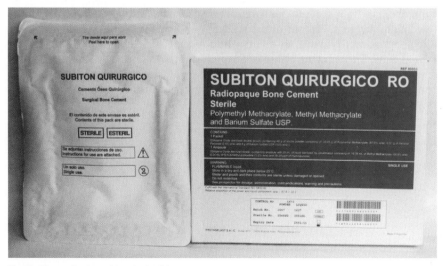

Fig. 99. The packaging of Surgical Subiton RO

pack has a typical sealing pattern (waffle design). In the case of the peel-off pouch and inner pouch, Tyvek is used in addition to polyethylene. The unprinted peel-off pouch has a green ethylene oxide indicator that is not clearly explained on the packing. The inner pouch and the peel-off pouch are made of the same packaging material. It seems that trilateral sealed pouches (which are manually closed after filling) are used. The printed paper side of the inner pouch contains indications regarding the batch number and expiration date.

In the case of one package of Surgical Subiton RO, it was observed that the expiration date on the outer carton was listed as November 2001.The inner pouch of the powder (batch number 1607), however, listed an expiration date of October 2001; the liquid (batch number 1627) had the expiration date November 2001. The expiration date on the outer carton, therefore, was indicated incorrectly.

The white polymer powder of Surgical Subiton RO contains 87.6% PMMA, 2.4% BPO and 10.0% barium sulfate (as an opacifier; Fig. 100) according to the manufacturer. However, analysis shows that the polymer also contains approximately 20% n-butyl methacrylate.

The blister pack contains the brown glass ampoule, which lies in a molded piece of PVC covered with medical paper. The medical paper is printed and contains (similar to the inner pouch of the powder) all the necessary information for the liquid. The ampoule itself is printed with a white color. The colorless monomer liquid of Surgical Subiton RO mainly consists of MMA (98.8%), 1.2% DmpT and approximately 70 ppm hydroquinone (Fig. 100).

There is no opening aid for opening the brown glass ampoule; the polymer pouch should be opened with a scissors. The polymer powder may be easily poured out of the pouch into the mixing vessel.

Before mixing the cement components, all the powder is put into the mixing vessel, as indicated by the manufacturer. The liquid is then added to the polymer powder, and the clock is started. In a few seconds, a low-viscosity, homogeneous dough arises. The viscosity slowly increases, depending on the temperature of the components with respect to the temperature of the operating room. For example, the dough may be taken out of the mixing vessel in a non-sticky state after between approximately 2 min 45 s and 3 min if the components and the room are kept at 23°C. The working phase of Surgical Subiton RO is very short (~2 min). After between approximately 4 min 40 s and 5 min, the cement can no longer be handled. By that time, the cement is already very warm. The hardening of the

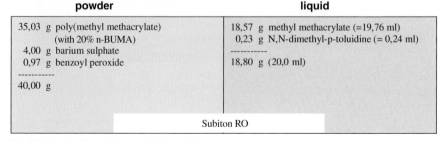

powder	liquid
35,03 g poly(methyl methacrylate) (with 20% n-BUMA)	18,57 g methyl methacrylate (=19,76 ml)
4,00 g barium sulphate	0,23 g N,N-dimethyl-p-toluidine (= 0,24 ml)
0,97 g benzoyl peroxide	-----------
-----------	18,80 g (20,0 ml)
40,00 g	

Subiton RO

Fig. 100. Composition of Surgical Subiton RO

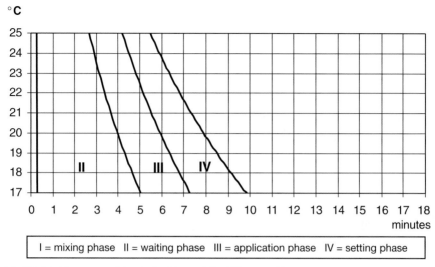

Fig. 101. Working curves of Surgical Subiton RO for different ambient/component temperatures

cement occurs 6 min after bringing together the components. Surgical Subiton RO, therefore, has to be regarded as a medium-viscosity cement (Fig. 101).

The mechanical data are very low and do not always correspond to the standard. In case of the tested batches, the bending strengths (determined according to ISO 5833 protocols) and the bending modulus were always less than the limit. The values determined according to DIN 53435 protocols were always very low (Table 65).

The setting time (as determined according to ISO 5833 protocols) is 9 min 50 s. The polymerization temperature of Surgical Subiton RO is very low. We found a value of 60.9°C.

The residual monomer content is very high (more than 6% after curing); the same applies to the residual monomer release (Fig. 102). The BPO percentage is comparatively high in the case of this cement, whereas the DmpT percentage is slightly more than 1%. This results in an initiator ratio of four.

It is striking that the qualitative and quantitative compositions of the powder and liquid are only explicitly indicated on the outer carton and in the insert. A

Table 65. Mechanical strength according to ISO 5833 and German Industrial Standard DIN 53435 for Surgical Subiton RO

	ISO 5833 Bending strength (MPa)	Bending modulus (MPa)	Compressive strength (MPa)	DIN 53435 Bending strength (MPa)	Impact strength (kJ/m²)
Limit given in the standard	>50	>1800	>70		
Actual strength	45.6	1765	87.1	64.3	2.7

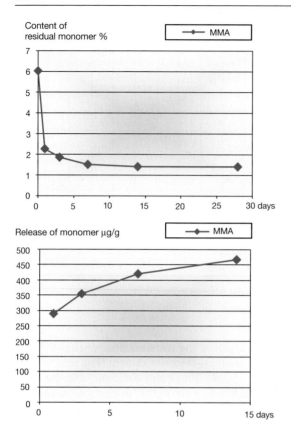

Fig. 102. Content and release of the residual monomer of Surgical Subiton RO with time

Table 66. ISO 5833 (1992) requirements for the packaging of Surgical Subiton RO

Requirements		Com-pliance	Location of information
General	Is the powder packed in a double-layered, sealed container?	+	–
	Is the liquid packed in a double-layered, sealed container?	+	–
Information regarding the powder ingredients	Qualitative	+	FS, PB
	Quantitative	+	FS, PB
Information regarding the liquid ingredients	Qualitative	+	FS, PB
	Quantitative	+	FS, PB
	Warning that the package contains flammable liquid	+	A, AB, FS
	Instructions for storage (≤25°C, darkness)	+	A, FS, PB
	Statement of the sterility of the contents	+	GB, FS
	Warning against reusing the package	–	–
	Batch number(s)	+	FS, AB
	Expiration date	+	FS, AB
	Name/address of the manufacturer/ distributor	+	IB, FS, PB
	Number and date of the standard	+	FS

Table 66. Continued

Requirements		Com-pliance	Location of information
Information in the package insert	Detailed instructions for handling the components and preparing the cement	+	PB
	A statement drawing attention to the dangers for the patient	+	PB
	Recommendations for using the cement (syringe/dough state)	+	PB
	A statement regarding the influence of the temperature on working times	+	PB
	Graphical representation of the effects of temperature on the length of the phases of cement curing	+	PB

+, complies; –, does not comply; *A*, ampoule; *AB*, ampoule blister; *FS*, carton; *GB*, shared blister; *IB*, primary pouch; *PB*, package insert

Table 67. The key characteristics of Surgical Subiton RO

Medium viscosity
Barium sulfate is the radiopaque medium
The powder contains a BuMA copolymer
The polymer is ethylene oxide sterilized
The powder and ampoule are packed separately
Mixing sequence: powder, then monomer
Working time: short
ISO 5833 is not completely fulfilled
Molecular weight greater than 350,000 Da
Low bending strength
Low impact strength

BuMA, butyl methacrylate

notice regarding the prohibition of reuse is missing. There are no indications concerning the batch number and expiration date on the primary vessels. A notice regarding the valid ISO 5833 standard (Table 66) exists but, for this cement, some mechanical tests executed according to this standard were outside the ISO requirements. The key characteristics of Surgical Subiton RO are listed in Table 67.

3.2.1.22
Zimmer Dough-Type Radiopaque Cement

Zimmer dough-type radiopaque cement is sold in an elongated, large, rectangular outer carton that closely resembles that of Osteobond (Fig. 103). The printing on the outer carton complies with ISO packaging regulations. Indications regarding the batch number of the polymer components are printed on a label attached to one side of the outer carton. Separate notices concerning the liquid are not included. The compositions of the powder and liquid are indicated on the blue-

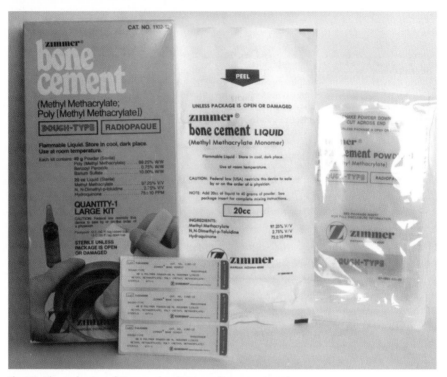

Fig. 103. The packaging of Zimmer dough-type radiopaque cement

colored upper side of the outer carton. The batch number printed on it is valid for both cement components. The expiration date on the additional label is indicated in the usual EC manner of writing and in normal written form.

This is the only notice regarding the EC characterization of the material, because all other packing components inside the outer carton do not have such information. The name of the distributor is clearly visible.

This outer carton for Zimmer dough-type bone cement has also two compartments; there is a greater compartment, in which the liquid ampoule is located, and a smaller one, in which the polymer pouch is located. In addition to the insert, one can find four information labels on one sheet; these may easily be taken off and which may be used for patients' records.

The inner pouch (which contains the polymer powder) is enclosed by a peel-off pouch. This pouch consists of a blue printed Tyvek side and an unprinted polyethylene side. The peel-off pouch may be easily opened without tearing the paper. The polyethylene pouch inside the peel-off pouch is placed with its blue printed side under the unprinted polyethylene side of the peel-off pouch so that the printing may be read through the peel-off pouch. The batch number and expiration date of the polymer are printed on the peel-off pouch but not on the inner pouch itself. The inner pouch can only be opened with a scissors. The poly-

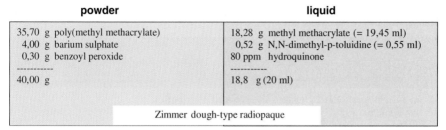

powder	liquid
35,70 g poly(methyl methacrylate) 4,00 g barium sulphate 0,30 g benzoyl peroxide ---------- 40,00 g	18,28 g methyl methacrylate (= 19,45 ml) 0,52 g N,N-dimethyl-p-toluidine (= 0,55 ml) 80 ppm hydroquinone ---------- 18,8 g (20 ml)
	Zimmer dough-type radiopaque

Fig. 104. Composition of Zimmer dough-type radiopaque cement

mer powder consists of 88.75% PMMA, 0.75% BPO and 10.0% barium sulfate (as an opacifier; Fig. 104).

The monomer ampoule is packed in the same way as Osteobond, i.e., like the polymer powder. The brown glass ampoule is enclosed by a peel-off pouch. This pouch consists of a printed Tyvek side and an unprinted polyethylene side. The peel-off pouch may be easily opened without tearing the paper. The inner pouch also consists of a Tyvek side and a polyethylene side and contains the ampoule; like the peel-off pouch, it is also printed on its paper side. The indicated information is identical to that on the peel-off pouch. The batch number and expiration date of the liquid are indicated on both packing units on the paper side. The inner pouch is packed in the peel-off pouch in such a way that one can clearly recognize the ampoule through the unprinted polyethylene side. The inner pouch is slightly attached to the peel-off pouch, so drawing out the inner pouch can be difficult.

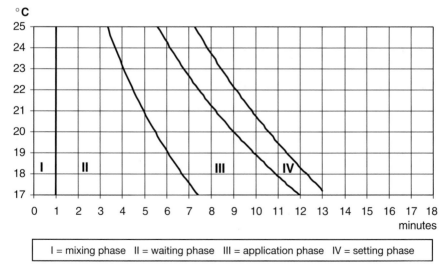

I = mixing phase   II = waiting phase   III = application phase   IV = setting phase

Fig. 105. Working curves of Zimmer dough-type radiopaque cement for different ambient/component temperatures

Table 68. Mechanical strength according to ISO 5833 and German Industrial Standard DIN 53435 for Zimmer dough-type radiopaque cement

	ISO 5833 Bending strength (MPa)	Bending modulus (MPa)	Compressive strength (MPa)	DIN 53435 Bending strength (MPa)	Impact strength (kJ/m²)
Limit given in the standard	>50	>1800	>70		
Actual strength	62.5	2454	75.4	77	5.02

The ampoule itself is printed with a white color and has an opening aid. The monomer liquid of Zimmer dough-type radiopaque cement mainly consists of MMA (97.23%), DmpT (2.77%) and 80 ppm hydroquinone (as a stabilizer; Fig. 104).

There is an opening aid on the brown glass ampoule; the polymer pouch should be opened with a scissors. The polymer powder can easily be poured out of the pouch into the bowl.

To mix the dough, the powder component is put into the mixing vessel. Due to the large volume of the powder, one should use a comparatively large vessel. After adding the liquid, it does not initially appear that the powder is wetted by the

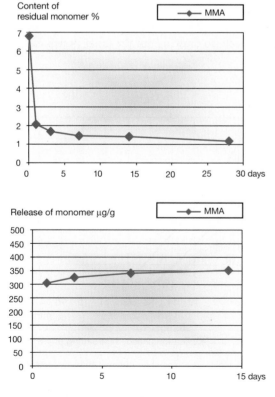

Fig. 106. Content and release of the residual monomer of Zimmer dough-type radiopaque cement with time

Table 69. ISO 5833 (1992) requirements for the packaging of Zimmer dough-type radiopaque cement

Requirements		Com-pliance	Location of information
General	Is the powder packed in a double-layered, sealed container?	+	–
	Is the liquid packed in a double-layered, sealed container?	+	–
Information regarding the powder ingredients	Qualitative	+	POB, FS, PB
	Quantitative	+	POB, FS, PB
Information regarding the liquid ingredients	Qualitative	+	A, POB, FS, PB
	Quantitative	+	A, POB, FS, PB
	Warning that the package contains flammable liquid	+	A, POB, FS
	Instructions for storage (≤25°C, darkness)	+	A, POB, FS
	Statement of the sterility of the contents	+	POB, IB, FS
	Warning against reusing the package	-	PB
	Batch number(s)	+	FS, POB
	Expiration date	+	FS, POB
	Name/address of the manufacturer/distributor	+	IB, FS, POB, PB
	Number and date of the standard	–	–
Information in the package insert	Detailed instructions for handling the components and preparing the cement	+	PB
	A statement drawing attention to the dangers for the patient	+	PB
	Recommendations for using the cement (syringe/dough state)	+	PB
	A statement regarding the influence of the temperature on working times	+	PB
	Graphical representation of the effects of temperature on the length of the phases of cement curing	–	–

+, complies; –, does not comply; A, ampoule; FS, carton; IB, primary pouch; PB, package insert; POB peel-off pouch

monomer. The mixing is, therefore, extremely difficult. After approximately 35–40 s, a quite homogeneous mass results from the mixing; after 60 s, the mass becomes a homogeneous dough that reaches the end of the sticky phase after 4 min. The viscosity of Zimmer dough-type radiopaque cement is always higher than that of Osteobond. The working phase ends after 6 min 40 s. During the working phase of the dough, the viscosity is also comparatively high. The hardening of the dough is finished 8 min 30 s after starting to mix (Fig. 105). Due to the cement properties, this variant has to be regarded as a low-viscosity cement.

The mechanical data completely fulfill the standards. The bending strength (determined according to the ISO 5833 protocol) is rather low (62.5 MPa; Table 68).

The setting time (as determined according to ISO 5833 protocols) is 12 min 40 s. The polymerization temperature of Zimmer dough-type radiopaque is 66.3°C.

This cement variant showed the highest residual monomer content of all the tested samples (Fig. 106). The percentage DmpT content is the highest for this cement and Simplex P. In contrast to the percentage DmpT content, the BPO content is rather low. This results in an extremely low initiator ratio (0.5).

The inner pouch of the polymer has no indications of the qualitative and quantitative composition; the ampoules, however, bear this information. On the primary vessels, there is no information regarding the batch number and expiration date. A notice concerning the presently valid ISO standard (Table 69) is missing. Moreover, in the insert, there is no graphic representation of the influence of temperature on the handling properties. The key characteristics of Zimmer dough-type radiopaque cement are listed in Table 70.

Table 70. The key characteristics of Zimmer dough-type radiopaque cement

Low viscosity
Barium sulfate is the radiopaque medium
The polymer is γ irradiated
The powder and ampoule are packed separately
Mixing sequence: powder, then monomer
Working time: long
ISO 5833 is fulfilled
Molecular weight less than 350,000 Da
Low bending strength
Low bending modulus

3.2.2
Comparison of Plain Cements

3.2.2.1
Setting Time and Temperature

Having described in detail the plain cements and their packaging, we want to compare them in terms of some important criteria of International Standards Organization (ISO) standard 5833. We found that the lowest temperatures were for Palavit Low Viscosity (LV) and Palavit High Viscosity (HV), obviously due to their unusual formulation for the monomer; terpinolene delays the polymerization. The Cemex cements, having a powder/liquid ratio of almost three (different from that of all others; Fig. 11), ought to have low temperatures, but this is not observed. The manufacturer claims peak temperatures of approximately 55°C because of the special powder/liquid ratio. Simplex P, Osteobond and Durus H, C-ment 1 and C-ment 3, and CMW 1 and CMW 3 show temperatures clearly above 80°C (Fig. 107).

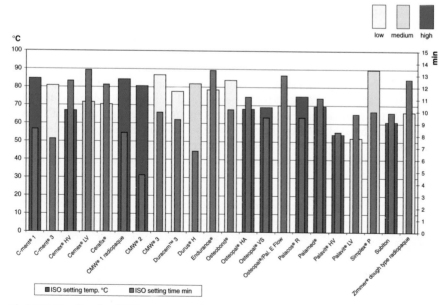

Fig. 107. Setting data for plain bone cements, determined according to ISO 5833 protocols

The relatively low polymerization temperature of Zimmer dough-type cement has been reported as 54°C (Edwards and Thomasz 1981) and 69.5°C (Hansen and Jensen 1990; Kindt-Larsen et al. 1995). The first two authors found the lowest temperatures; maybe their sample mass or thickness was different. Meyer et al. (1973) found a setting temperature of 60°C with 3-mm-thick specimens of Simplex P, and 107°C with 10-mm samples.

Hansen and Jensen (1990) tested nine different cements and found polymerization temperatures (determined using ISO 5833 protocols and 6-mm samples) of 66–82.5°C. Our results for Cerafix (66°C), Palacos E-Flow (73°C) and Zimmer dough-type cement (69.5°C) correspond to their results.

However, our results for CMW 3 (77.5°C), Simplex P (81.5°C), CMW 1 (76.5°C) and Palacos R (82.5°C) differ from theirs. Hansen and Jensen (1990) found temperatures approximately 10°C lower than ours for CMW cements and Simplex P and approximately 10°C higher than ours for Palacos, though the method used was the same (ISO 5833). Similar deviations were found between our setting times and those found by Hansen and Jensen (1990). A good correspondence, however, was found between our setting times and those reported by Edwards and Thomasz (1981).

3.2.2.2
Compressive Strength

Compressive strength was the only mechanical criterion implemented by American Society for Testing and Materials standards in the USA in 1978 and by ISO 5833 world wide. Ungethüm and Hinterberger (1978) tested the cements on the marketplace at that time (Table 71).

In terms of the compressive strengths, their results correspond well with ours. They followed the instructions given in the standard precisely, as did we.

Based on our results we can divide the cements in two groups: those that have compressive strengths of above 100 MPa and those that are not much more than the lower limit (70 MPa). Palavit LV, Osteobond, C-ment 3, Palavit HV, Endurance, Durus H, CMW 1, CMW 2, CMW 3, Cerafix and Cemex HV belong to the first group. Many of them have a low viscosity (Fig. 108). The high values of Palavit cements can be explained by their special cross-linking ingredient, ethylene glycol dimethacrylate. This yields a polymer matrix that is more rigid when exposed to a compressive influence. The material is more brittle than cements with a high

Table 71. Comparison of mechanical data in terms of ISO 5833/1 (Ungethüm and Hinterberger 1978)

Cement	Compressive strength (MPa)	Impact strength (kJ/m²)
Palacos R	82.8±6.1	2.83
Refobacin-Palacos R	86.3±6.2	2.45
Sulfix 6	103.6±7.8	2.62
Simplex	92.3±3.7	2.42
CMW	91.3±5.6	2.17

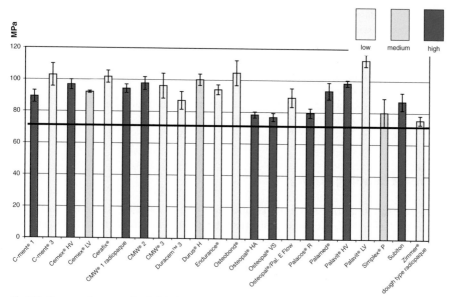

Fig. 108. Compressive strength of plain bone cements, determined according to ISO 5833 protocols

modulus and may break more easily under stress. Thus, a high compressive strength and a high modulus of elasticity seem to be disadvantageous in surgery in terms of the cement's function as an elastically buffering interface. An upper limit for the compressive strength should be demanded in the standard.

Compressive strengths above 100 MPa are reported for Sulfix 6 in the literature (Edwards and Thomasz 1981). Similar data for other low-viscosity cements are reported by Hansen and Jensen (1992), e.g., for CMW 3 (100–104 MPa). Krause et al. (1980), however, found a compressive strength of only 73 MPa for Zimmer dough, and Bargar et al. (1983) found a compressive strength of 81 MPa for the same cement, despite its low viscosity.

Some manufacturers advertise the high compressive strengths of their products. For instance, the distributor's results for Cerafix (107 MPa) correspond well with the data found by us. For Cemex cements, compressive strengths above 120 MPa and moduli far greater than 3000 MPa are claimed. This would result in considerable brittleness. We did not find such high values.

Osteopal HA, Osteopal VS, Palacos R, Simplex P and Zimmer dough-type cement belong to the second group of cements. The low compressive strengths of Osteopal VS and Osteopal HA may be explained by their high content of filler.

Our results correspond to those of Hansen et al. (1992) and Kindt and Larsen (1995), who found that the compressive strengths of high-viscosity cements were below 90 MPa. Different results were sometimes found, especially for Simplex P. While we found an average compressive strength of approximately 80 MPa, Kindt and Larsen (1995) found a value of almost 100 MPa, independent of the mixing technique. Edwards and Thomasz (1981) came to the same conclusion. The high compressive strengths of low-viscosity cements compared with high-viscosity variants were confirmed by our study.

In addition to the preparation of the test specimens and their storage, the test parameters are of decisive importance, as Lee et al. (1978) have already pointed out. We want to cite the importance of the »strain rate«, which leads to values of between 80 MPa and 122 MPa for the compressive strength. The strain rate is also important for the modulus (Lee et al. 1978).

3.2.2.3
Dynstat Bending Strength

The Dynstat bending strength is not part of the relevant standard for bone cements (ISO 5833). Moreover, the specimens are very small (15 x 10 x 3.3 mm). The fundamental requirements for normal stress distribution may not be fulfilled for specimens of that size. That is why Dynstat results should not be stressed too much. Small inhomogeneities may lead to dramatically low results. Thus, both the data and the standard deviations should be considered.

Palamed, Palacos, Osteopal and the Cemex cements have the highest bending-strength values (Fig. 109). An overview of Dynstat mechanics [German Industrial Standard (DIN) 53435] and the modulus (DIN 13907) is given by Ege (1994).

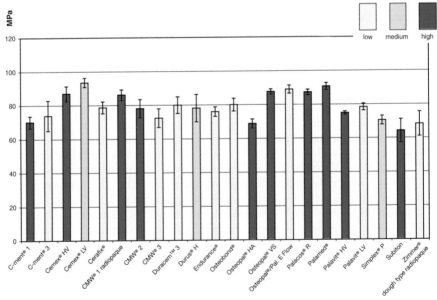

Fig. 109. Dynstat bending strength of all plain cements, determined according to German Industrial Standard 53435 protocols

3.2.2.4
Dynstat Impact Strength

The impact strength is often used as a parameter to describe properties of materials exposed to large, fast impacts (for example, plastic materials for cars). Thus, its importance for bone cements is not evident, and the small dimensions cause a problem (Sect. 3.2.2.3). For the »true« measurement of the impact strength, specimens of the same dimensions as for ISO 5833 are used (3.3 x 10 x 75 mm). Interestingly, Ungethüm and Hinterberger tested the impact strength in 1978 using a pendulum, thus facilitating comparison with our results.

Despite the questionable suitability of the test, we found interesting results for the different bone cements, in addition to those found by Ungethüm and Hinterberger (1978). C-ment 3, Cemex LV, Osteopal cements, Palacos, Palamed and Palavit cements have values greater than 5 kJ/m² (Fig. 110). CMW 3, Duracem, Subiton and Zimmer, however, have impact strengths clearly less than 3 kJ/m².

Ege (1992) also found a low impact strength for Zimmer dough-type cement. His report showed extremely high impact strengths for some low-viscosity cements. Our study shows that this high strength cannot be assigned to all of these cements, however.

Ungethüm and Hinterberger (1978) essentially came to the same conclusions we did: materials with methylacrylate–methyl methacrylate copolymers (all Palacos, Palamed and Osteopal products) have significantly higher impact strengths

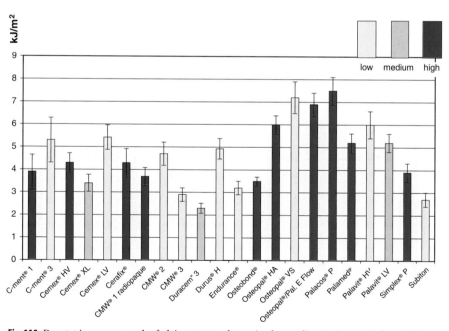

Fig. 110. Dynstat impact strength of plain cements, determined according to German Industrial Standard 53435 protocols

than those based on polymethyl methacrylate (CMW cements), butyl methacrylate (Duracem 3) or styrene (Simplex P). Older studies of Sulfix 6 and Sulfix (precursors of Duracem 3) also show low impact strengths.

Another assay for interpretation of the differences found for the impact strength could be the differing degree of post-polymerization. The specimens are tested dry after at least 16 h of dry storage. By that time, the materials are certainly at different levels of post-polymerization. Cements with a favorable benzoyl peroxide/dimethyl-p-toluidine ratio might have an advantage in this case. A faster post-polymerization should be an advantage, because the cement reaches the final state earlier.

3.2.2.5
ISO Bending Strength

Unlike the case for the Dynstat tests, the test specimens defined in the relevant standard are used in the ISO bending-strength tests. Moreover, the specimens have to be stored for 50 h in water or Ringer solution at 37°C. Because of the water storage, the possibility of water absorption must be considered which depends very much on the used copolymers.

It is notable that the Cemex products have low strengths and that the values for all the Subiton samples are below the limit in the standard (Fig. 111). From the literature, the low bending strength of Zimmer cements is known [56 MPa, according to Weber and Bargar (1983); 48 MPa, according to Hansen and Jensen (1992)]. All other cements have bending-strength values of approximately

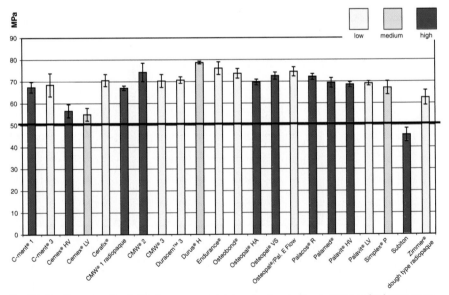

Fig. 111. Bending strength of plain bone cements, determined according to ISO standard 5833 protocols

70 MPa. Unlike Hansen and Jensen (1992), who reported a high result for Simplex P (74 MPa), we always found a low value. Moreover, CMW cements and Palacos have higher strengths in our study than in the study by Hansen and Jensen (1992).

3.2.2.6
Modulus of Elasticity

The modulus of elasticity is known to be a measure of the stiffness of a material. It tells how much a material is deformed by stress. The higher the modulus, the less the material is deformed. The stiffness depends on the amount of absorbed water. Thus, the ISO 5833 standard requires a defined method and duration of storage before testing. Lee et al. (1978) describe other influences.

All moduli found in our study (except the one for Subiton) fulfil the requirements of the standard. We also tested ISO specimens that were stored dry for at least 16 h (Dynstat storage, different from the ISO method) to determine the influence of water uptake in detail. The water-stored samples had moduli that were as much as 500 MPa lower (Fig. 112).

However, all values were clearly above the lower limit of 1800 MPa (ISO 5833). The bending strength, however, was not significantly different whether it was tested after being stored dry for 16 h or in 37°C water for 50 h (Table 72).

In Table 72, the extreme deviations of Simplex P are interesting. While the regular test resulted in a bending strength of approximately 70 MPa, the samples tested in the different manner only resulted in a bending strength of 50.5 MPa.

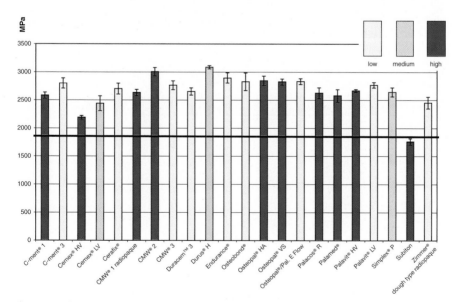

Fig. 112. Bending moduli of plain bone cements, determined according to ISO 5833 protocols

Table 72. Comparison of the bending moduli and the bending strengths of ISO test specimens stored dry for 16 h at 37°C or wet for 50 h at 37°C (Kühn and Ege 1999)

Material	Batch	Four-point bending modulus (dry, 16 h) (MPa)	Four-point bending modulus (wet, 50 h) (MPa)	Four-point bending strength (dry, 16 h) (MPa)	Four-point bending strength (wet, 50 h) (MPa)
Simplex P	148DD/822DD	2915	2665	51.7	50.5
Palacos R	8909	3075	2697	71.7	68.3
CMW 1	XO79R40	2964	2682	68.2	70.8
CMW 3	YOO9L40	3275	2875	73.7	72.8
Osteopal	9035	3049	2795	77.1	73.6

We also checked the influence of water storage at 37°C for different times on the bending strength and impact strength (Table 73). We found that the mechanical strength of the specimens after 2 h of water storage at 37°C was comparable to that of specimens stored for 4 weeks in the same manner. In our experience, there were no further deviations after longer periods of time. An explanation could be that, during post-polymerization, there is an initial increase of mechanical strength. However, there is also a plasticizing effect; further water uptake is the reason for the decrease (Table 73).

Table 73. Bending and impact strengths (according to German Industrial Standard 53435) of Palacos test specimens after storage dry or in water at 37°C

Storage	Time of test (after making the specimens)	Dynstat bending strength (MPa)	Dynstat impact strength (kJ/m^2)
Dry	1 h	66.87	4.41
Water (37°C)	2 h	77.38	4.95
Water (37°C)	5 h	79.64	5.07
Water (37°C)	16 h	88.24	4.90
Water (37°C)	2 weeks	81.64	4.39
Water (37°C)	4 weeks	76.24	4.58

3.2.3
Antibiotic-Loaded Cements

We will now describe all antibiotic cements on the market. To our knowledge, there are 18 different cements. In most cases the manufacturers make their antibiotic cements by simply mixing antibiotic to a plain cement version they have. Allofix G, according to the manufacturer, is not produced any more; however, it is still sold in some countries. Some antibiotic cements seem to exist only in the brochures of the manufacturers. For example, despite our efforts, we could not get Durus HA or Durus LA for our study. According to the package insert, a separate pouch of antibiotic to be mixed with Durus powder can be ordered.

Most cements contain the antibiotic gentamicin (as gentamicin sulfate) in different concentrations. Only Antibiotic Simplex (= AKZ) is different; it uses erythromycin-glucoheptonate and colistin-methane sulfonate sodium salt. Copal contains both gentamicin sulfate and clindamicin hydrochloride. This cement is to be used particularly for revisions of infected hips. As with the plain cements, we tested at least three different batches of each cement.

We described and tested the packages available for clinics in Germany (Table 74). In other countries, there may be other variants that could not be taken into consideration here.

Table 74. Antibiotic cements on the market

Name	Responsible Manufacturer	Viscosity type	Powder sterilization	Market
AKZ	Howmedica	Medium	γ irradiated	World-wide
Allofix-G	Sulzer	Low	Formaldehyde	Central Europe, CH
Cemex-Genta HV	Tecres	High	Ethylene oxide	South Europe, I
Cemex-Genta LV	Tecres	Medium	Ethylene oxide	South Europe, I
Cerafixgenta	Ceraver Osteal	Low	γ irradiated	South Europe, F
CMW 1 Gentamicin	DePuy	High	γ irradiated	World-wide
CMW 2 G	DePuy	High	γ irradiated	World-wide
CMW 2000 Gentamicin	DePuy	High	γ irradiated	World-wide
CMW 3 Gentamicin	DePuy	Low	γ irradiated	World-wide
Copal	Merck	High	Ethylene oxide	World-wide
Genta C-ment 1	E.M.C.M.B.V.	High	Ethylene oxide	Central Europe, G
Genta C-ment 3	E.M.C.M.B.V.	Low	Ethylene oxide	Central Europe, G
Osteopal G	Merck	Low	Ethylene oxide	World-wide
Palacos LV + G/E Flow with G.	Schering Plough	Low	Ethylene oxide	World-wide
Palacos R with Gentamicin	Schering Plough	High	Ethylene oxide	World-wide
Palamed G	Merck	High	Ethylene oxide	World-wide
Refobacin-Palacos R	Merck	High	Ethylene oxide	World-wide
Subiton G	Prothoplast	High	Ethylene oxide	Argentina

F, France; *G*, Germany; *I*, Italy; *CH*, Switzerland

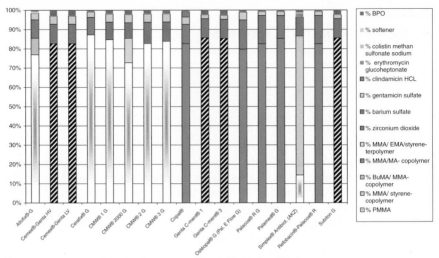

Fig. 113. Composition of the powder components of all tested antibiotic cements

The composition of the polymer powders showed significant differences, as could be observed for the plain cements. Again, there were some differences between the ingredients found by us and those declared on the packages.

The Cemex Genta cements contain approximately 3% styrene, the Subiton G approximately 20% n-butyl methacrylate. The Genta C-ment cements show even two extra co-monomers besides MMA: methyl acrylate and ethyl acrylate. All these were not declared on the labels (see special marking **NNN** for the declared PMMA in Fig. 113). The precise percentages could not be determined. These cements contain both pure polymethyl methacrylate (PMMA) and co-polymers.

Only a few manufacturers offer more than one antibiotic cement variant. Again, the variants made by one manufacturer have a very similar chemical basis. The active substances are simply added to the basic powder. We never found indications regarding the different qualities of the antibiotics; obviously, they comply with the requirements given in the pharmacopeia. All antibiotic-loaded materials produced by Heraeus-Kulzer are based on nearly identical green polymers.

The liquids (Fig. 114) were not different from those of the plain cements. They are all based on methyl methacrylate (MMA) and dimethyl-*p*-toluidine (DmpT). For CMW 2000 G, however, as the only bone cement, we found a great deviation between the DmpT content given by the manufacturer and the content determined by us. We found in many ampoules 99,3°% MMA and 0,7°% DmpT, whereas the manufacturer declares 98°% MMA and 2,0°% DmpT. For our comparisons we used the data of the manufacturer. Four of them also contain BuMA (in addition to MMA) in the monomer: Allofix G, Cerafixgenta, Genta C-ment 1 and Genta C-ment 3.

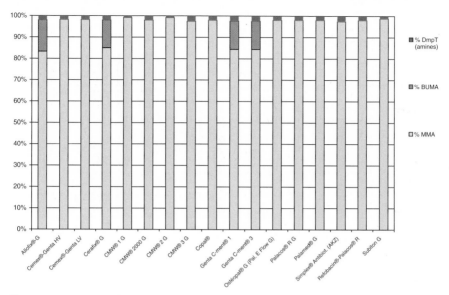

Fig. 114. Composition of the liquid components of all tested antibiotic cements

Though cross-linking monomers that improve the performance of cements are mentioned in the literature, we could not find any in the liquids. Figure 115 shows the percentages of the initiators in the powder and liquid and shows the ratio in the ready mixture.

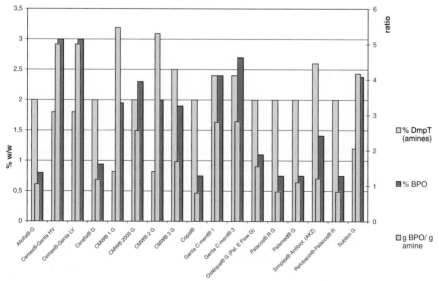

Fig. 115. Initiator/activator ratios for antibiotic cements

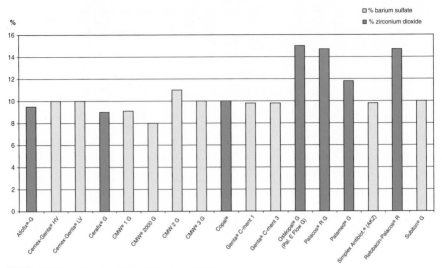

Fig. 116. Content of radiopaque media in antibiotic cements

Again, zirconium dioxide and barium sulfate are the radiopaque media used (Fig. 116). The lowest amount of radiopaque medium is found in CMW 2000 G (8%) followed by Cerafixgenta and Allofix G. For CMW products, we found 10% for CMW 3 G, 11% for CMW 2 G and only 9% for CMW 1 G. The highest amounts of radiopaque medium were in Osteopal G/Palacos LV/E Flow + G and Refobacin-Palacos R (14–15%). Palamed G only contains approximately 12%.

Approximately 10% is the most common content of radiopaque medium. This is a bit lower than for the plain cements.

3.2.3.1
Antibiotic Simplex (= AKZ)

The components of AKZ are packaged in a simple, flat outer carton that can be opened at the side by a marked flap (Fig. 117). The printed front sides feature all relevant information. An additional label features the batch number, sterilization date and expiration date of polymer and monomer and an extra control number. Moreover, there are two barcodes on it. The outer carton is not printed directly. The information given totally conforms to the ISO 5833 packaging regulations. The back side of the outer carton of AKZ features additional information normally presented on the package insert (contraindications, warnings and precautions). The name of the manufacturer is also given.

The outer cartons of AKZ do not contain a cardboard tray. An additional partition in the carton keeps the blistered ampoule away from the doubly packaged polymer pouch. There are four chart labels for the patients' documentation; these allow traceability via the control number.

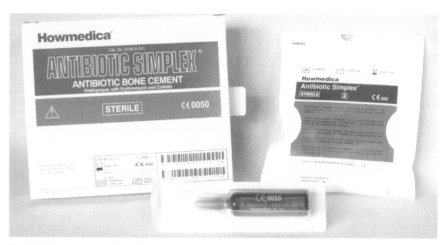

Fig. 117. The packaging of Antibiotic Simplex

The polyethylene (PE) peel-off pouch of the polymer, which is printed on one side, is opened via a Tyvek flap. The inner pouch can then be taken out easily. The PE peel-off pouch gives instructions for use. There is an adhesive, dark-red indicator dot, but no clear explanation of its use is given on the package. The Tyvek opening flap on the transparent back side of the peel-off pouch extends half the length of the pouch. The information on the inner pouch (batch number, sterilization number and expiration date) can easily be read through the transparent PE foil. This information is not on the printed part of the peel-off pouch.

The polymer powder consists of 15.0% PMMA, 75.0% MMA-styrene co-polymer, 1.5% benzoyl peroxide (BPO) and 10.0% barium sulfate (as an opacifier). The content of BPO is not given on the package, but it is obviously a part of the polymer (Fig. 118).

The ampoule blister consists of molded polyvinyl chloride (PVC) and Tyvek. The printed Tyvek part features all necessary information, such as batch number, expiration date and sterilization number. Unlike the powder pouch, the blister features a warning not to use the ampoule if the four indicator points are blue. The colorless liquid consists of 97.4% MMA, 2.6% DmpT and 80 ppm hydro-

powder	liquid
29,51 g poly(methyl methacrylate, styrene) 5,91 g poly(methyl methacrylate) 4,00 g barium sulphate 0,58 g benzoyl peroxide 0,73 g erythromycin-gluco heptonate (0,5 g base) 0,24 g colistin-methane sulfonate-sodium (=3000000 I.E.) ---------- 40,97 g	18,31 g methyl methacrylate (= 19,50 ml) 0,48 g N,N-dimethyl-p-toluidine (= 0,50 ml) 1,5 mg hydroquinone ---------- 18,79 g (20 ml)
AKZ (Antibiotic Simplex)	

Fig. 118. Composition of Antibiotic Simplex

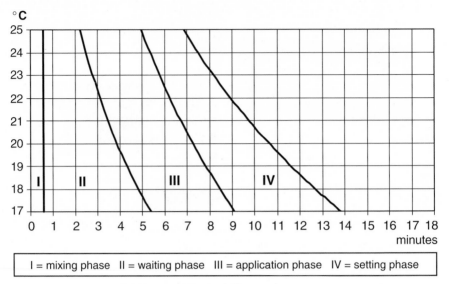

°C

I = mixing phase   II = waiting phase   III = application phase   IV = setting phase

Fig. 119. Working curves of Antibiotic Simplex for different ambient/component temperatures

quinone (Fig. 96). Therefore, there is no difference between the composition of Simplex P and that of AKZ.

The ampoule has a opening aid; the polymer pouch should be opened using scissors. Due to the very bulky structure of the powder, it cannot be poured out easily.

The powder is put into a bowl; the bowl should be big because of the volume of the powder. The monomer liquid is added, and the stopwatch is started. At first, it appears that the amount of liquid will not be sufficient to wet all of the powder. Thus, stirring has to be done very carefully. After 15–20 s, the powder breaks down abruptly, and total wetting is achieved. The relatively low viscosity then allows easy homogenization of the dough. At 23°C (room and components), it can be taken out of the mixing vessel after 2 min 45 s without sticking to the gloves. The working time of AKZ is between 3 min and 6 min. The viscosity, however, is already quite high after between 4 min and 4 min 30 s, thus preventing further handling. Hardening occurs after between 7 min 45 s and 8 min. AKZ must be classified as a medium-viscosity cement (Fig. 119).

Table 75. Mechanical strength according to ISO 5833 and German Industrial Standard DIN 53435 for Antibiotic Simplex

	ISO 5833			DIN 53435	
	Bending strength (MPa)	Bending modulus (MPa)	Compressive strength (MPa)	Bending strength (MPa)	Impact strength (kJ/m²)
Limit given in the standard	>50	>1800	>70		
Actual strength	66.6	2506	91.5	68.5	3.9

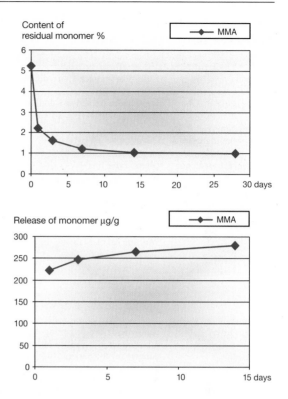

Fig. 120. Content and release of the residual monomer of Antibiotic Simplex with time

The mechanical properties of AKZ are not very good (Table 75). The bending strength determined according to both the ISO 5833 and German Industrial Standard (DIN) 53435 protocols are comparatively low. The impact strength determined according to the DIN 53435 protocol is also low (3.9 kJ/m^2). The setting time (determined according to the ISO 5833 protocol) is 10 min, and the polymerization temperature is 89.7°C.

The content of residual monomer immediately after hardening is slightly above 5% (Fig. 120). The DmpT content (>2.5%) is one of the highest, together with those of Surgical Simplex P and Zimmer dough-type cement. The BPO percentage is only 1.5%, resulting in a favorable initiator ratio of 1.5.

Information regarding the compositions of the powder and liquid are only given on the carton and on the package insert (Table 76). The ampoule blister features the batch number and expiration date; the inner polymer pouch has none of these data. The symbols of the applicable product standard are used; the number of the standard, however, is not given. A graphical representation of the temperature dependence of the working time is not presented. The key characteristics of AKZ are listed in Table 77.

Table 76. ISO 5833 (1992) requirements for the packaging of Antibiotic Simplex

Requirements		Compliance	Location of information
General	Is the powder packed in a double-layered, sealed container?	+	–
	Is the liquid packed in a double-layered, sealed container?	+	–
Information regarding the powder ingredients	Qualitative	+	FS, PB
	Quantitative	+	FS, PB
Information regarding the liquid ingredients	Qualitative	+	FS, PB
	Quantitative	+	FS, PB
	Warning that the package contains flammable liquid	+	A, AB, FS
	Instructions for storage (≤25°C, darkness)	+	A, FS, IB, PB
	Statement of the sterility of the contents	+	A, AB, POB, FS, PB
	Warning against reusing the package	+	AB, POB
	Batch number(s)	+	FS, AB, POB
	Expiration date	+	FS, AB, POB
	Name/address of the manufacturer/distributor	+	AB, POB, FS, PB
	Number and date of the standard	–	–
Information in the package insert	Detailed instructions for handling the components and preparing the cement	+	PB
	A statement drawing attention to the dangers for the patient	+	PB
	Recommendations for using the cement (syringe/dough state)	+	PB
	A statement regarding the influence of the temperature on working times	+	PB
	Graphical representation of the effects of temperature on the length of the phases of cement curing	–	–

+, complies; –, does not comply; *A*, ampoule; *AB*, ampoule blister; *FS*, carton; *IB*, primary pouch; *PB*, package insert; *POB* peel-off pouch

Table 77. The key characteristics of Antibiotic Simplex

Medium viscosity
Barium sulfate is the radiopaque medium
The polymer contains a styrene co-polymer
The polymer is γ irradiated
The powder and ampoule are packed separately
Mixing sequence: powder, then monomer
Working time: long, but the viscosity is relatively high
ISO 5833 is fulfilled
Molecular weight less than 350,000 Da
The used antibiotics are only bacteriostatic, not bactericid

3.2.3.2
Allofix G

Allofix G is no longer produced, but it is still sold in various markets. Therefore, we included Allofix G in our investigation.

As is the case for Duracem 3, the polymer powder and monomer liquid of Allofix G are packed in a small outer carton (Fig. 121). Only doubly packed units of Allofix G could be obtained. The outer carton may be easily opened via its upper side; a transparent label is then removed and cut through.

The outer carton itself is printed with the most important information. In comparison to Duracem 3, detailed information concerning the composition of the powder and liquid is given on the outer carton of Allofix G. On one narrow side, a white label that contains information regarding the batch numbers, expiration date, institution for registration and distributor is attached.

The outer carton contains a PE pouch that encloses a blister pack. This blister pack contains the powder in a glass bottle and a monomer ampoule. Furthermore, one can find the insert and three chart stickers for patients' records. The packing of the polymer powder in a brown glass ampoule is characteristic of all cements of Sulzer Medica.

The transparent, unprinted PE pouch can easily be opened. The blister pack consists of transparent PVC and is closed with printed Tyvek. This pack has no indications concerning the batch number and expiration date. This information may be easily read through the PVC, as both of the brown glass bottles have a printed label.

The blister pack can easily be opened by means of a paper flap. Inside the blister, there is a packed formaldehyde tablet (which obviously guarantees the

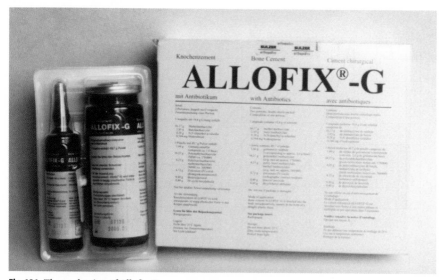

Fig. 121. The packaging of Allofix G

powder	liquid
38,27 g poly(methyl methacrylate) 4,25 g poly(butyl methacrylate) 4,72 g zirconium dioxide 0,40 g benzoyl peroxide 0,40 g di-cyclo-hexyl phthalate 1,66 g gentamicin sulphate (=1,0 g base) ------------ 49,70 g	16,17 g methyl methacrylate (=17,20 ml) 2,85 g butyl methacrylate (=3,17 ml) 0,38 g N,N-dimethyl-p-toluidine (=0,404 ml) 0,54 mg hydroquinone ------------- 19,40 g (20,77 ml)
Allofix-G	

Fig. 122. Composition of Allofix G

sterility of the blister contents). A notice giving an explanation of the purpose of the tablet is missing. The user could believe that this is an element that is to be added to the cement.

The polymer powder is packed in a brown glass bottle. It bears a label that indicates the batch number, expiration date and sterilization process procedure. Consequently the powder is sterilized by means of formaldehyde. It seems that only the surface of the brown glass bottle is sterilized by the formaldehyde tablet packed in the blister. The opening of the brown glass bottle is somewhat problematic. Often, the metal ring could not be completely removed, which sometimes led to injury of the medical staff.

The white polymer powder contains 77% PMMA, 8.6% poly(BuMA/MMA), 0.8% BPO, 3.3% gentamicin sulfate (2.0% gentamicin base), 0.8% dicyclo-hexylphthalate (as a plasticizer) and 9.5% zirconium dioxide (as an opacifier; Fig. 122). A printed paper label that contains all necessary information is also

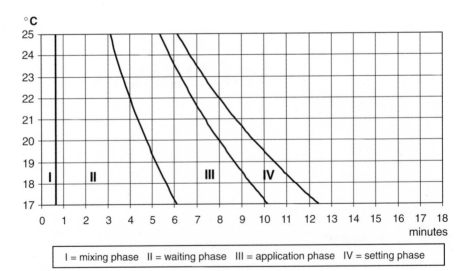

I = mixing phase   II = waiting phase   III = application phase   IV = setting phase

Fig. 123. Working curves of Allofix G for different ambient/component temperatures

Table 78. Mechanical strength according to ISO 5833 and German Industrial Standard DIN 53435 for Allofix G

	ISO 5833 Bending strength (MPa)	Bending modulus (MPa)	Compressive strength (MPa)	DIN 53435 Bending strength (MPa)	Impact strength (kJ/m^2)
Limit given in the standard	>50	>1800	>70		
Actual strength	63	2378	91.8	79.2	5.5

attached to the liquid ampoule. A notice concerning the sterile filtration of the monomer liquid is printed. The liquid consists of two different methacrylates (83.3% MMA and 14.6% BuMA), 2.0% DmpT and approximately 0.54 mg hydroquinone (as a stabilizer; Fig. 122). The interesting thing concerning the composition of the liquid is the use DmpT instead of DMAPE, as was observed in the case of Duracem 3. Therefore, the liquid composition of Allofix G is quite different from that of Duracem 3 (Fig. 122).

Before mixing the dough, the liquid is put into the mixing vessel; the voluminous powder is then added. The wetting is very slow. It initially appears as though the quantity of liquid is not sufficient. After approximately 25–30 s, a liquid dough that is completely homogeneous arises. The end of the sticky phase is after 3 min 30 s. The dough may then be taken out of the mixing vessel. The end of the working phase is at 6 min 15 s. However, the dough is already very warm after between 5 min 45 s and 6 min. Hardening takes place after 7 min (Fig. 123).

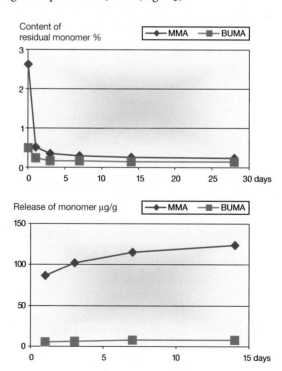

Fig. 124. Content and release of the residual monomers of Allofix G with time

The manufacturer recommends only syringe application in the use of Allofix G, whereas the working criteria indicated in the insert refer only to hand application. However, there should be no important change of the handling properties in cases of application by syringe. Due to the above-mentioned properties, Allofix G has to be regarded as a low-viscosity bone cement. The manufacturer points out that the material is only suitable for application by syringe.

The mechanical data correspond to the standards and exhibit quasi-static results. A high impact strength of 5.5 kJ/m^2 (compared with 2.3 kJ/m^2 for Duracem 3) could be observed (Table 78). The setting time (determined according to ISO 5833 protocols) showed values of 9 min 20 s, and the polymerization temperature was 77.5°C.

The residual monomer content is similar to that for Cerafixgenta (Fig. 124). The liquid also contains BuMA (~15%). The ratio of initiators is also comparable (a bit more than one), although Allofix G contains less BPO and DmpT. A comparison with cements containing a pure MMA liquid is not given.

Only the insert features qualitative and quantitative indications concerning the ingredients of the polymer and monomer. A notice regarding the valid ISO

Table 79. ISO 5833 (1992) requirements for the packaging of Allofix G

Requirements		Com-pliance	Location of information
General	Is the powder packed in a double-layered, sealed container?	+	–
	Is the liquid packed in a double-layered, sealed container?	+	–
Information regarding the powder ingredients	Qualitative	+	PB
	Quantitative	+	PB
Information regarding the liquid ingredients	Qualitative	+	PB
	Quantitative	+	PB
	Warning that the package contains flammable liquid	+	A
	Instructions for storage (≤ 25°C, darkness)	+	PB, FS
	Statement of the sterility of the contents	+	PF, A, GB, FS, PB
	Warning against reusing the package	+	PB, FS
	Batch number(s)	+	A, PF, FS
	Expiration date	+	A, PF, FS
	Name/address of the manufacturer/distributor	+	A, PF, FS, PB
	Number and date of the standard	–	–
Information in the package insert	Detailed instructions for handling the components and preparing the cement	+	PB
	A statement drawing attention to the dangers for the patient	+	PB
	Recommendations for using the cement (syringe/dough state)	+	PB
	A statement regarding the influence of the temperature on working times	+	PB
	Graphical representation of the effects of temperature on the length of the phases of cement curing	+	PB

+, complies; –, does not comply; *A*, ampoule; *FS*, carton; *GB*, shared blister; *PB*, package insert; *PF* powder bottle

Table 80. The key characteristics of Allofix G

Low viscosity
The monomer contains BuMA
The polymer contains BuMA (as a copolymer) and dicyclohexylphthalate
Zirconium dioxide is the radiopaque medium
The polymer is treated with formaldehyde
The polymer is in a brown glass bottle
The polymer bottle and monomer ampoule are packed in one blister
Mixing sequence: powder, then monomer
Working time: medium
ISO 5833 is fulfilled
Molecular weight less than 350,000 Da
High impact strength
High gentamicin content, low release

BuMA, butyl methacrylate

standard 5833 is missing (Table 79). The key characteristics of Allofix G are listed in Table 80.

3.2.3.3
Cemex-Genta HV

The cement components of Cemex-Genta HV are packed in a little, rectangular, navy-blue, marked outer carton (Fig. 125). This carton is printed on all sides except the lower front side. On the back of the outer carton, the composition of

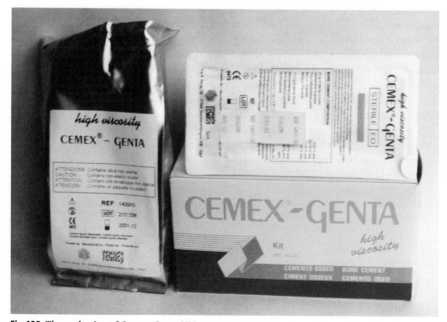

Fig. 125. The packaging of Cemex-Genta HV

the components and storage advice are included. A little label on one of the front sides gives the necessary information regarding the batch number and expiration date. This label also contains all necessary EC indications.

The distributor and the manufacturer are clearly indicated. The outer carton may only be opened on one side. Inside the carton, there is an insert and a blister pack that contains the polymer pouch and the monomer ampoule.

The molded PVC part is covered by printed Tyvek. This side features all necessary product information, such as the composition, batch number and expiration date. The indications regarding batch number and expiration date are not directly printed but are printed on chart stickers on the Tyvek. These labels can later be used for documentation in the patients' records. In case of older blister packs, a large, completely printed label was used. Furthermore, a brown indicator strip that documents successful sterilization is prominent. A notice explaining when this indicator indeed indicates the sterility is not included.

The Tyvek may be separated from the PVC lower part so that the single components may be taken out easily. First, the polymer inner pouch, which itself consists of a paper side and a polyester side, may be seen. It is striking that the inner pouch is completely unprinted, i.e., it contains no information. A marking indicates where the pouch should be opened. The pouch may easily be opened with the opening aid. The white, slightly rose-colored polymer powder consists of 82.8% PMMA (which certainly contains approximately 3% styrene, in the form of a co-polymer), 3.0% BPO, 4.2% gentamicin sulfate (2.5% gentamicin base) and 10.0% barium sulfate (as an opacifier; Fig. 126)

The monomer ampoule lies under the inner pouch in a special space in the PVC molding foil. The brown glass ampoule is printed with a white color. The information on the ampoule is extremely sparse; there is only the storage notice and information concerning how to inject the material. The batch number and expiration date are completely missing. It is remarkable that the monomer composition of Cemex-Genta HV is different from that of the plain high-viscosity version of the cement. The monomer ampoule contains the colorless monomer, which consists of 98.2% MMA, 1.8% DmpT and approximately 75 ppm hydroquinone (as a stabilizer). Therefore, the material contains twice the amount of DmpT contained by the plain monomer.

It is remarkable that only one batch number and one expiration date are indicated on the packing unit. Consequently, the liquid and the powder have both the same batch number and the same expiration date.

powder	liquid
33,11 g poly(methyl methacrylate) (with 3% styrene)	13,06 g methyl methacrylate (=13,89 ml)
4,00 g barium sulphate	0,24 g N,N-dimethyl-p-toluidine (=0,255 ml)
1,20 g benzoyl peroxide	75 ppm hydroquinone
1,69 g gentamicin sulphate (1,0 g base)	---------
---------	13,30 g (14,2 ml)
40,00 g	
	Cemex-Genta HV

Fig. 126. Composition of Cemex-Genta HV

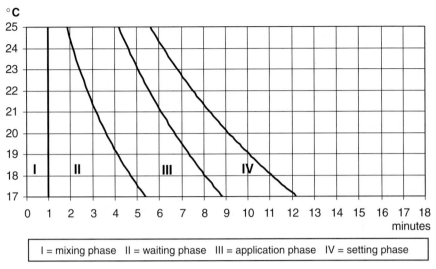

I = mixing phase   II = waiting phase   III = application phase   IV = setting phase

Fig. 127. Working curves of Cemex-Genta HV for different ambient/component temperatures

To mix the dough, the liquid is put into the mixing vessel first, then the powder is added. After adding the powder, one obtains an extremely dry dough that may not be homogenized at first. The great excess of polymer powder compared with the monomer liquid hinders easy mixing. It initially appears that the monomer is missing and that wetting of the polymer by the monomer will not be possible. While trying to homogenize the dough with the help of a mixing spatula, one has to be especially cautious, because material can easily be thrown out of the mixing vessel.

After approximately 50 s, one obtains a rather homogeneous dough that flows slowly together. The viscosity at the beginning is strikingly high, but the end of the sticky phase of the dough (at 23°C) is reached after only 2 min 15 s (Fig. 127). The end of the working phase occurred after 4 min 45 s in the tests we carried out; complete hardening could be observed after 6 min 45 s. The cement may be regarded as high-viscosity with a low working phase, because the viscosity seems to be extremely high very early and, therefore, considerably hinders the fixation of the prosthesis.

The mechanical strengths correspond to those specified in the standard (Table 81). It is remarkable that the ISO bending strength (67.1 MPa) is higher

Table 81. Mechanical strength according to ISO 5833 and German Industrial Standard DIN 53435 for Cemex-Genta HV

	ISO 5833 Bending strength (MPa)	Bending modulus (MPa)	Compressive strength (MPa)	DIN 53435 Bending strength (MPa)	Impact strength (kJ/m²)
Limit given in the standard	>50	>1800	>70		
Actual strength	67.1	2767	87.8	75.3	3.4

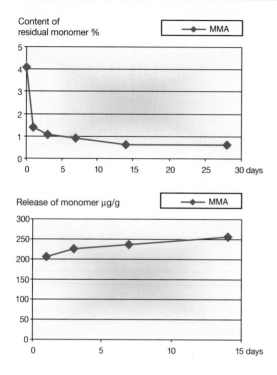

Fig. 128. Content and release of the residual monomer of Cemex-Genta HV with time

than in the case of the plain material tested. The ISO bending strength and the bending strength determined according to Dynstat protocols do not differ significantly.

On the outer packing, the manufacturer advertises a low polymerization temperature, as the component ratio of powder to liquid is 3:1. The determined hardening temperature (determined according to ISO protocols) is 76.8°C. This demonstrates that the temperatures determined by us are essentially not lower than those of other bone cements. The setting time (determined according to ISO 5833 protocols) is 9 min 35 s.

The residual monomer content was at first determined to be lower than 5% (Fig. 128), although the high amount of BPO should have a positive influence on the complete monomer reaction. The differences in the monomer composition lead to a lower residual monomer content compared with the plain version of Cemex HV examined. Sufficient starting radicals for polymerization and chains may first be built but, due to the quick increase of viscosity, a further build-up of chains is deferred. Also, the small portion of liquid used when mixing the dough should lead to a lower residual monomer content.

The qualitative and quantitative indications regarding the components of the powder and liquid are not printed directly on the polymer pouch or on the ampoule itself. Nevertheless, the blister pack contains all this information. Additionally, the batch number and the expiration date are not directly indicated on the primary packed polymer and monomer components. Apparently, one should

Table 82. ISO 5833 (1992) requirements for the packaging of Cemex-Genta HV

Requirements		Com-pliance	Location of information
General	Is the powder packed in a double-layered, sealed container?	+	–
	Is the liquid packed in a double-layered, sealed container?	+	–
Information regarding the powder ingredients	Qualitative	+	GB, FS, PB
	Quantitative	+	GB, FS, PB
Information regarding the liquid ingredients	Qualitative	+	GB, FS, PB
	Quantitative	+	GB, FS, PB
	Warning that the package contains flammable liquid	+	FS, PB, A, GB, Alu
	Instructions for storage (≤25°C, darkness)	+	FS, A, PB
	Statement of the sterility of the contents	+	FS, GB, PB, Alu
	Warning against reusing the package	+	FS, GB, PB, Alu
	Batch number(s)	+	FS, GB, Alu
	Expiration date	+	FS, GB, Alu
	Name/address of the manufacturer/distributor	+	GB, FS, A, PB, Alu
	Number and date of the standard	–	–
Information in the package insert	Detailed instructions for handling the components and preparing the cement	+	PB
	A statement drawing attention to the dangers for the patient	+	PB
	Recommendations for using the cement (syringe/dough state)	+	PB
	A statement regarding the influence of the temperature on working times	+	PB
	Graphical representation of the effects of temperature on the length of the phases of cement curing	+	PB

+, complies; –, does not comply; *A*, ampoule; *Alu*, aluminum pouch; *FS*, carton; *GB*, shared blister; *PB*, package insert

avoid storing the single components separately. A graphical representation of the influence of temperature on the handling properties of the material is not found on the insert. Furthermore, a reference to the presently valid ISO 5833 standard is missing on all packing units (Table 82). The key characteristics of Cemex Genta HV are listed in Table 83.

Table 83. The key characteristics of Cemex-Genta HV

High viscosity
The polymer contains styrene
Barium sulfate is the radiopaque medium
The polymer is γ irradiated
The polymer is in a brown glass bottle
The polymer bottle and monomer ampoule are packed in one blister
Mixing sequence: monomer, then powder
Working time: short
ISO 5833 is fulfilled
Molecular weight less than 350,000 Da
High gentamicin content, low release

3.2.3.4
Cemex-Genta LV

The cement components of Cemex-Genta LV are packed in a little, rectangular, red, marked outer carton (Fig. 129). This carton is printed on all sides except the lower front side. On the back of the outer carton, the composition of the components and storage advice are included. A little label on one of the front sides gives the necessary information regarding the batch number and expiration date. This label also contains all necessary EC indications.

The distributor and the manufacturer are clearly indicated. The outer carton may only be opened on one side. Inside the carton, there is an insert and a blister pack that contains the polymer pouch and the monomer ampoule.

The molded PVC part is covered by printed Tyvek. This side features all necessary product information, such as the composition, batch number and expiration date. The indications regarding batch number and expiration date are not directly printed but are printed on chart stickers on the Tyvek. These labels can later be used for documentation in the patients' records. In case of older blister packs a large, completely printed label was used. Furthermore, a brown indicator strip that documents successful sterilization is prominent. A notice explaining when this indicator indeed indicates the sterility is not included.

The Tyvek foil may be separated from the PVC lower part so that the single components may be taken out easily. First, the polymer inner pouch, which itself consists of a paper side and a polyester side, may be seen. It is striking that the inner pouch is completely unprinted, i.e., it contains no information. A marking indicates where the pouch should be opened. The pouch may easily be opened with the opening aid. The white, slight rose-colored polymer powder consists of

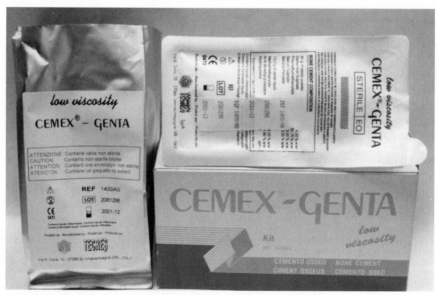

Fig. 129. The packaging of Cemex-Genta LV

powder	liquid
33,11 g poly(methyl methacrylate) (with 3% styrenel)	13,06 g methyl methacrylate (=13,89 ml)
4,00 g barium sulphate	0,24 g N,N-dimethyl-p-toluidine (=0,255 ml)
1,20 g benzoyl peroxide	75 ppm hydroquinone
1,69 g gentamicin sulphate (1,0 g base)	---------
---------	13,30 g (14,2 ml)
40,00 g	
	Cemex-Genta LV

Fig. 130. Composition of Cemex-Genta LV

82.8% PMMA (which certainly contains approximately 3% styrene, in the form of a co-polymer), 3.0% BPO, 4.2% gentamicin sulfate (2.5% gentamicin base) and 10.0% barium sulfate (as an opacifier; Fig. 130).

The monomer ampoule lies under the inner pouch in a special space in the PVC molding foil. The brown glass ampoule is printed with a white color. The information on the ampoule is extremely sparse; there is only the storage notice and indication concerning how to inject the material. The batch number and expiration date are completely missing. The composition of the monomer ampoule is the same as in the case of the high-viscosity material. The ampoule contains the colorless monomer, which consists of 98.2% MMA, 1.8% DmpT and approximately 75 ppm hydroquinone (as a stabilizer).

It is remarkable that only one batch number and one expiration date are indicated on the packing unit. Consequently, the liquid and the powder have both the same batch number and the same expiration date.

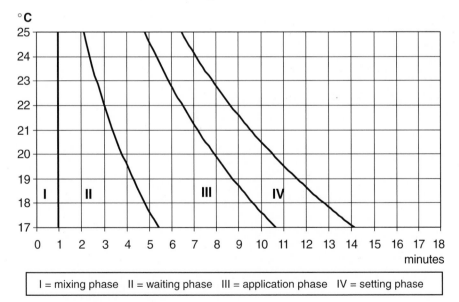

I = mixing phase   II = waiting phase   III = application phase   IV = setting phase

Fig. 131. Working curves of Cemex-Genta LV for different ambient/component temperatures

Table 84. Mechanical strength according to ISO 5833 and German Industrial Standard DIN 53435 for Cemex-Genta LV

	ISO 5833 Bending strength (MPa)	Bending modulus (MPa)	Compressive strength (MPa)	DIN 53435 Bending strength (MPa)	Impact strength (kJ/m²)
Limit given in the standard	>50	>1800	>70		
Actual strength	64.9	2694	88.1	80.1	3.3

To mix the dough, the liquid is put into the mixing vessel first, then the powder is added. After adding the powder, one obtains an extremely dry dough that may not be homogenized at first. The great excess of polymer powder compared with the monomer liquid hinders easy mixing. It initially appears that the monomer is missing and that wetting of the polymer by the monomer will not be possible. While trying to homogenize the dough with the help of a mixing spatula, one has to be especially cautious, because material can easily be thrown out of the mixing vessel.

After approximately 45–50 s, one obtains a rather homogeneous dough that flows slowly together. The viscosity at the beginning is lower than in the case of the high-viscosity version of the cement, and the end of the sticky phase of the dough (at 23°C) is reached after only 3 min (Fig. 131). The end of the working

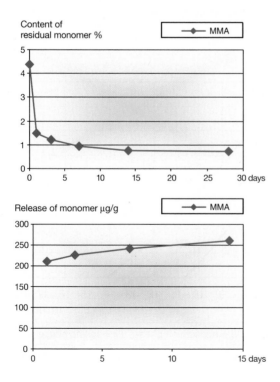

Fig. 132. Content and release of the residual monomer of Cemex-Genta LV with time

phase occurred after 5 min 45 s in the tests we carried out; complete hardening could be observed after 8 min 15 s. The cement may be regarded as medium-viscosity, with a working phase that has a high viscosity very early and, therefore, considerably hinders the fixation of the prosthesis. Additionally, implantation by syringes may be extremely difficult.

The mechanical strengths correspond to those specified in the standard (Table 84). It is remarkable that the ISO bending strength (64.9 MPa) is higher than in the case of the plain material. The ISO bending strength and the bending strength determined according to Dynstat protocols (80.1 MPa) differ significantly. A low impact strength can also be observed.

Also, in the case of Cemex-Genta LV, the manufacturer advertises a low polymerization temperature on the outer packing, as the component ratio of powder to liquid is 3:1. The determined hardening temperature (determined according to ISO protocols) is 75.4°C. This demonstrates that the temperatures determined by us are essentially not lower than those of other bone cements. The setting time (determined according to ISO 5833 protocols) is 11 min 5 s.

Table 85. ISO 5833 (1992) requirements for the packaging of Cemex-Genta LV

Requirements		Compliance	Location of information
General	Is the powder packed in a double-layered, sealed container?	+	–
	Is the liquid packed in a double-layered, sealed container?	+	–
Information regarding the powder ingredients	Qualitative	+	GB, FS, PB
	Quantitative	+	GB, FS, PB
Information regarding the liquid ingredients	Qualitative	+	GB, FS, PB
	Quantitative	+	GB, FS, PB
	Warning that the package contains flammable liquid	+	FS, PB, A, GB, Alu
	Instructions for storage (≤25°C, darkness)	+	FS, A, PB
	Statement of the sterility of the contents	+	FS, GB, PB, Alu
	Warning against reusing the package	+	FS, GB, PB, Alu
	Batch number(s)	+	FS, GB, Alu
	Expiration date	+	FS, GB, Alu
	Name/address of the manufacturer/distributor	+	GB, FS, A, PB, Alu
	Number and date of the standard	–	–
Information in the package insert	Detailed instructions for handling the components and preparing the cement	+	PB
	A statement drawing attention to the dangers for the patient	+	PB
	Recommendations for using the cement (syringe/dough state)	+	PB
	A statement regarding the influence of the temperature on working times	+	PB
	Graphical representation of the effects of temperature on the length of the phases of cement curing	+	PB

+, complies; –, does not comply; *A*, ampoule; *Alu*, aluminum pouch; *FS*, carton; *GB*, shared blister; *PB*, package insert

The residual monomer content was at first determined to be lower than 5% (Fig. 132), although the high amount of BPO should have a positive influence on the complete monomer reaction. The differences in the monomer composition lead to a lower residual monomer content compared with the plain version of Cemex LV examined. Sufficient starting radicals for polymerization and chains may first be built but, due to the quick increase of viscosity, a further building up of chains is deferred. Also, the small portion of liquid used when mixing the dough should lead to a lower residual monomer content.

The qualitative and quantitative indications regarding the components of the powder and liquid are not printed on the primary container. Nevertheless, the blister pack contains all this information.

The batch number and the expiration date are not directly indicated on the primary container. Apparently, one should avoid storing the single components separately.

A graphical representation of the influence of temperature on the handling properties of the material is not found on the insert. Furthermore, a reference to the presently valid ISO 5833 standard is missing on all packing units (Table 85). The key characteristics of Cemex-Genta LV are listed in Table 86.

Table 86. The key characteristics of Cemex-Genta LV

Medium viscosity
The polymer contains styrene
Barium sulfate is the radiopaque medium
The polymer is γ irradiated
The polymer is in a brown glass bottle
The polymer bottle and monomer ampoule are packed in one blister
Mixing sequence: monomer, then powder
Working time: long
ISO 5833 is fulfilled
Molecular weight less than 350,000 Da
High Dynstat bending strength
High gentamicin content, low release

3.2.3.5
Cerafixgenta

The different components of Cerafixgenta are packed in a simple, rectangular, blue outer carton that may be easily opened on the front side (Fig. 133). In the outer carton, there is a plastic tray that has a space for the blister pack. On the ampoule blister pack, there is a doubly packed powder pouch and, over it, an insert in the form of a brochure. Additionally, in the outer carton, there is a label that may be attached to the patients' records for documentation.

The outer carton is printed on all sides. On its back, the composition of the cement components is indicated in four different languages. The layout of the outer carton and the packaging components comply with the ISO packaging regulation. However, the necessary information about the batch number and expiration date and the CE characterization are only printed on a label that was

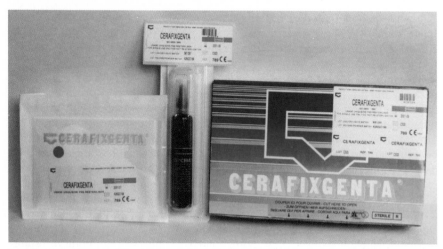

Fig. 133. The packaging of Cerafixgenta

obviously attached to the outer carton after packing. Moreover, it is remarkable that the typical ISO standard symbols (for example, for the batch number or for the expiration date) are not yet used. On the additional label on the outer carton, there is a notice that the material complies with the ISO 5833 standard for the cements.

The polymer inner pouch is enclosed by a peel-off pouch that consists of an unprinted, transparent PE side and a Tyvek side. On the Tyvek, there is a sterilization indicator that indicates the success of sterilization with its red color. A corresponding notice is printed on the label. It that a trilateral closed pouch is used; this pouch is closed manually on its fourth side after adding the inner pouch. This suggests that the pouch is manually filled. The inner pouch itself bears only the brand of the product. There is an additional red sterilization-indicating dot. A paper label that contains indications regarding the batch number and expiration date is attached to the pouch. The printing on the inner pouch may be recognized through the transparent polyester side of the peel-off pouch. There is no notice of the composition of the polymer on the peel-off pouch or on the inner pouch. Further remarks (for example warnings) are completely missing.

powder	liquid
41,75 g poly(methyl methacrylate) 4,30 g zirconium dioxide 0,45 g benzoyl peroxide 1,33 g gentamicin sulphate (= 0,8 g base) ----------- 47,83 g	15,88 g methyl methacrylate (=16,91 ml) 2,43 g n-butyl methacrylate (=2,69 ml) 0,38 g N,N-dimethyl-p-toluidine (=0,4 ml) 45 ppm hydroquinone ----------- 18,69 g (20 ml)
Cerafixgenta	

Fig. 134. Composition of Cerafixgenta

The white polymer powder consists of 87.3% PMMA, 0.9% BPO, 2.87% genta-micin sulfate (1.7% gentamicin base) and 9.0% zirconium dioxide (as an opa-cifier; Fig. 134). We tested the powder for possible co-polymers but could not find further components.

The ampoule blister pack, which is located in a plastic tray, contains a doubly packed ampoule. Both blister packs are made of molded PVC and are covered by unprinted Tyvek. The outer blister pack contains a little label with the batch number and expiration date and a notice regarding the sterilization procedure. The function of the green stripe on the label is not clearly described. It seems to be a further sterilization indicator. The second blister pack has a green-colored dot on its side, where the pack may be opened. The dot is clearly displayed; in all probability, it is a sterilization indicator. The brown glass ampoule is printed in white and has a plastic opening aid. Neither the packing unit nor the ampoule itself has information about the composition of the colorless liquid. This liquid contains 98.0% of two different methacrylates (85.1% MMA and 12.9% BuMA) and 2.0% DmpT. It also contains approximately 45 ppm hydroquinone as a stabi-lizer. Therefore, there is no difference between the liquid composition of the plain material and the antibiotic-loaded material.

According to the instructions of the manufacturer, the powder is put into the bowl first, and then the liquid is added. Mixing results in a liquid homogeneous dough after approximately 10–15 s. This dough shows a faint, cream-like coloring. The dough remains liquid and sticky for a long time. The dough may be taken out of the mixing vessel rather non-sticky after only 4 min 30 s. The sticky phase of the components was sometimes longer than 5 min. The working phase seems to be rather short, as the viscosity of the dough increases quickly and, after 6 min 30 s, is already so high that the fixation of the prosthesis may no longer be exe-

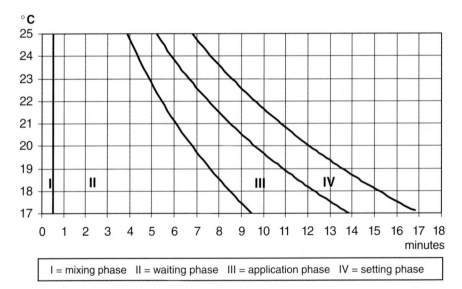

I = mixing phase   II = waiting phase   III = application phase   IV = setting phase

Fig. 135. Working curves of Cerafixgenta for different ambient/component temperatures

Table 87. Mechanical strength according to ISO 5833 and German Industrial Standard DIN 53435 for Cerafixgenta

	ISO 5833 Bending strength (MPa)	Bending modulus (MPa)	Compressive strength (MPa)	DIN 53435 Bending strength (MPa)	Impact strength (kJ/m²)
Limit given in the standard	>50	>1800	>70		
Actual strength	63	2378	91.8	78.7	4

cuted without risk for the patient. The complete hardening of the dough is finished after 8 min 15 s.

Due to the liquid starting phase and the short working phase, manual processing is not advisable. The cement has to be regarded as a low-viscosity one (Fig. 135).

The mechanical characteristics all fulfil the standard (Table 87). A lower compressive strength of 91.8 MPa, compared with that of the plain material (101.9 MPa), could be found. The setting time (determined according to ISO 5833 protocols) was 11 min 35 s, and the polymerization temperature was clearly under 80°C (it had a value of 65°C).

The determined residual monomer content is remarkably low (Fig. 136). However, in addition to MMA, BuMA (~13) is used in the liquid. A comparison with other liquids exclusively containing MMA is not possible. Regarding the initiator ratio, the rather low BPO content and the comparatively high DmpT

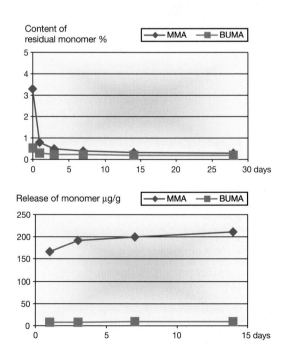

Fig. 136. Content and release of the residual monomers of Cerafixgenta with time

content are noteworthy. These conditions should have a positive influence on the extent of polymerization and thereby should cause a low residual monomer content.

Qualitative and quantitative indications regarding the powder and liquid constituents are found only on the outer carton and in the insert. Such information

Table 88. ISO 5833 (1992) requirements for the packaging of Cerafixgenta

Requirements		Compliance	Location of information
General	Is the powder packed in a double-layered, sealed container?	+	–
	Is the liquid packed in a double-layered, sealed container?	+	–
Information regarding the powder ingredients	Qualitative	+	FS, PB
	Quantitative	+	FS, PB
Information regarding the liquid ingredients	Qualitative	+	FS, PB
	Quantitative	+	FS, PB
	Warning that the package contains flammable liquid	+	FS, A
	Instructions for storage (≤25°C, darkness)	+	FS, PB
	Statement of the sterility of the contents	+	AB, IB, POB, FS, PB
	Warning against reusing the package	+	IB
	Batch number(s)	+	FS, AB, IB
	Expiration date	+	FS, AB, IB
	Name/address of the manufacturer/ distributor	+	IB, FS, PB
	Number and date of the standard	+	FS
Information in the package insert	Detailed instructions for handling the components and preparing the cement	+	PB
	A statement drawing attention to the dangers for the patient	+	PB
	Recommendations for using the cement (syringe/dough state)	+	PB
	A statement regarding the influence of the temperature on working times	+	PB
	Graphical representation of the effects of temperature on the length of the phases of cement curing	+	PB

+, complies; –, does not comply; *A*, ampoule; *AB*, ampoule blister; *FS*, carton; *IB*, primary pouch; *PB*, package insert;

Table 89. The key characteristics of Cerafixgenta

Low viscosity
The monomer contains BuMA
Zirconium dioxide is the radiopaque medium
The polymer is γ irradiated
The powder and ampoule are packed separately
Mixing sequence: powder, then monomer
Working time: short
ISO 5833 is fulfilled
Molecular weight less than 350,000 Da
Medium gentamicin content, low release

BuMA, butyl methacrylate

is, therefore, not printed on the primary vessels. The batch number and expiration date are not directly indicated on the primary vessel. Apparently, one should avoid storing the single components separately. On its outer carton, Cerafixgenta features a notice regarding the presently valid ISO 5833 standard (Table 88), information which is missing in the case of almost all other distributors. The key characteristics of Cerafixgenta are listed in Table 89.

3.2.3.6
CMW 1 G

All the cement components of CMW 1 G are packed in a rectangular outer carton that may be easily opened with the help of a perforated opening aid (Fig. 137). One of the front sides of the outer carton now serves as a cover under which the cement components are packed. The printing on the outer carton corresponds in every respect to the valid ISO packaging regulations. The indications regarding the batch number and expiration date are not printed on the front side of the carton but on its lower part. The name of the distributor is easily recognizable.

The outer carton contains a cardboard tray in which one space is left for the ampoule-containing blister pack. Above and below the space is an opening that makes it easier to the take out the tray. The same tray has two such spaces on its lower part so that the same unit can be used for two ampoule-containing blister packs.

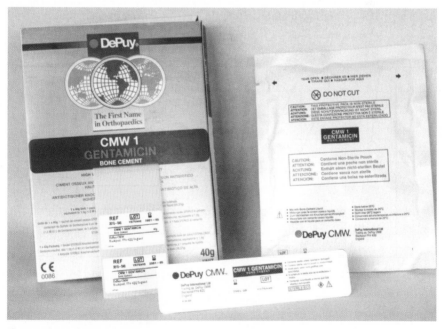

Fig. 137. The packaging of CMW 1 G

powder	**liquid**
33,89 g poly(methyl methacrylate) 1,69 g gentamicin sulphate (= 1 g base) 3,60 g barium sulphate 0,82 g benzoyl peroxide ---------- 40,00 g	18,22 g methyl methacrylate (=19,36 ml) 0,15 g N,N-dimethyl-p-toluidine (=0,16 ml) 25 ppm hydroquinone ---------- 18,37 g (19,57 ml)
	CMW 1 Gentamicin

Fig. 138. Composition of CMW 1 G

The insert and an aluminum protective pouch (alu-pouch) that contains the polymer-containing pouch are attached to the blister-packed monomer ampoule. In the outer carton, there are also six stickers that may be attached to patients' records.

The alu-pouch, which is printed on both sides, should expressly not be opened with a scissors; instead, it should be opened at the mark specially provided for this purpose. The alu-pouch is also printed with the batch number and the expiration date of the material. The inner surface of the alu-pouch is completely laminated with PE. In the alu-pouch, there is a folded peel-off pouch, which is printed on its Tyvek side and which contains a sterilization-indicating dot. When opening the enclosing pouch, it is striking that the seal of the pouch has a distinct sealing pattern (waffle design).

The inner pouch can be easily distinguished through the unprinted, transparent PE side, and the printing of the inner pouch can easily be read. The PE inner pouch is printed with black letters (in a script font). The batch number and

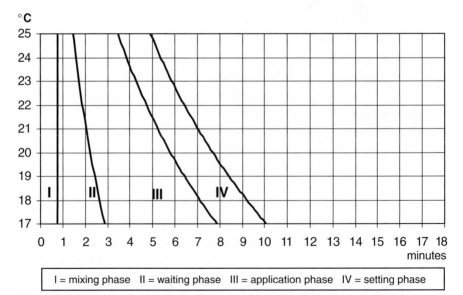

I = mixing phase   II = waiting phase   III = application phase   IV = setting phase

Fig. 139. Working curves of CMW 1 G for different ambient/component temperatures

Table 90. Mechanical strength according to ISO 5833 and German Industrial Standard DIN 53435 for CMW 1 G

	ISO 5833 Bending strength (MPa)	Bending modulus (MPa)	Compressive strength (MPa)	DIN 53435 Bending strength (MPa)	Impact strength (kJ/m²)
Limit given in the standard	>50	>1800	>70		
Actual strength	66.9	2468	85.7	72.8	3.5

expiration date are printed on the lower part, outside the seal. The polymer powder consists of 84.7% PMMA, 2.05% BPO, 4.2% gentamicin sulfate (2.5% gentamicin base) and 9.0% barium sulfate (as an opacifier; Fig. 138).

The ampoule, which is packed in a blister pack, has the same batch number and the same expiration date as the powder. These indications are on the Tyvek side of the blister pack, which also contains all necessary caution notices (warning symbols). The brown glass ampoule is in the molded PVC part of the blister pack. A label that contains all necessary information is attached to it.

It seems that there was a change in the composition of the monomer in August 1997; earlier, the ampoules contained 0.17 g ethanol (as a plasticizer) and 0.004 g ascorbic acid (as an additional stabilizer). At the present, the colorless monomer liquid consists of 99.18% MMA and 0.82% DmpT. As a stabilizer, approximately 25 ppm hydroquinone may be found.

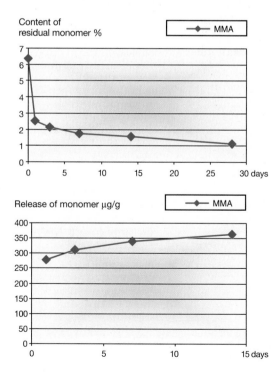

Fig. 140. Content and release of the residual monomer of CMW 1 G with time

There is no opening help included for the opening of the brown glass ampoule. The polymer pouch should be opened with the help of a scissors. The polymer powder can easily be poured out of the pouch into the mixing vessel.

The polymer is first put into the bowl for mixing; the monomer is then added. The wetting is remarkably slow. Initially, it appears as if the quantity of the liquid is not sufficient. The result is a dry dough that, after 30 s, suddenly flows together and may then be described as a homogeneous mass. The sudden falling of the dough during the wetting phase is typical of all CMW cements with gentamicin.

CMW 1 G reaches the end of the sticky phase after between 1 min 20 s and 1 min 30 s. The end of the working phase occurs after 4 min 15 s. At the end of the working phase, the dough becomes remarkably warm. Complete setting may be observed after 5 min 45 s. Because of its handling behavior, CMW 1 G can be regarded as a high-viscosity bone cement (Fig. 139).

The quasi-static mechanical strength clearly corresponds to the standard (Table 90). It may be observed that the bending strengths determined according

Table 91. ISO 5833 (1992) requirements for the packaging of CMW 1 G

Requirements		Com-pliance	Location of information
General	Is the powder packed in a double-layered, sealed container?	+	–
	Is the liquid packed in a double-layered, sealed container?	+	–
Information regarding the powder ingredients	Qualitative	+	PB
	Quantitative	+	PB
Information regarding the liquid ingredients	Qualitative	+	PB
	Quantitative	+	PB
	Warning that the package contains flammable liquid	+	A, AB, FS
	Instructions for storage (≤25°C, darkness)	+	IB, Alu, FS
	Statement of the sterility of the contents	+	IB, POB, A, AB, FS, Alu
	Warning against reusing the package	+	–
	Batch number(s)	+	IB, A, AB, FS, Alu
	Expiration date	+	IB, A, AB, FS, Alu
	Name/address of the manufacturer/distributor	+	IB, A, AB, FS, Alu, PB
	Number and date of the standard	–	–
Information in the package insert	Detailed instructions for handling the components and preparing the cement	+	PB
	A statement drawing attention to the dangers for the patient	+	PB
	Recommendations for using the cement (syringe/dough state)	+	PB
	A statement regarding the influence of the temperature on working times	+	PB
	Graphical representation of the effects of temperature on the length of the phases of cement curing	+	PB

+, complies; –, does not comply; *A*, ampoule; *AB*, ampoule blister; *Alu*, aluminum pouch; *FS*, carton; *IB*, primary pouch; *PB*, package insert; *POB* peel-off pouch

Table 92. The key characteristics of CMW 1 G

High viscosity
Barium sulfate is the radiopaque medium
The polymer is γ irradiated
The powder and ampoule are packed separately
Mixing sequence: powder, then monomer
Working time: short
ISO 5833 is fulfilled
Molecular weight less than 350,000 Da
High bending strength
High gentamicin content, low release

to ISO 5833 and DIN 53435 protocols hardly differ from each other. Moreover, the compressive strength (85.7 MPa) is significantly lower than that of the plain version. The setting time (determined according to ISO 5833 protocols) is 8 min 10 s, and the polymerization temperature is 84.3°C.

The BPO content is lower than the DmpT content, so the ratio is higher than five. The residual monomer content was higher than 6% and, therefore, was higher in the case of CMW 3 G (Fig. 140). The change in the composition of the liquid in CMW 1 G probably leads to worse values compared with those of the low-viscosity types.

According to the requirements of the ISO 5833 standard, the qualitative and quantitative indications regarding the ingredients of the cement components can only be found on the insert. An instruction prohibiting reuse is not included. Furthermore, a graphical representation of the influence of the temperature on the handling properties of the cement is not found on the insert. A reference to the presently valid ISO standard is also missing (Table 91). The key characteristics of CMW 1 G are listed in Table 92.

3.2.3.7
CMW 2 G

All the cement components of CMW 2 G are packed in a rectangular outer carton that may be easily opened with the help of a perforated opening aid (Fig. 141). One of the front sides of the outer carton now serves as a cover under which the cement components are packed. The printing on the outer carton corresponds in every respect to the valid ISO packaging regulations. The indications regarding the batch number and expiration date are not printed on the front side of the carton but on its lower part. The name of the distributor is easily recognizable.

The outer carton contains a cardboard tray in which one space is left for the ampoule-containing blister pack. Above and below the space is an opening that makes it easier to the take out the tray. The same tray has two such spaces on its lower part so that the same unit can be used for two ampoule-containing blister packs.

The insert and an alu-pouch that contains the polymer-containing pouch are attached to the blister-packed monomer ampoule. In the outer carton, there are also six stickers that may be attached to patients' records.

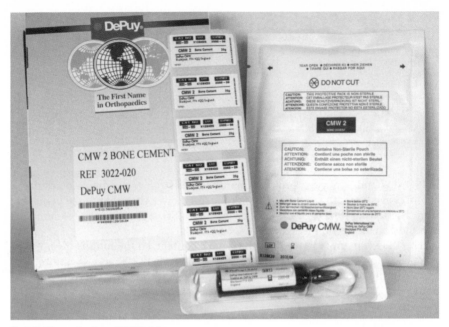

Fig. 141. The packaging of CMW 2 G

The alu-pouch, which is printed on both sides, should expressly not be opened with a scissors; instead, it should be opened at the mark specially provided for this purpose. The alu-pouch is also printed with the batch number and the expiration date of the material. The inner surface of the alu-pouch is completely laminated with PE. In the alu-pouch, there is a folded peel-off pouch, which is printed on its Tyvek side and which contains a sterilization-indicating dot. When opening the enclosing pouch, it is striking that the seal of the pouch has a distinct sealing pattern (waffle design).

The inner pouch can be easily distinguished through the unprinted, transparent PE side, and the printing of the inner pouch can easily be read. The PE inner pouch is printed with black letters. The batch number and expiration date are printed on the lower part, outside the seal. The polymer powder consists of

powder	liquid
33,11 g poly(methyl methacrylate)	18,22 g methyl methacrylate (=19,36 ml)
0,80 g benzoyl peroxide	0,15 g N,N-dimethyl-p-toluidine (=0,16 ml)
4,40 g barium sulphate	25 ppm hydroquinone
1,69 g gentamicin sulphate (=1g base)	----------
---------	18,37 g (19,57 ml)
40,00 g	
CMW 2 Gentamicin	

Fig. 142. Composition of CMW 2 G

82.8% PMMA, 2.0% BPO, 4.2% gentamicin sulfate (2.5% gentamicin base) and 11.3% barium sulfate (as an opacifier; Fig. 142).

The ampoule, which is packed in a blister pack, has the same batch number and the same expiration date as the powder. These indications are on the Tyvek side of the blister pack, which also contains all necessary caution notices (warning symbols). The brown glass ampoule is in the molded PVC part of the blister pack. A label that contains all necessary information is attached to it.

It seems that there was a change in the composition of the monomer in August 1997; earlier, the ampoules contained 0.17 g ethanol (as a plasticizer) and 0.004 g ascorbic acid (as an additional stabilizer). At the present, the colorless monomer liquid consists of 99.18% MMA and 0.82% DmpT. As a stabilizer, approximately 25 ppm hydroquinone may be found. Thus, the liquids of CMW 2 G and CMW 1 G have the same composition.

There is no opening help installed for the opening of the brown glass ampoule. The polymer pouch should be opened with the help of a scissors. The polymer powder can easily be poured out of the pouch into the mixing vessel.

The polymer is first put into the bowl for mixing; the monomer is then added. The wetting is extremely slow. Initially, it appears as if the quantity of the liquid is not sufficient. The result is a very dry dough that, after 30–35 s, suddenly flows together and may then be described as a homogeneous mass. The sudden falling of the dough during the wetting phase is typical of CMW 2 G.

CMW 2 G reaches the end of the sticky phase 45–50 s after wetting. The very short working phase ends after 2 min 45 s, whereas the dough becomes remarkably warm at the end of the working phase (after 2 min). Complete setting may be observed after 3 min 30 s (Fig. 143).

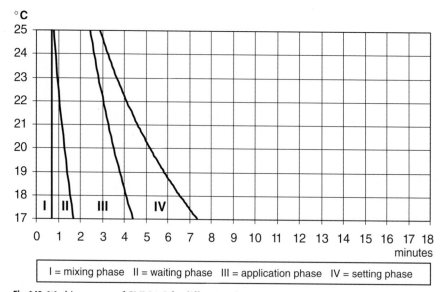

Fig. 143. Working curves of CMW 2 G for different ambient/component temperatures

Table 93. Mechanical strength according to ISO 5833 and German Industrial Standard DIN 53435 for CMW 2 G

	ISO 5833 Bending strength (MPa)	Bending modulus (MPa)	Compressive strength (MPa)	DIN 53435 Bending strength (MPa)	Impact strength (kJ/m²)
Limit given in the standard	>50	>1800	>70		
Actual strength	68.9	2636	92.9	73.3	2.9

The manufacturer indicates that this high-viscosity material is not suitable for mixing under a vacuum or application with syringes. Therefore, the high-viscosity CMW 2 G should not be used for total hip replacements. The quasi-static mechanical strength clearly corresponds to that described in the standard; the low impact strength is remarkable (Table 93).

The setting time (determined according to ISO 5833 protocols) is 4 min 50 s, and the polymerization temperature is higher than for the plain version. We found values of approximately 75.7°C.

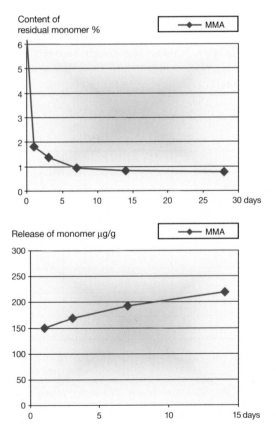

Fig. 144. Content and release of the residual monomer of CMW 2 G with time

Table 94. ISO 5833 (1992) requirements for the packaging of CMW 2 G

Requirements		Com-pliance	Location of information
General	Is the powder packed in a double-layered, sealed container?	+	–
	Is the liquid packed in a double-layered, sealed container?	+	–
Information regarding the powder ingredients	Qualitative	+	PB
	Quantitative	+	PB
Information regarding the liquid ingredients	Qualitative	+	PB
	Quantitative	+	PB
	Warning that the package contains flammable liquid	+	A, AB, FS
	Instructions for storage (≤25°C, darkness)	+	IB, Alu, FS
	Statement of the sterility of the contents	+	IB, POB, A, AB, FS, Alu
	Warning against reusing the package	+	–
	Batch number(s)	+	IB, A, AB, FS, Alu
	Expiration date	+	IB, A, AB, FS, Alu
	Name/address of the manufacturer/distributor	+	IB, A, AB, FS, Alu, PB
	Number and date of the standard	–	–
Information in the package insert	Detailed instructions for handling the components and preparing the cement	+	PB
	A statement drawing attention to the dangers for the patient	+	PB
	Recommendations for using the cement (syringe/dough state)	+	PB
	A statement regarding the influence of the temperature on working times	+	PB
	Graphical representation of the effects of temperature on the length of the phases of cement curing	–	–

+, complies; –, does not comply; *A*, ampoule; *AB*, ampoule blister; *Alu*, aluminum pouch; *FS*, carton; *IB*, primary pouch; *PB*, package insert; *POB* peel-off pouch

The BPO content is lower than the DmpT content, so the ratio is higher than five. The residual monomer content was higher than 6%; therefore, it was higher than in the case of CMW 3 G but was comparable to the value for CMW 1 G (Fig. 144). The change in the compositions of the liquids in CMW 1 G and CMW 2 G probably leads to worse values compared with those of the low-viscosity types.

According to the requirements of the ISO 5833 standard, the qualitative and quantitative indications regarding the ingredients of the cement components can only be found on the insert. An instruction prohibiting reuse is not included. Furthermore, a graphical representation of the influence of the temperature on the handling properties of the cement is not found on the insert. A reference to the presently valid ISO standard is also missing (Table 94). The key characteristics of CMW 2 G are listed in Table 95.

Table 95. The key characteristics of CMW 2 G

High viscosity
Barium sulfate is the radiopaque medium
The polymer is γ irradiated
The powder and ampoule are packed separately
Mixing sequence: powder, then monomer
Working time: short
ISO 5833 is fulfilled
Molecular weight less than 350,000 Da
High ISO bending strength
Low impact strength
High gentamicin content, low release

3.2.3.8
CMW 3 G

All the cement components of CMW 3 G are packed in a rectangular outer carton that may be easily opened with the help of a perforated opening aid (Fig. 145). One of the front sides of the outer carton now serves as a cover under which the cement components are packed. The printing on the outer carton corresponds in every respect to the valid ISO packaging regulations. The indications regarding the batch number and expiration date are not printed on the front side of the carton but on its lower part. The name of the distributor is easily recognizable.

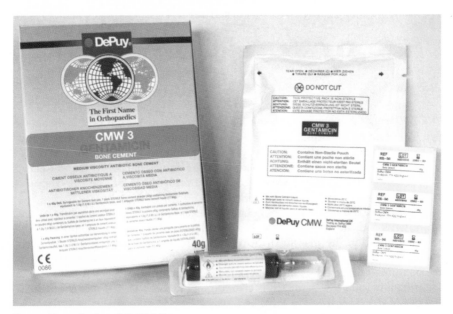

Fig. 145. The packaging of CMW 3 G

The outer carton contains a cardboard tray in which one space is left for the ampoule-containing blister pack. Above and below the space is an opening that makes it easier to the take out the tray. The same tray has two such spaces on its lower part so that the same unit can be used for two ampoule-containing blister packs.

The insert and an alu-pouch that contains the polymer-containing pouch are attached to the blister-packed monomer ampoule. In the outer carton, there are also six stickers that may be attached to patients' records.

The alu-pouch, which is printed on both sides, should expressly not be opened with a scissors; instead, it should be opened at the mark specially provided for this purpose. The alu-pouch is also printed with the batch number and the expiration date of the material. The inner surface of the alu-pouch is completely laminated with PE. In the alu-pouch, there is a folded peel-off pouch, which is printed on its Tyvek side and which contains a sterilization-indicating dot. When opening the enclosing pouch, it is striking that the seal of the pouch has a distinct sealing pattern (waffle design).

The inner pouch may be easily distinguished through the unprinted and transparent PE side, and the printing of the inner pouch can easily be read. The PE inner pouch is printed with black letters. The batch number and expiration date are printed on the lower part, outside the seal. The polymer powder consists of 83.8% PMMA, 1.9% BPO, 4.2% gentamicin sulfate (2.5% gentamicin base) and 10.0% barium sulfate (as an opacifier; Fig. 146).

The ampoule, which is packed in a blister pack, has the same batch number and the same expiration date as the powder. These indications are on the Tyvek side of the blister pack, which also contains all necessary caution notices (warning symbols). The brown glass ampoule is in the molded PVC part of the blister pack. A label that contains all necessary information is attached to it.

It seems as if there was been a change in the composition of the monomer in August 1997; earlier, the ampoules contained 0.17 g ethanol (as a plasticizer) and 0.004 g ascorbic acid (as an additional stabilizer). At the present, the colorless monomer liquid consists of 97.50% MMA and 2.50% DmpT. As a stabilizer approximately 25 ppm hydroquinone may be found. Therefore, CMW 3 G obviously does not have the same liquid composition as CWM 1 G or CMW 2 G.

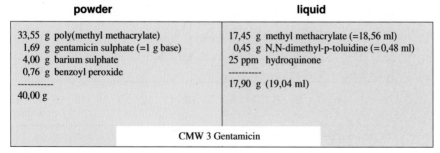

powder	liquid
33,55 g poly(methyl methacrylate)	17,45 g methyl methacrylate (=18,56 ml)
1,69 g gentamicin sulphate (=1 g base)	0,45 g N,N-dimethyl-p-toluidine (=0,48 ml)
4,00 g barium sulphate	25 ppm hydroquinone
0,76 g benzoyl peroxide	----------
----------	17,90 g (19,04 ml)
40,00 g	
CMW 3 Gentamicin	

Fig. 146. Composition of CMW 3 G

There is no opening help installed for the opening of the brown glass ampoule. The polymer pouch should be opened with the help of a scissors. The polymer powder can easily be poured out of the pouch into the mixing vessel.

The polymer is first put into the bowl for mixing; the monomer is then added. The wetting is slow but is considerably better than for CMW 1 G and CMW 2 G. Initially, it appears as if the quantity of the liquid is not sufficient. The result is a dry dough that, after 30 s, suddenly flows together and may then be described as a liquid, homogeneous mass. In this case, the sudden falling of the dough is not as distinct as in the cases of the high-viscosity antibiotic-loaded CMW cements.

CMW 3 G reaches the end of the sticky phase after between 3 min 40 s and 3 min 45 s. The end of the working phase occurs after 6 min 45 s. Complete setting may be observed after 7 min 45 s. Furthermore, the low-viscosity CMW types show very clearly that the dough already feels warm at the end of the working phase (after approximately 6 min 45 s; Fig. 147).

The quasi-static mechanical strength clearly corresponds to that described in the standard; the low impact strength is remarkable (Table 96). Furthermore, it may be observed that the bending strength determined according to ISO 5833 protocols (70.3 MPa) and DIN 53435 protocols (74.4 MPa) hardly differ from each other. Moreover, the compressive strength is quite high (100.8 MPa).

The setting time (determined according to ISO 5833 protocols) of 9 min 55 s is clearly higher in the case of CMW 3 G than in the cases of CMW 1 G and CMW 2 G. The polymerization (determined according to ISO 5833 protocols) is 86.7°C.

In contrast to the both variants described before, CMW 3 G has a uniform distribution of the initiators and therefore has a ratio of a little more than one. The

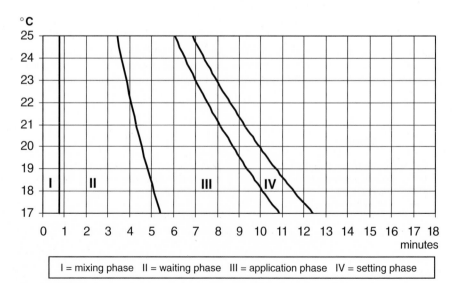

Fig. 147. Working curves of CMW 3 G for different ambient/component temperatures

Table 96. Mechanical strength according to ISO 5833 and German Industrial Standard DIN 53435 for CMW 3 G

	ISO 5833 Bending strength (MPa)	Bending modulus (MPa)	Compressive strength (MPa)	DIN 53435 Bending strength (MPa)	Impact strength (kJ/m²)
Limit given in the standard	>50	>1800	>70		
Actual strength	70.3	2764	100.8	74.4	3

residual monomer content was always below 5% and, therefore, was lower than in the cases of CMW 1 G and CMW 2 G (Fig. 148). The change in the composition of the liquid in the case of CMW 3 G probably leads to better values than those of the high-viscosity types.

According to the requirements of the ISO 5833 standard, the qualitative and quantitative indications regarding the ingredients of the cement components can only be found on the insert. An instruction prohibiting reuse is not included. Furthermore, a graphical representation of the influence of the temperature on the handling properties of the cement is not found on the insert. A reference to the presently valid ISO standard is also missing (Table 97). The key characteristics of CMW 3 G are listed in Table 98.

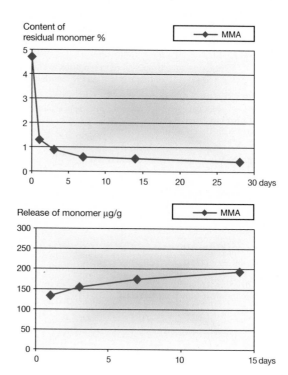

Fig. 148. Content and release of the residual monomer of CMW 3 G with time

Table 97. ISO 5833 (1992) requirements for the packaging of CMW 3 G

Requirements		Compliance	Location of information
General	Is the powder packed in a double-layered, sealed container?	+	–
	Is the liquid packed in a double-layered, sealed container?	+	–
Information regarding the powder ingredients	Qualitative	+	PB
	Quantitative	+	PB
Information regarding the liquid ingredients	Qualitative	+	PB
	Quantitative	+	PB
	Warning that the package contains flammable liquid	+	A, AB, FS
	Instructions for storage (≤25°C, darkness)	+	IB, Alu, FS
	Statement of the sterility of the contents	+	IB, POB, A, AB, FS, Alu
	Warning against reusing the package	+	–
	Batch number(s)	+	IB, A, AB, FS, Alu
	Expiration date	+	IB, A, AB, FS, Alu
	Name/address of the manufacturer/ distributor	+	IB, A, AB, FS, Alu, PB
	Number and date of the standard	–	–
Information in the package insert	Detailed instructions for handling the components and preparing the cement	+	PB
	A statement drawing attention to the dangers for the patient	+	PB
	Recommendations for using the cement (syringe/dough state)	+	PB
	A statement regarding the influence of the temperature on working times	+	PB
	Graphical representation of the effects of temperature on the length of the phases of cement curing	+	PB

+, complies; –, does not comply; *A*, ampoule; *AB*, ampoule blister; *Alu*, aluminum pouch; *FS*, carton; *IB*, primary pouch; *PB*, package insert; *POB* peel-off pouch

Table 98. The key characteristics of CMW 3 G

Low viscosity
Barium sulfate is the radiopaque medium
The polymer is γ irradiated
The powder and ampoule are packed separately
Mixing sequence: powder, then monomer
Working time: long
ISO 5833 is fulfilled
Molecular weight less than 350,000 Da
High compressive strength
High bending strength
High gentamicin content, low release

3.2.3.9
CMW 2000 Gentamicin

All the cement components of CMW 2000 Gentamicin are packed in a rectangular outer carton that may be easily opened with the help of a perforated opening aid (Fig. 149). One of the front sides of the outer carton now serves as a cover under which the cement components are packed. The printing on the outer carton corresponds in every respect to the valid ISO packaging regulations. The indications regarding the batch number and expiration date are not printed on the front side of the carton but on its lower part. The name of the distributor is easily recognizable.

The outer carton contains a cardboard tray in which one space is left for the ampoule-containing blister pack. Above and below the space is an opening that makes easier the taking out of the tray. The same tray has two such spaces on its lower part so that the same unit can be used for two ampoule-containing blister packs.

The insert and an alu-pouch that contains the polymer-containing pouch are attached to the blister-packed monomer ampoule. In the outer carton, there are also six stickers that may be attached to patients' records.

The alu-pouch, which is printed on both sides, should expressly not be opened with a scissors; instead, it should be opened at the mark specially provided for this purpose. The alu-pouch is also printed with the batch number and the expiration date of the material. The inner surface of the alu-pouch is completely lami-

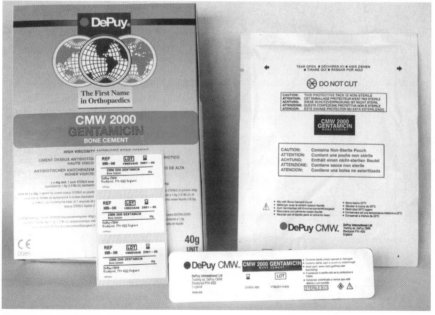

Fig. 149. The packaging of CMW 2000 Gentamicin

powder	liquid
29,06 g poly(methyl methacrylate) 5,13 g poly(methyl methacrylate,ethyl methacrylate,styrene) 1,69 g gentamicin sulphate (=1 g base) 3,20 g barium sulphate 0,92 g benzoyl peroxide ---------- 40,00 g	17,64 g methyl methacrylate (=18,76 ml) 0,36 g N,N-dimethyl-p-toluidine (=0,38ml) 75 ppm hydroquinone ---------- 18 g (19,15 ml)

CMW 2000 Gentamicin

Fig. 150. Composition of CMW 2000 Gentamicin

nated with PE. In the alu-pouch, there is a folded peel-off pouch, which is printed on its Tyvek side and which contains a sterilization-indicating dot. When opening the enclosing pouch, it is striking that the seal of the pouch has a distinct sealing pattern (waffle design).

The inner pouch can be easily distinguished through the unprinted, transparent PE side, and the printing of the inner pouch can easily be read. The PE inner pouch is printed with black letters. The batch number and expiration date are printed on the lower part, outside the seal. The polymer powder has a composition completely different from all the CMW bone cements described before. The polymer of CMW 2000 Gentamicin consists of 72.65% PMMA, 12.8% MMA-ethyl methacrylate-styrene terpolymer, 4.2% gentamicin sulfate (2.5% gentamicin base), 2.3% BPO and 8.0% barium sulfate (as an opacifier; Fig. 150).

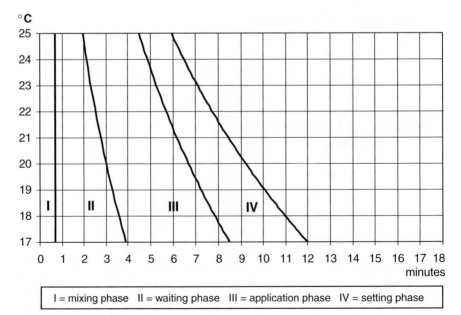

I = mixing phase   II = waiting phase   III = application phase   IV = setting phase

Fig. 151. Working curves of CMW 2000 Gentamicin for different ambient/component temperatures

Table 99. Mechanical strength according to ISO 5833 and German Industrial Standard DIN 53435 for CMW 2000 Gentamicin

	ISO 5833 Bending strength (MPa)	Bending modulus (MPa)	Compressive strength (MPa)	DIN 53435 Bending strength (MPa)	Impact strength (kJ/m²)
Limit given in the standard	>50	>1800	>70		
Actual strength	69	2546	94	82.5	3.8

The ampoule, which is packed in a blister pack, has the same batch number and the same expiration date as the powder. These indications are on the Tyvek side of the blister pack, which also contains all necessary caution notices (warning symbols). The brown glass ampoule is in the molded PVC part of the blister pack. A label that contains all necessary information is attached to it.

At the present, the colorless monomer liquid consists of 98% MMA and 2% DmpT. As a stabilizer, approximately 75 ppm hydroquinone may be found.

There is no opening help installed for the opening of the brown glass ampoule. The polymer pouch should be opened with the help of a scissors. The polymer powder can easily be poured out of the pouch into the mixing vessel.

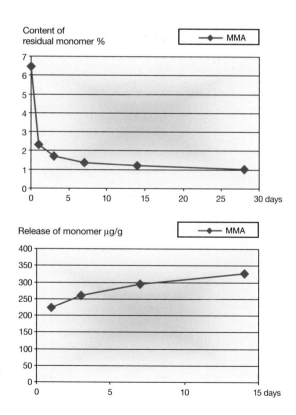

Fig. 152. Content and release of the residual monomer of CMW 2000 Gentamicin with time

The polymer is first put into the bowl for mixing; the monomer is then added. The wetting is remarkably slow. Initially, it appears as if the quantity of the liquid is not sufficient. The result is a dry dough that, after 30–35 s, suddenly flows together and may then be described as a homogeneous mass. The sudden falling of the dough during the wetting phase is typical of all CMW cements with gentamicin.

CMW 2000 Gentamicin reaches the end of the sticky phase after 2 min 15 s (Fig. 151). The end of the working phase occurs after 5 min 15 s. The viscosity of the dough during the sticky phase and the working phase is distinctly higher than that of the high-viscosity CMW 1 G. At the end of the working phase, the dough becomes remarkably warm. Complete setting may be observed after 7 min. Because of its handling behavior, CMW 2000 Gentamicin can be regarded as a high-viscosity bone cement, due to its relatively long sticky phase, which is remarkable for medium-viscosity bone cement types.

The quasi-static mechanical strength clearly corresponds to that described in the standard (Table 99). It may be observed that the bending strengths deter-

Table 100. ISO 5833 (1992) requirements for the packaging of CMW 2000 Gentamicin

Requirements		Com-pliance	Location of information
General	Is the powder packed in a double-layered, sealed container?	+	–
	Is the liquid packed in a double-layered, sealed container?	+	–
Information regarding the powder ingredients	Qualitative	+	PB
	Quantitative	+	PB
Information regarding the liquid ingredients	Qualitative	+	PB
	Quantitative	+	PB
	Warning that the package contains flammable liquid	+	A, AB, FS
	Instructions for storage (≤25°C, darkness)	+	IB, Alu, FS
	Statement of the sterility of the contents	+	IB, POB, A, AB, FS, Alu
	Warning against reusing the package	+	–
	Batch number(s)	+	IB, A, AB, FS, Alu
	Expiration date	+	IB, A, AB, FS, Alu
	Name/address of the manufacturer/distributor	+	IB, A, AB, FS, Alu, PB
	Number and date of the standard	–	–
Information in the package insert	Detailed instructions for handling the components and preparing the cement	+	PB
	A statement drawing attention to the dangers for the patient	+	PB
	Recommendations for using the cement (syringe/dough state)	+	PB
	A statement regarding the influence of the temperature on working times	+	PB
	Graphical representation of the effects of temperature on the length of the phases of cement curing	+	PB

+, complies; –, does not comply; *A*, ampoule; *AB*, ampoule blister; *Alu*, aluminum pouch; *FS*, carton; *IB*, primary pouch; *PB*, package insert; *POB* peel-off pouch

mined according to ISO 5833 and DIN 53435 protocols hardly differ from each other. The setting time (determined according to ISO 5833 protocols) is 11 min, and the polymerization temperature is 83°C.

The BPO content is lower than the DmpT content, so the ratio is higher than two. The residual monomer content was higher than 6%; therefore, it was higher than in any other CMW version tested in this study (Fig. 152). The change in the composition of the liquid in the case of CMW 2000 Gentamicin probably leads to worse values compared with those of all the other CMW types.

According to the requirements of the ISO 5833 standard, the qualitative and quantitative indications regarding the ingredients of the cement components can only be found on the insert. An instruction prohibiting reuse is not included. A reference to the presently valid ISO standard is also missing (Table 100). The key characteristics of CMW 2000 Gentamicin are listed in Table 101.

Table 101. The key characteristics of CMW 2000 G

High viscosity
Barium sulfate is the radiopaque medium
The polymer contains a MMA/EMA/styrene terpolymer
The polymer is γ irradiated
The powder and ampoule are packed separately
Mixing sequence: powder, then monomer
Working time: long
ISO 5833 is fulfilled
Molecular weight less than 350,000 Da
High bending strength
High gentamicin content, low release

MMA, methyl methacrylate/*EMA*, ethyl methacrylate

3.2.3.10
Copal

All the cement components of Copal are packed in a rectangular outer carton that may be easily opened at the upper, narrow side (Fig. 153). The printing on the outer cartons corresponds in every respect to the valid ISO packaging regulations. The indications regarding the batch number and expiration date are not printed on the front side of the carton but on one of the two unprinted small sides. The names of the distributor and manufacturer are easily recognizable.

The outer carton contains a cardboard tray in which two spaces are left for the secure packaging of the ampoule-containing blister pack; therefore, only single versions of the bone cement can be found. Usually, the insert, four to six chart stickers and an alu-pouch that contains an inner pouch with polymer powder are attached to the monomer ampoule, which is located in one of the two spaces of the cardboard tray. The folded, doubly packed inner pouch within the alu-pouch contains the sterile pouches in which the polymer powder is located.

The inner pouch of the polymer is printed on the paper side and contains important information regarding handling and storage. Furthermore, the batch number and the expiration date are located noticeably on the printed front side,

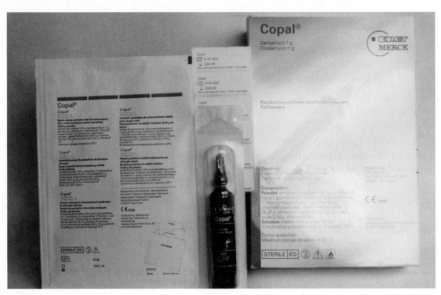

Fig. 153. The packaging of Copal

as prescribed by the standards. The back of the inner pouch is made of polyester and, therefore, is transparent.

The green-pigmented polymer powder, which is well known and is characteristic of Palacos-like products, is clearly visible. The polymer powder is sterilized by ethylene oxide. The composition of the polymer powder is 82.6% MMA-methylacrylate co-polymer, 0.75% BPO, 3.8% gentamicin sulfate (2.2% gentamicin base), 2.8% clindamicin hydrochloride and 10.0% zirconium dioxide (as an opacifier; Fig. 154).

The sterile inner pouch is enclosed by an unprinted peel-off-pouch, which contains an inner pouch with a paper side and a PE side. Because the transparent PE side encloses the printed paper side of the inner pouch, the printing on the inner pouch can be clearly read through the outer pouch. A sterile label is located on the outer pouch; this label is obviously put on the pouch after successful sterilization. Usually, one folded peel-off pouch is packed in an alu-pouch that has

powder	liquid
35,20 g poly(methyl acrylate, methyl methacrylate)	18,40 g methyl methacrylate (=19,57 ml)
	0,38 g N,N-dimethyl-p-toluidine (=0,43 ml)
4,27 g zirconium dioxide	0,4 mg chlorophyllin
0,32 g benzoyl peroxide	---------
1,60 g gentamicin sulphate (=1,0 g base)	18,78 g (20 ml)
1,20 g clindamicin hydrochloride (=1,0 g base)	

42,59 g	
Copal	

Fig. 154. Composition of Copal

printing on one side. The print contains all the necessary information, including the batch number and expiration date.

The ampoule, which is located in the cardboard tray, is protected in the wrapping by the blister pack and by the alu-pouch located above it. The blister pack itself consists of transparent, molded PVC and a paper side. A printed ampoule label is attached to the paper side; this label contains all necessary information, especially the batch number and the expiration date of the liquid monomer. A brown glass ampoule contains the sterile, filtered green monomer, which is typical of Palacos R. Each ampoule has a translucent label. The blister pack is also sterilized by ethylene oxide. The monomer consists of 98.0% MMA, 2.0% DmpT and approximately 60 ppm hydroquinone. Thus, no differences in the composition of Copal and Palacos R liquid can be observed.

For the opening of the brown glass ampoule, no opening aid is included; the polymer pouch should be opened with the help of a scissors. The polymer powder can easily be poured out of the pouch into the mixing vessel.

Before mixing the cement components of Copal, the liquid is first poured into the bowl. The polymer powder is then added to the monomer, and the clock is started. In a few seconds, a homogeneous dough can easily be produced. The viscosity of the dough increases very quickly, depending on the temperature of the components with respect to the temperature of the operating room. For example, the dough may be taken out of the mixing vessel non-sticky after approximately 1 min at 23°C (Fig. 155). The working phase of Copal varies from 3 min 30 s to 4 min and usually ends approximately 4 min 30 s to 5 min after the start of mixing. The cement hardens after approximately 6–7 min. Therefore, Copal is characterized as a high-viscosity PMMA bone cement.

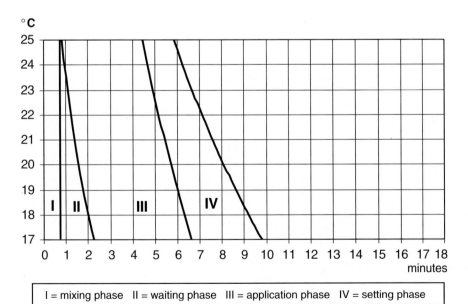

I = mixing phase   II = waiting phase   III = application phase   IV = setting phase

Fig. 155. Working curves of Copal for different ambient/component temperatures

Table 102. Mechanical strength according to ISO standard 5833 and German Industrial Standard DIN 53435 for Copal

	ISO 5833 Bending strength (MPa)	Bending modulus (MPa)	Compressive strength (MPa)	DIN 53435 Bending strength (MPa)	Impact strength (kJ/m²)
Limit given in the standard	>50	>1800	>70		
Actual strength	63.8	2160	78.9	70.3	3.7

All mechanical parameters fulfil the ISO and DIN standards (Table 102). The hardening temperature (determined according to ISO 5833 protocols) was 81.5°C. The setting time is 11 min 5 s.

The residual monomer content of the specimens is less than 5% after setting (Fig. 156). The BPO content of these cements is clearly lower than the proportion of DmpT. The ratio of the initiator to the activator is distinctly less than one. In contrast to the low- and medium-viscosity cements of this manufacturer, the high-viscosity cements have a low BPO content. The residual monomer content is not significantly lower than those of the low- and medium-viscosity cement types. The same applies to the residual monomer release.

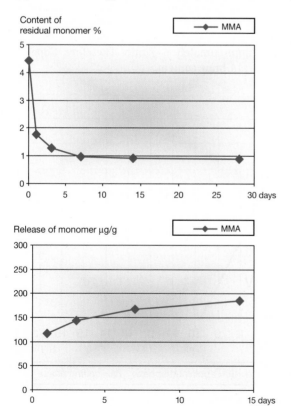

Fig. 156. Content and release of the residual monomer of Copal with time

Table 103. ISO 5833 (1992) requirements for the packaging of Copal

Requirements		Com-pliance	Location of information
General	Is the powder packed in a double-layered, sealed container?	+	–
	Is the liquid packed in a double-layered, sealed container?	+	–
Information regarding the powder ingredients	Qualitative	+	IB, Alu, FS, PB
	Quantitative	+	IB, Alu, FS, PB
Information regarding the liquid ingredients	Qualitative	+	A, AB, PB
	Quantitative	+	AB, PB
	Warning that the package contains flammable liquid	+	A, AB, FS, PB
	Instructions for storage (≤25°C, darkness)	+	IB, Alu, FS, AB, PB
	Statement of the sterility of the contents	+	IB, Alu, FS, AB, PB
	Warning against reusing the package	+	IB, Alu, FS, AB, PB
	Batch number(s)	+	IB, Alu, FS, A, PB
	Expiration date	+	IB, Alu, FS, AB
	Name/address of the manufacturer/ distributor	+	IB, Alu, FS, A, AB, PB
	Number and date of the standard	–	–
Information in the package insert	Detailed instructions for handling the components and preparing the cement	+	PB
	A statement drawing attention to the dangers for the patient	+	PB
	Recommendations for using the cement (syringe/dough state)	+	PB
	A statement regarding the influence of the temperature on working times	+	PB
	Graphical representation of the effects of temperature on the length of the phases of cement curing	+	PB

+, complies; –, does not comply; *A*, ampoule; *AB*, ampoule blister; *Alu*, aluminum pouch; *FS*, carton; *IB*, primary pouch; *PB*, package insert

The residual monomer content of the specimens is under 5% after setting. A reference to the presently valid ISO standard is missing on the packaging units of this type of bone cement (Table 103). The key characteristics of Copal are listed in Table 104.

Table 104. The key characteristics of Copal

High viscosity
Zirconium dioxide is the radiopaque medium
The polymer contains a MMA/MA co-polymer
The polymer is ethylene oxide sterilized
The powder and ampoule are packed separately
Mixing sequence: monomer, then polymer
Working time: long
ISO 5833 is fulfilled
Molecular weight greater than 350,000 Da
High fatigue strength
High gentamicin/clindamicin content, very high release

MMA/MA, methyl methacrylate/methyl acrylate

3.2.3.11
Genta C-ment 1

The polymer powder and monomer liquid of Genta C-ment 1 are packed in a rather small and very solid outer carton (Fig. 157). The carton may be easily opened on the upper side. The outer carton itself is printed with the most important information (for example, the composition of the powder and liquid). Two small, separate labels show the batch number and the expiration date. Indications regarding the registration and the distributor may also be clearly displayed.

The outside of the packing contains a PE pouch that encloses a blister pack. This blister pack contains the powder (in a glass bottle) and the monomer (in an ampoule). Furthermore, there is an insert and four chart stickers for patients' records. To our knowledge, this type of packing of the polymer powder (i.e., in a brown glass bottle) is otherwise only used by the company Sulzer for the cements Allofix G and Duracem 3.

The peel-off pouch consists of a Tyvek side and a transparent PE side. On the paper side, there is a label that indicates the composition of both cement components, the expiration date and the batch number.

The peel-off pouch may be easily opened. The blister pack contained in it consists of transparent, molded PVC and is sealed with unprinted Tyvek. The powder bottle and the monomer ampoule may be well visualized through the PVC. The blister pack may be easily opened. Both primary packed materials bear a batch number related to the product; this number is not identical to the number on the peel-off pouch on the outer carton. An expiration date is missing on the polymer bottle and the monomer ampoule. The brown glass bottle that contains the poly-

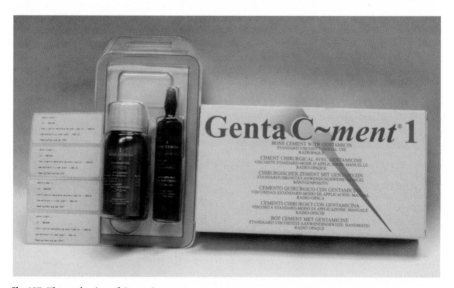

Fig. 157. The packaging of Genta C-ment 1

powder	**liquid**
34,97 g poly(methyl methacrylate) containing some % of methyl acrylate and ethyl acrylate 0,98 g benzoyl peroxide 4,00 g barium sulphate 0,80 g gentamicin sulphate (= 0,5 g base) ------------ 40,80 g	12,15 g methyl methacrylate (=12,93 ml) 1,90 g butyl methacrylate (= 2,12 ml) 0,35 g N,N-dimethyl-p-toluidine (= 0,37 ml) 20 ppm hydroquinone ------------ 14,40 g (15,42 ml)
	Genta C-ment 1

Fig. 158. Composition of Genta C-ment 1

mer powder is a screw-cap bottle. The lock is different from those of the powder bottles of Allofix G and Duracem 3.

A stopper made of plastic serves as a locking aid on the bottle. This bottle is printed with white letters. Instructions are given regarding sterilization by means of X-rays, and the composition, batch number and manufacturer are listed. The polymer powder contains 85.8% PMMA, 2.4% BPO, 2% gentamicin sulfate (1.2% gentamicin base) and 9.8% barium sulfate (as an opacifier; Fig. 158) as declared by the manufacturer. However, analysis shows that the polymer also contains a low percentage of methyl acrylate and ethyl acrylate.

The ampoule is also printed like the polymer bottle. The top of the ampoule features a white point, which shows the breaking shaft.

In addition to monomer quantity and composition, the batch number and manufacturer are given as information. The liquid consists of two different methacrylates – 84.4% MMA and 13.2% BuMA – in addition to 2.4% DmpT and approximately 20 ppm hydroquinone (as a stabilizer).

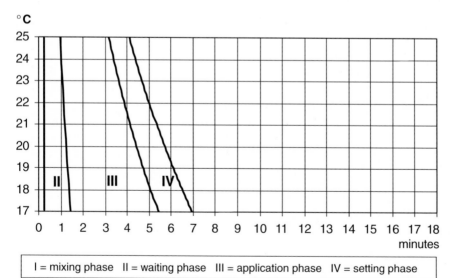

I = mixing phase   II = waiting phase   III = application phase   IV = setting phase

Fig. 159. Working curves of Genta C-ment 1 for different ambient/component temperatures

Table 105. Mechanical strength according to ISO 5833 and German Industrial Standard DIN 53435 for Genta C-ment 1

| | ISO 5833 | | | DIN 53435 | |
	Bending strength (MPa)	Bending modulus (MPa)	Compressive strength (MPa)	Bending strength (MPa)	Impact strength (kJ/m²)
Limit given in the standard	>50	>1800	>70		
Actual strength	63	2514	84.7	66.5	2.9

To mix the dough, the powder is put into the vessel, and the liquid is then added. The wetting occurs very quickly, although it often seems that the material is too dry at first. However, after approximately 15–20 s, the dough is rather viscous and completely homogeneous. From the beginning, the cement shows a high viscosity and may be taken out of the vessel after less than 1 min, and processing may be continued. This viscosity is so high that processing without problems is not easy. After 3 min 30 s, the dough can no longer be handled. After 4 min, warming may be detected. After between 4 min 50 s and 5 min, the dough is completely harden-ed (Fig. 159). Due to these properties, Genta C-ment 1 has to be regarded as a high-viscosity cement.

The mechanical strengths all correspond to those listed in the ISO standard (Table 105). The low impact strength (2.9 kJ/m²) and bending strength and the slight deviations between the bending strengths determined according to Dynstat (66.5 MPa) and ISO 5833 (63 MPa) protocols are striking.

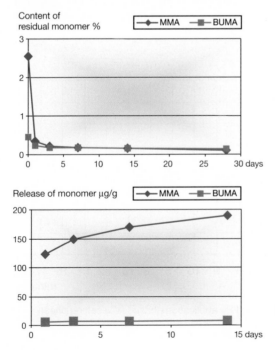

Fig. 160. Content and release of the residual monomers of Genta C-ment 1 with time

The hardening temperature (determined according to ISO protocols) was 80.8°C. Thus, this material has a high polymerization temperature, which is

Table 106. ISO 5833 (1992) requirements for the packaging of Genta C-ment 1

Requirements		Com-pliance	Location of information
General	Is the powder packed in a double-layered, sealed container?	+	–
	Is the liquid packed in a double-layered, sealed container?	+	–
Information regarding the powder ingredients	Qualitative	+	PF, FS, POB, PB
	Quantitative	+	PF, FS, POB, PB
Information regarding the liquid ingredients	Qualitative	+	A, POB, FS, PB
	Quantitative	+	A, POB, FS, PB
	Warning that the package contains flammable liquid	+	PB, A, FS
	Instructions for storage (≤25°C, darkness)	+	FS, POB
	Statement of the sterility of the contents	+	A, PF, FS, PB, POB
	Warning against reusing the package	+	FS, POB, PB, PF
	Batch number(s)	+	A, PF, FS, POB
	Expiration date	+	FS, POB
	Name/address of the manufacturer/distributor	+	A, PF, POB, FS, PB
	Number and date of the standard	–	–
Information in the package insert	Detailed instructions for handling the components and preparing the cement	+	PB
	A statement drawing attention to the dangers for the patient	+	PB
	Recommendations for using the cement (syringe/dough state)	+	PB
	A statement regarding the influence of the temperature on working times	+	PB
	Graphical representation of the effects of temperature on the length of the phases of cement curing	+	PB

+, complies; –, does not comply; A, ampoule; FS, carton; PB, package insert; PF, powder bottle; POB peel-off pouch

Table 107. The key characteristics of Genta C-ment 1

High viscosity
The monomer contains BuMA
Barium sulfate is the radiopaque medium
The polymer is γ irradiated
The polymer is in a brown glass bottle
The polymer bottle and monomer ampoule are packed in one blister
Mixing sequence: powder, then monomer
Working time: short
ISO 5833 is fulfilled
Molecular weight less than 350,000 Da
Low bending strength
Low impact strength
Low gentamicin content, low release

BuMA, butyl methcrylate

expected, due to the favorable powder/liquid ratio (Fig. 11). The residual mono-mer (Fig. 160) has not been considered in the comparison; both MMA and BuMA monomers are contained in the liquid.

Regarding the packing components and their printing, it is striking that the batch number is only printed on the primary container; an expiration date is completely missing. Moreover, a notice regarding the present standard (ISO 5833; Table 106) is missing. The key characteristics of Genta C-ment 1 are listed in Table 107.

3.2.3.12
Genta C-ment 3

The polymer powder and monomer liquid of Genta C-ment 3 are packed in a rather small and very solid outer carton (Fig. 161). The carton may be easily open-ed on the upper side. The outer carton itself is printed with the most important information (for example, the composition of the powder and liquid). Two small, separate labels show the batch number and the expiration date. Indications regar-ding the registration and the distributor may also be clearly displayed.

The outside of the packing contains a PE pouch that encloses a blister pack. This blister pack contains the powder (in a glass bottle) and the monomer (in an ampoule). Furthermore, there is an insert and four chart stickers for patients' records. To our knowledge, this type of packing of the polymer powder (i.e., in a brown glass bottle) is otherwise only used by the company Sulzer for the cements Allofix G and Duracem 3.

The peel-off pouch consists of a Tyvek side and a transparent PE side. On the paper side, there is a label that indicates the composition of both cement com-

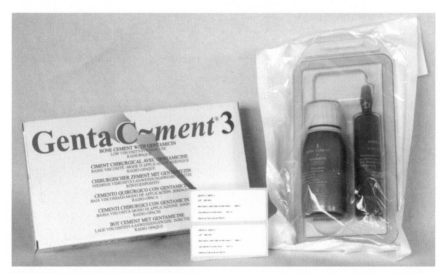

Fig. 161. The packaging of Genta C-ment 3

powder	liquid
34,90 g poly(methyl methacrylate) containing some % of methyl acrylate and ethyl acrylate 1,10 g benzoyl peroxide 4,00 g barium sulphate 0,80 g gentamicin sulphate (= 0,5 g base) ------------ 40,80 g	13,85 g methyl methacrylate (=14,73 ml) 2,16 g butyl methacrylate (= 2,42 ml) 0,39 g N,N-dimethyl-p-toluidine (= 0,42 ml) 20 ppm hydroquinone ----------- 16,40 g (17,57 ml)

Genta C-ment 3

Fig. 162. Composition of Genta C-ment 3

ponents, the expiration date and the batch number. The peel-off pouch may be easily opened. The blister pack contained in it consists of a transparent, molded PVC and is sealed with unprinted Tyvek. The powder bottle and the monomer ampoule may be well visualized through the PVC. The blister pack may be easily opened. Both primary packed materials bear a batch number related to the product; this number is not identical to the number indicated on the peel-off pouch on the outer carton. An expiration date is missing on the polymer bottle and the monomer ampoule. The brown glass bottle that contains the polymer powder is a screw-cap bottle. The lock is different from those of the powder bottles of Allofix G and Duracem 3.

A stopper made of plastic serves as a locking aid on the bottle. This bottle is printed with white letters. Instructions are given regarding sterilization by means of X-rays, and the composition, batch number and manufacturer are listed. The polymer powder contains 85.5% PMMA, 2.7% BPO, 2% gentamicin sulfate (1.2% gentamicin base) and 9.8% barium sulfate (as an opacifier; Fig. 162) as declared by the manufacturer. However, analysis shows that the polymer also contains a low percentage of methyl acrylate and ethyl acrylate.

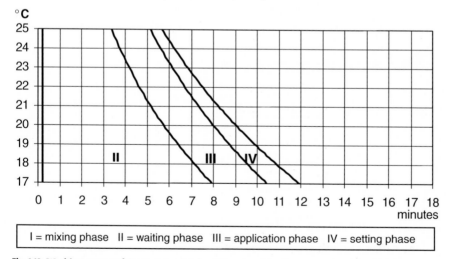

I = mixing phase   II = waiting phase   III = application phase   IV = setting phase

Fig. 163. Working curves of Genta C-ment 3 for different ambient/component temperatures

Table 108. Mechanical strength according to ISO 5833 and German Industrial Standard DIN 53435 for Genta C-ment 3

	ISO 5833 Bending strength (MPa)	Bending modulus (MPa)	Compressive strength (MPa)	DIN 53435 Bending strength (MPa)	Impact strength (kJ/m^2)
Limit given in the standard	>50	>1800	>70		
Actual strength	68	2699	97.9	75.7	3.5

The ampoule is also printed like the polymer bottle. The top of the ampoule features a white point, which shows the breaking shaft.

In addition to monomer quantity and composition, the batch number and manufacturer are given as information. The liquid consists of two different methacrylates – 84.4% MMA and 13.2% BuMA – in addition to 2.4% DmpT and approximately 20 ppm hydroquinone (as a stabilizer). It can be seen that the liquid monomers of Genta C-ment 1 and Genta C-ment 3 do not differ from each other, but different amounts of monomer are used (14.4 g for Genta C-ment 1 and 16.4 g for Genta C-ment 3).

To mix the dough, the powder is put into the vessel, and the liquid is then added. The wetting occurs very quickly; after approximately 15–20 s, the dough

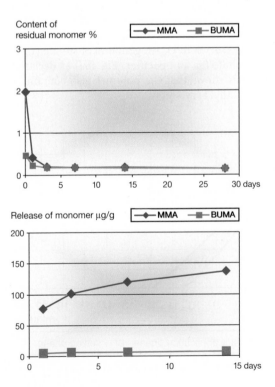

Fig. 164. Content and release of the residual monomers of Genta C-ment 3 with time

has a rather low-viscosity and is completely homogeneous. The end of the sticky phase is reached after 4 min, and processing may then be continued. After 6 min, the dough can no longer be handled. The material has a very short working phase.

After 5 min 30 s, warming may be detected. After between 6 min 40 s and 6 min 45 s, the dough is completely hardened (Fig. 163). Due to these handling properties, Genta C-ment 3 has to be regarded as a low-viscosity cement.

The mechanical strengths all correspond to those listed in the ISO standard (Table 108). A high compressive strength and a low impact strength can be observed.

The hardening temperature (determined according to ISO protocols) was 80.8°C. Thus, this material has a high polymerization temperature, which is expected, due to the favorable powder/liquid ratio. The setting time has a value of approximately 7 min 40 s. The residual monomer has not been considered in the comparison (Fig. 164); both MMA and BuMA are contained in the liquid.

Regarding the packing components and their printing, it is striking that the batch number is only printed on the primary container; an expiration date is completely missing. Moreover, a notice regarding the present standard (ISO 5833;

Table 109. ISO 5833 (1992) requirements for the packaging of Genta C-ment 3

Requirements		Com-pliance	Location of information
General	Is the powder packed in a double-layered, sealed container?	+	–
	Is the liquid packed in a double-layered, sealed container?	+	–
Information regarding the powder ingredients	Qualitative	+	PF, FS, POB, PB
	Quantitative	+	PF, FS, POB, PB
Information regarding the liquid ingredients	Qualitative	+	A, POB, FS, PB
	Quantitative	+	A, POB, FS, PB
	Warning that the package contains flammable liquid	+	PB, A, FS
	Instructions for storage (≤25°C, darkness)	+	FS, POB
	Statement of the sterility of the contents	+	A, PF, FS, PB, POB
	Warning against reusing the package	+	FS, POB, PB, PF
	Batch number(s)	+	A, PF, FS, POB
	Expiration date	+	FS, POB
	Name/address of the manufacturer/distributor	+	A, PF, POB, FS, PB
	Number and date of the standard	–	–
Information in the package insert	Detailed instructions for handling the components and preparing the cement	+	PB
	A statement drawing attention to the dangers for the patient	+	PB
	Recommendations for using the cement (syringe/dough state)	+	PB
	A statement regarding the influence of the temperature on working times	+	PB
	Graphical representation of the effects of temperature on the length of the phases of cement curing	+	PB

+, complies; –, does not comply; A, ampoule; FS, carton; PB, package insert; PF, powder bottle; POB peel-off pouch

Table 110. The key characteristics of Genta C-ment 3

Low viscosity
The monomer contains BuMA
Barium sulfate is the radiopaque medium
The polymer is γ irradiated
The polymer is in a brown glass bottle
The polymer bottle and monomer ampoule are packed in one blister
Mixing sequence: powder, then monomer
Working time: short
ISO 5833 is fulfilled
Molecular weight less than 350,000 Da
Low gentamicin content, low release

BuMA, butyl methacrylate

Table 109) is missing. The key characteristics of Genta C-ment 3 are listed in Table 110.

3.2.3.13
Osteopal G and Palacos LV + G/E Flow with Gentamicin

Osteopal G and Palacos LV with Gentamicin are sold by different distributors under different trade names, but the material in each case is exactly the same (Fig. 165). All the cement components of Osteopal G or Palacos LV with Gentamicin are packed in a rectangular outer carton that may be easily opened at the upper, narrow side. The printing on the outer cartons corresponds in every respect to the valid ISO packaging regulations. The indications regarding the batch number and expiration date are not printed on the front side of the carton but on one of the two unprinted small sides. The names of the distributor and manufacturer are easily recognizable.

The outer carton contains a cardboard tray in which two spaces are left for the secure packaging of both of the ampoule containing blister packs; in single versions of the bone cements, only one blister packed ampoule is located there. Usually, the insert, four to six chart stickers and an alu-pouch that contains two inner pouches with polymer powder are attached to the two monomer ampoules, which are located in the spaces of the cardboard tray. Each of the two folded, doubly packed inner pouches within the alu-pouch contains the sterile pouches in which the polymer powder is located.

The inner pouch of the polymer is printed on the paper side and contains important information regarding handling and storage. Furthermore, the batch number and the expiration date are located noticeably on the printed front side, as prescribed by the standards. The back of the inner pouch is made of polyester and, therefore, is transparent.

The green pigmented polymer powder, which is well known and is characteristic of such Palacos-like products, is clearly visible. The polymer powder is sterilized by ethylene oxide. The composition of the polymer powder is 79.5% MMA-methylacrylate co-polymer, 1.5% BPO, 4.0% gentamicin sulfate

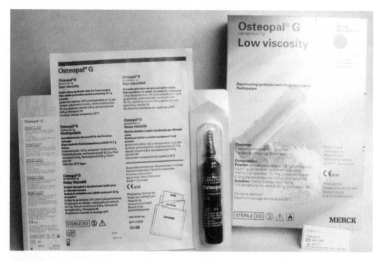

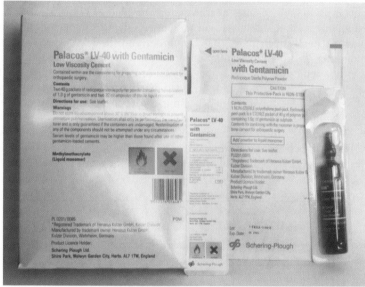

Fig. 165. The packaging of Osteopal G/Palacos LV + G

(2.4% gentamicin base), 1 mg chlorophyll and 15.0% zirconium dioxide (as an opacifier; Fig. 166).

The sterile inner pouch is enclosed by an unprinted peel-off-pouch, which contains an inner pouch with a paper side and a PE side. Because the transparent PE side encloses the printed paper side of the inner pouch, the printing on the inner pouch can be clearly read through the outer pouch. A sterile label is located on the outer pouch; this label is obviously put on the pouch after successful sterilization. Usually, two folded peel-off pouches are packed in an alu-pouch that has

powder	liquid
33,14 g poly(methyl acrylate, methyl methacrylate) 6,26 g zirconium dioxide 0,63 g benzoyl peroxide 1 mg chlorophyllin 1,67 g gentamicin sulphate (=1,0 g base) ----------- 41,70 g	18,40 g methyl methacrylate (=19,57 ml) 0,38 g N,N-dimethyl-p-toluidine (= 0,43 ml) 0,4 mg chlorophyllin --------- 18,78 g (20 ml)
Osteopal G/Palacos LV + G	

Fig. 166. Composition of Osteopal G/Palacos LV + G

printing on one side. The print contains all the necessary information, including the batch number and expiration date.

The two ampoules, which are located in the cardboard tray, are protected in the wrapping by the blister pack and by the alu-pouch located above it. The blister pack itself consists of transparent, molded PVC and a paper side. A printed ampoule label is attached on the paper side; this label contains all necessary information, especially the batch number and the expiration date of the liquid monomer. A brown glass ampoule contains the sterile, filtered green monomer, which is typical of Osteopal and Palacos brands. Each ampoule has a translucent label. The blister pack is also sterilized by ethylene oxide. The monomer consists of 98.0% MMA, 2.0% DmpT, 0.4 mg chlorophyll and approximately 60 ppm hydroquinone (Fig. 166).

For the opening of the brown glass ampoule, no opening aid is included; the polymer pouch should be opened with the help of a scissors. The polymer powder can easily be poured out of the pouch into the mixing vessel.

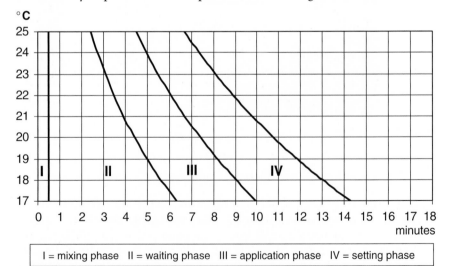

I = mixing phase   II = waiting phase   III = application phase   IV = setting phase

Fig. 167. Working curves of Osteopal G/Palacos LV + G for different ambient/component temperatures

Table 111. Mechanical strength according to ISO 5833 and German Industrial Standard DIN 53435 for Osteopal G

	ISO 5833 Bending strength (MPa)	Bending modulus (MPa)	Compressive strength (MPa)	DIN 53435 Bending strength (MPa)	Impact strength (kJ/m²)
Limit given in the standard	>50	>1800	>70		
Actual strength	72.8	2490	97	81.4	5.7

Before mixing the cement components of Osteopal G/Palacos LV with Gentamicin, the liquid is first poured into the bowl. The polymer powder is then added to the monomer, and the clock is started. In a few seconds, a very liquid, low-viscosity, homogeneous dough can easily be produced. The viscosity of the dough increases very slowly, depending on the temperature of the components with respect to the temperature of the operating room. For example, the dough may be taken out of the mixing vessel non-sticky after approximately 3 min at 23°C (Fig. 167). The working phase of Osteopal G or Palacos LV with gentamicin varies from 2 min 30 s to 3 min and usually ends approximately 5–6 min after the start of mixing. The cement hardens after approximately 7–8 min. Therefore, Osteopal G and Palacos LV with Gentamicin are characterized as low-viscosity PMMA bone cements.

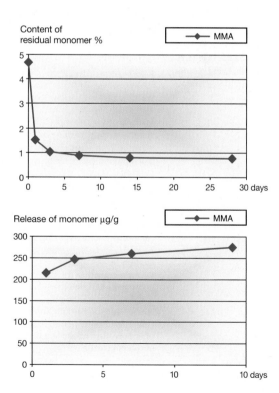

Fig. 168. Content and release of the residual monomer of Osteopal G/Palacos LV + G with time

The mechanical testing results have good values, especially for the bending strength. The bending strength determined according to ISO 5833 protocols is remarkably high (72.8 MPa), and that determined according to DIN 53435 protocols is 81.4 MPa (Table 111). Additionally, the impact strength has a high value (>5 kJ/m^2).

The hardening temperature (determined according to ISO 5833 protocols) had significant lower values than that displayed by the plain material. We found a value of 69.5°C for the antibiotic-loaded cements instead of 83.9°C, as found for the plain material. The setting time is 11 min 20 s, instead of 10 min 15 s as found for the plain material.

The residual monomer content of the specimens is less than 5% after setting (Fig. 168). The BPO content of these cements is clearly lower than the proportion of DmpT. The ratio of the initiator to the activator is distinctly less than two. In contrast to the high- and medium-viscosity cements of this manufacturer, the low-viscosity cement has a high BPO content. The residual monomer content is

Table 112. ISO 5833 (1992) requirements for the packaging of Osteopal G and Palacos LV + G

Requirements		Com-pliance	Location of information
General	Is the powder packed in a double-layered, sealed container?	+	–
	Is the liquid packed in a double-layered, sealed container?	+	–
Information regarding the powder ingredients	Qualitative	+	IB, Alu, FS, PB
	Quantitative	+	IB, Alu, FS, PB
Information regarding the liquid ingredients	Qualitative	+	A, AB, PB
	Quantitative	+	AB, PB
	Warning that the package contains flammable liquid	+	A, AB, FS, PB
	Instructions for storage (≤25°C, darkness)	+	IB, Alu, FS, AB, PB
	Statement of the sterility of the contents	+	IB, Alu, FS, AB, PB
	Warning against reusing the package	+	IB, Alu, FS, AB, PB
	Batch number(s)	+	IB, Alu, FS, A, PB
	Expiration date	+	IB, Alu, FS, AB
	Name/address of the manufacturer/distributor	+	IB, Alu, FS, A, AB, PB
	Number and date of the standard	–	–
Information in the package insert	Detailed instructions for handling the components and preparing the cement	+	PB
	A statement drawing attention to the dangers for the patient	+	PB
	Recommendations for using the cement (syringe/dough state)	+	PB
	A statement regarding the influence of the temperature on working times	+	PB
	Graphical representation of the effects of temperature on the length of the phases of cement curing	+	PB

+, complies; –, does not comply; A, ampoule; AB, ampoule blister; Alu, aluminum pouch; FS, carton; IB, primary pouch; PB, package insert

Table 113. The key characteristics of Osteopal G and Palacos LV + G

Low viscosity
Zirconium dioxide is the radiopaque medium
The polymer contains a MMA/MA co-polymer
The polymer is ethylene oxide sterilized
The powder and ampoule are packed separately
Mixing sequence: monomer, then polymer
Working time: long
ISO 5833 is fulfilled
Molecular weight greater than 350,000 Da
Very high fatigue strength
High bending strength
High impact strength
Osteopal G: high gentamicin content, very high gentamicin release
Palacos LV + G: high gentamicin content, high gentamicin release

MMA/MA, methyl methacrylate/methyl acrylate

not significantly higher than those of the high- and medium-viscosity cement types. The same applies to the residual monomer release. A notice regarding the presently valid ISO standard is missing on the packaging units of this type of bone cement (Table 112). The key characteristics of Osteopal G and Palacos LV with Gentamicin are listed in Table 113.

3.2.3.14
Refobacin-Palacos R and Palacos R with Gentamicin

These two cements are basing on the same plain powder (Palacos R). Because of the usage of gentamicin of different sources and different kind of processing the cements are not identical and sold under different trade names by different companies.

All the cement components of Refobacin-Palacos R and Palacos R with Gentamicin are packed in a rectangular outer carton that may be easily opened at the upper, narrow side (Fig. 169). The printing on the outer cartons corresponds in every respect to the valid ISO packaging regulations. The indications regarding the batch number and expiration date are not printed on the front side of the carton but on one of the two unprinted small sides. The names of the distributor and manufacturer are easily recognizable.

The outer carton contains a cardboard tray in which two spaces are left for the secure packaging of both of the ampoule containing blister packs; in single versions of the bone cements, only one blister packed ampoule is located there. Usually, the insert, four to six chart stickers and an alu-pouch that contains two inner pouches with polymer powder are attached to the two monomer ampoules, which are located in the spaces of the cardboard tray. Each of the two folded, doubly packed inner pouches within the alu-pouch contains the sterile pouches in which the polymer powder is located.

The inner pouch for the polymer is printed on the paper side and contains important information regarding handling and storage. Furthermore, the batch number and the expiration date are located noticeably on the printed front side,

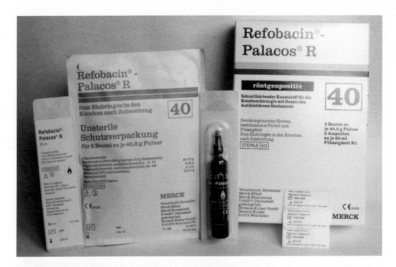

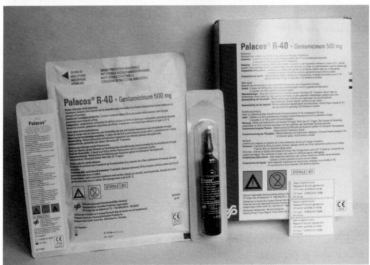

Fig. 169. The packaging of Refobacin-Palacos R or Palacos R with Gentamicin

as prescribed by the standards. The back of the inner pouch is made of polyester and, therefore, is transparent.

The green pigmented polymer powder, which is well known and is characteristic of such products, is clearly visible. The polymer powder is sterilized by ethylene oxide. The composition of the polymer powder is 82.1% MMA-methylacrylate co-polymer, 0.8% BPO, 2% gentamicin sulfate (1.2% gentamicin base) and 15.0% zirconium dioxide (as an opacifier; Fig. 170).

The sterile inner pouch is enclosed by an unprinted peel-off-pouch, which contains an inner pouch with a paper side and a PE side. Because the transparent PE side encloses the printed paper side of the inner pouch, the printing on the

powder	liquid
33,55 g poly(methyl acrylate, methyl methacrylate) 6,13 g zirconium dioxide 0,32 g benzoyl peroxide 1 mg chlorophyllin 0,84 g gentamicin sulphate (= 0,5 g base) --------- 40,84 g	18,40 g methyl methacrylate (=19,57 ml) 0,38 g N,N-dimethyl-p-toluidine (=0,43 ml) 0,4 mg chlorophyllin --------- 18,78 g (20 ml)
	Refobacin-Palacos R/Palacos R + G

Fig. 170. Composition of Refobacin-Palacos R or Palacos R with Gentamicin

inner pouch can be clearly read through the outer pouch. A sterile label is located on the outer pouch; this label is obviously put on the pouch after successful sterilization. Usually, two folded peel-off-pouches are packed in an alu-pouch that has printing on one side. The print contains all the necessary information, including the batch number and expiration date.

The two ampoules, which are located in the cardboard tray, are protected in the wrapping by the blister pack and by the alu-pouch located above it. The blister pack itself consists of transparent, molded PVC and a paper side. A printed ampoule label is attached on the paper side; this label contains all necessary information, especially the batch number and the expiration date of the liquid monomer. A brown glass ampoule contains the sterile, filtered green monomer, which is typical of Palacos R with Gentamicin and Refobacin-Palacos R. Each ampoule has a translucent label. The blister pack is also sterilized by ethylene oxide. The monomer consists of 98.0% MMA, 2.0% DmpT and approximately

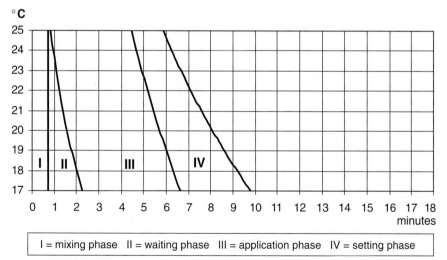

I = mixing phase   II = waiting phase   III = application phase   IV = setting phase

Fig. 171. Working curves of Refobacin-Palacos R or Palacos R with Gentamicin for different ambient/component temperatures

Table 114. Mechanical strength according to ISO 5833 and German Industrial Standard DIN 53435 for Refobacin-Palacos R and Palacos R with Gentamicin

	ISO 5833 Bending strength (MPa)	Bending modulus (MPa)	Compressive strength (MPa)	DIN 53435 Bending strength (MPa)	Impact strength (kJ/m²)
Limit given in the standard	>50	>1800	>70		
Actual strength	69.9	2680	97	82.9	4.7

60 ppm hydroquinone (Fig. 170). Thus, the monomer of Refobacin-Palacos R and Palacos R with Gentamicin does not contain an antibiotic.

For the opening of the brown glass ampoule, no opening aid is included; the polymer pouch should be opened with the help of a scissors. The polymer powder can easily be poured out of the pouch into the mixing vessel.

Before mixing the cement components of Palacos R with Gentamicin and Refobacin-Palacos R, the liquid is first poured into the bowl. The polymer powder is then added to the monomer, and the clock is started. In a few seconds, a homogeneous dough can easily be produced. The viscosity of the dough increases very quickly, depending on the temperature of the components with respect to the temperature of the operating room. For example, the dough may be taken out of the mixing vessel non-sticky after approximately 1 min at 23°C (Fig. 171). The working phase of Palacos R varies from 3 min 30 s to 4 min and usually ends approximately

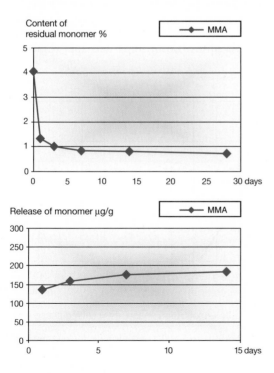

Fig. 172. Content and release of the residual monomer of Refobacin-Palacos R or Palacos R with Gentamicin with time

4 min 30 s to 5 min after the start of mixing. The cement hardens after approximately 6–7 min. Therefore, Palacos R with Gentamicin and Refobacin-Palacos R are
characterized as high-viscosity PMMA bone cements.

One has to take into consideration that chilled Palacos R with Gentamicin and
Refobacin-Palacos R have completely different working characteristics. The
mechanical testing results have good values, especially for the bending strength.
The bending strength determined according to ISO 5833 protocols is remarkably
high (69.9 MPa), and that determined according to DIN 53435 protocols is
82.9 MPa. The impact strength is 4.7 kJ/m^2 (Table 114).

The hardening temperature (determined according to ISO 5833 protocols) is
83°C. The setting time is 11 min 10 s.

The residual monomer content of the specimens is less than 5% after setting
(Fig. 172). The BPO content of these cements is clearly lower than the proportion
of DmpT. The ratio of the initiator to the activator is distinctly less than one. In
contrast to the low- and medium-viscosity cements of this manufacturer, the
high-viscosity cements have a low BPO content. The residual monomer content is

Table 115. ISO 5833 (1992) requirements for the packaging of Refobacin-Palacos R and Palacos R with
Gentamicin

Requirements		Com-pliance	Location of information
General	Is the powder packed in a double-layered, sealed container?	+	–
	Is the liquid packed in a double-layered, sealed container?	+	–
Information regarding the powder ingredients	Qualitative	+	IB, Alu, FS, PB
	Quantitative	+	IB, Alu, FS, PB
Information regarding the liquid ingredients	Qualitative	+	A, AB, PB
	Quantitative	+	AB, PB
	Warning that the package contains flammable liquid	+	A, AB, FS, PB
	Instructions for storage (≤25°C, darkness)	+	IB, Alu, FS, AB, PB
	Statement of the sterility of the contents	+	IB, Alu, FS, AB, PB
	Warning against reusing the package	+	IB, Alu, FS, AB, PB
	Batch number(s)	+	IB, Alu, FS, A, PB
	Expiration date	+	IB, Alu, FS, AB
	Name/address of the manufacturer/ distributor	+	IB, Alu, FS, A, AB, PB
	Number and date of the standard	–	–
Information in the package insert	Detailed instructions for handling the components and preparing the cement	+	PB
	A statement drawing attention to the dangers for the patient	+	PB
	Recommendations for using the cement (syringe/dough state)	+	PB
	A statement regarding the influence of the temperature on working times	+	PB
	Graphical representation of the effects of temperature on the length of the phases of cement curing	+	PB

+, complies; –, does not comply; *A*, ampoule; *AB*, ampoule blister; *Alu*, aluminum pouch; *FS*, carton; *IB*, primary
pouch; *PB*, package insert

Table 116. The key characteristics of Refobacin-Palacos R and Palacos R with Gentamicin

High viscosity
Zirconium dioxide is the radiopaque medium
The polymer contains a MMA/MA co-polymer
The polymer is ethylene oxide sterilized
The powder and ampoule are packed separately
Mixing sequence: monomer, then powder
Working time: long
ISO 5833 is fulfilled
Molecular weight greater than 350,000 Da
High fatigue strength
High bending strength
High impact strength
Refobacin-Palacos R has a low gentamicin content and a very high release
Palacos R with Gentamicin has a low gentamicin content and a high release

MMA/MA, methyl methacrylate/methyl acrylate

not significantly lower than those of the low- and medium-viscosity cement
types. The same applies to the residual monomer release. A notice regarding the
presently valid ISO standard is missing on the packaging units of this type of
bone cement (Table 115). The key characteristics of Refobacin-Palacos R and
Palacos R with Gentamicin are listed in Table 116.

3.2.3.15
Palamed G

All the cement components of Palamed G are packed in a rectangular outer carton that may be easily opened at the upper, narrow side (Fig. 173). The printing on

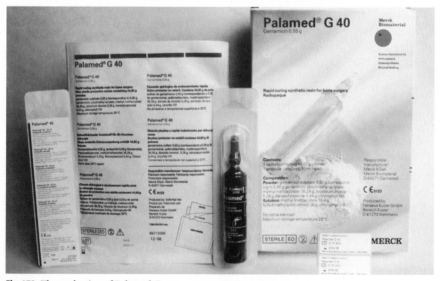

Fig. 173. The packaging of Palamed G

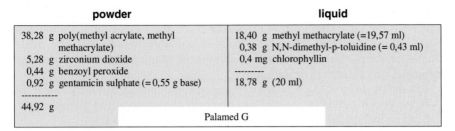

powder	liquid
38,28 g poly(methyl acrylate, methyl methacrylate) 5,28 g zirconium dioxide 0,44 g benzoyl peroxide 0,92 g gentamicin sulphate (= 0,55 g base) ---------- 44,92 g	18,40 g methyl methacrylate (=19,57 ml) 0,38 g N,N-dimethyl-p-toluidine (= 0,43 ml) 0,4 mg chlorophyllin --------- 18,78 g (20 ml)
Palamed G	

Fig. 174. Composition of Palamed G

the outer cartons corresponds in every respect to the valid ISO packaging regulations. The indications regarding the batch number and expiration date are not printed on the front side of the carton but on one of the two unprinted small sides. The names of the distributor and manufacturer are easily recognizable.

The outer carton contains a cardboard tray in which two spaces are left for the secure packaging of both of the ampoule containing blister packs; in single versions of the bone cements, only one blister packed ampoule is located there. Usually, a multilingual brochure, four to six chart stickers and an alu-pouch that contains two inner pouches with polymer powder are attached to the two monomer ampoules, which are located in the spaces of the cardboard tray. Each of the two folded, doubly packed inner pouches within the alu-pouch contains the sterile pouches in which the polymer powder is located.

The inner pouch for the polymer is printed on the paper side and contains important information regarding handling and storage. Furthermore, the batch number and the expiration date are located noticeably on the printed front side, as prescribed by the standards. The back of the inner pouch is made of polyester and, therefore, is transparent.

The green pigmented polymer powder, which is well known and is characteristic of Palacos R-like products, is clearly visible. The polymer powder is sterilized by ethylene oxide. The composition of the polymer powder is 85.3% MMA-methylacrylate co-polymer, 0.8% BPO, 2% gentamicin sulfate (1.2% gentamicin base) and 11.8% zirconium dioxide (as an opacifier; Fig. 174).

The sterile inner pouch is enclosed by an unprinted peel-off-pouch, which contains an inner pouch with a paper side and a PE side. Because the transparent PE side encloses the printed paper side of the inner pouch, the printing on the inner pouch can be clearly read through the outer pouch. A sterile label is located on the outer pouch; this label is obviously put on the pouch after successful sterilization. Usually, two folded peel-off pouches are packed in an alu-pouch that has printing on one side. The print contains all the necessary information, including the batch number and expiration date.

The two ampoules, which are located in the cardboard tray, are protected in the wrapping by the blister pack and by the alu-pouch located above it. The blister pack itself consists of transparent, molded PVC and a paper side. A printed ampoule label is attached on the paper side; this label contains all necessary information, especially the batch number and the expiration date of the liquid monomer. A brown glass ampoule contains the sterile, filtered green monomer, which has the same composition as Palacos R and plain Palamed. Each ampoule has a translucent label. The blister pack is also sterilized by ethylene oxide. Therefore, the monomer of Palamed G consists of 98.0% MMA, 2.0% DmpT and approximately 60 ppm hydroquinone.

For the opening of the brown glass ampoule, no opening aid is included; the polymer pouch should be opened with the help of a scissors. The polymer powder can easily be poured out of the pouch into the mixing vessel.

Before mixing the cement components of Palamed G, the liquid is first poured into the bowl. The polymer powder is then added to the monomer, and the clock is started. In a few seconds, a liquid, low-viscosity, homogeneous dough can easily be produced, depending on the temperature of the components with respect to the temperature of the operating room. For example, the dough may be taken out of the mixing vessel non-sticky after between approximately 1 min 30 s and 1 min 40 s at 23°C (Fig. 175). The working phase of Palamed G varies from 3.5 min to 4 min and usually ends approximately 5 min to 5 min 30 s after the start of mixing. Therefore, the working phases of Palamed G, Palamed and Palacos R are comparable. The cement hardens after approximately 6–8 min. Therefore, Palamed G is characterized as a high-viscosity PMMA bone cement with a liquid, low-viscosity wetting phase, comparable with Palacos R.

The mechanical testing results have good values, especially the bending strength determined according to DIN 53435 protocols (80.1 MPa; Table 117). The hardening temperature (determined according to ISO 5833 protocols) has low values of approximately 64°C. The setting time is 11 min 20 s.

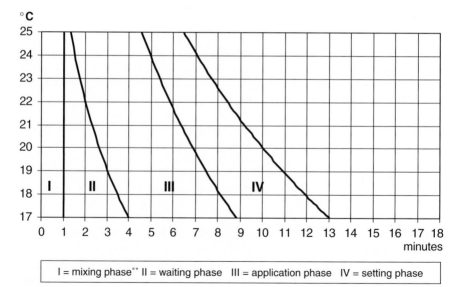

I = mixing phase°° II = waiting phase   III = application phase   IV = setting phase

Fig. 175. Working curves of Palamed G for different ambient/component temperatures

Table 117. Mechanical strength according to ISO 5833 and German Industrial Standard DIN 53435 for Palamed G

	ISO 5833 Bending strength (MPa)	Bending modulus (MPa)	Compressive strength (MPa)	DIN 53435 Bending strength (MPa)	Impact strength (kJ/m²)
Limit given in the standard	>50	>1800	>70		
Actual strength	62.7	2516	89.3	80.1	4.5

The residual monomer content of the specimens is less than 5% after setting (Fig. 176). The BPO content of these cements is clearly lower than the proportion of DmpT. The ratio of initiator to activator is near to one. In contrast to the high-viscosity cements of this manufacturer, the medium-viscosity cement has a higher BPO content but has a lower BPO content than the low-viscosity material. The residual monomer content is comparable to those of the high-viscosity and low-viscosity cement types. The same applies to the residual monomer release. A notice regarding the presently valid ISO standard is missing on the packaging units of this type of bone cement (Table 118). The key characteristics of Palamed G are listed in Table 119.

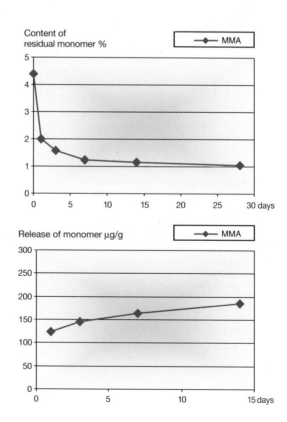

Fig. 176. Content and release of the residual monomer of Palamed G with time

Table 118. ISO 5833 (1992) requirements for the packaging of Palamed G

Requirements		Compliance	Location of information
General	Is the powder packed in a double-layered, sealed container?	+	–
	Is the liquid packed in a double-layered, sealed container?	+	–
Information regarding the powder ingredients	Qualitative	+	IB, Alu, FS, PB
	Quantitative	+	IB, Alu, FS, PB
Information regarding the liquid ingredients	Qualitative	+	A, AB, PB
	Quantitative	+	AB, PB
	Warning that the package contains flammable liquid	+	A, AB, FS, PB
	Instructions for storage (≤25°C, darkness)	+	IB, Alu, FS, AB, PB
	Statement of the sterility of the contents	+	IB, Alu, FS, AB, PB
	Warning against reusing the package	+	IB, Alu, FS, AB, PB
	Batch number(s)	+	IB, Alu, FS, A, PB
	Expiration date	+	IB, Alu, FS, AB
	Name/address of the manufacturer/ distributor	+	IB, Alu, FS, A, AB, PB
	Number and date of the standard	–	–
Information in the package insert	Detailed instructions for handling the components and preparing the cement	+	PB
	A statement drawing attention to the dangers for the patient	+	PB
	Recommendations for using the cement (syringe/dough state)	+	PB
	A statement regarding the influence of the temperature on working times	+	PB
	Graphical representation of the effects of temperature on the length of the phases of cement curing	+	PB

+, complies; –, does not comply; *A*, ampoule; *AB*, ampoule blister; *Alu*, aluminum pouch; *FS*, carton; *IB*, primary pouch; *PB*, package insert

Table 119. The key characteristics of Palamed G

High viscosity
Zirconium dioxide is the radiopaque medium
The polymer contains a MMA/MA co-polymer
The polymer is ethylene oxide sterilized
The powder and ampoule are packed separately
Mixing sequence: monomer, then polymer
Working time: long
ISO 5833 is fulfilled
Molecular weight greater than 350,000 Da
High DIN bending strength
High fatigue strength
Low gentamicin content, very high release

MMA/MA, methyl methacrylate/methyl acrylate

3.2.3.16
Surgical Subiton G

The cement components of Surgical Subiton G are packed in a flat, rectangular outer carton that may easily be opened on the upper, narrow sphere (Fig. 177). The printing on the green-colored outer carton corresponds to the valid ISO packaging regulations. Instructions concerning batch number and expiration date are printed on an additional attached label, not on the outer packing. A notice regarding the distributor may be clearly seen. The packing has an EC character, though the material is nearly exclusively sold in Argentina. A further notice on the outer packing indicates that the material fulfils ISO standard 5833 for bone cements.

In the outer carton, there is only a blister pack containing the polymer powder pouch and the monomer ampoule. The sterilization of the different components is obviously performed simultaneously inside this blister pack. An alu-pouch is not present. The molded PVC is designed in such a way that two ampoule blisters could be packed into it. In the middle of the blister pack is the doubly packed inner pouch. The printing on the inner pouch may be clearly read through the transparent PVC, but the back of the ampoule label cannot be identified on this package.

The back of the blister pack is made of medical paper on which some general information is indicated. A notice concerning the expiration date and the batch number is missing. The paper side cannot be easily separated from the PVC; usually, the paper becomes torn.

The doubly packed inner pouch slightly sticks to the laminated inner side of the paper of the outer blister. The paper that encloses the PVC molded blister pack has a typical sealing pattern (waffle design). In the case of the peel-off

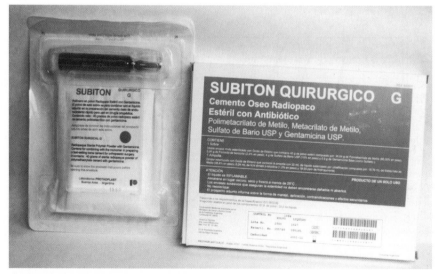

Fig. 177. The packaging of Surgical Subiton G

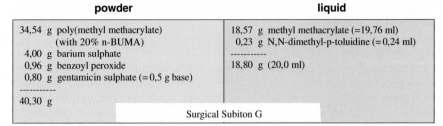

powder	liquid
34,54 g poly(methyl methacrylate) (with 20% n-BUMA) 4,00 g barium sulphate 0,96 g benzoyl peroxide 0,80 g gentamicin sulphate (=0,5 g base) ----------- 40,30 g	18,57 g methyl methacrylate (=19,76 ml) 0,23 g N,N-dimethyl-p-toluidine (=0,24 ml) ----------- 18,80 g (20,0 ml)

Surgical Subiton G

Fig. 178. Composition of Surgical Subiton G

pouch and inner pouch, Tyvek is used in addition to PE. In contrast to the plain version, a printed peel-off pouch is used by Surgical Subiton G. This pouch also has a green ethylene oxide indicator, which is not clearly indicated on the packing. The inner pouch and the peel-off pouch are made of the same packaging material. The printed paper side of the inner pouch features only an indication regarding the batch number. A notice referring to the expiration date is missing on all packaging components. The white polymer powder of Surgical Subiton G contains 85.7% PMMA, 2.4% BPO, 2.0% gentamicin sulfate (1.2% gentamicin base) and 10.0% barium sulfate (as an opacifier; Fig. 178) according to the manufacturer. However, analysis shows that the polymer also contains approximately 20% n-butyl methacrylate.

The blister pack contains the brown glass ampoule, which is located in molded PVC covered with medical paper. The medical paper is printed and contains (contrary to the case for the inner pouch for the powder) all the necessary information for the liquid. The ampoule itself is printed with a white color. There is no

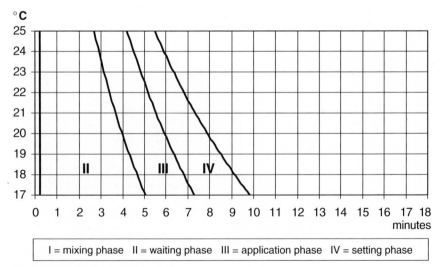

I = mixing phase   II = waiting phase   III = application phase   IV = setting phase

Fig. 179. Working curves of Surgical Subiton G for different ambient/component temperatures

Table 120. Mechanical strength according to ISO 5833 and German Industrial Standard DIN 53435 for Surgical Subiton G

	ISO 5833 Bending strength (MPa)	Bending modulus (MPa)	Compressive strength (MPa)	DIN 53435 Bending strength (MPa)	Impact strength (kJ/m²)
Limit given in the standard	>50	>1800	>70		
Actual strength	59.6	2269	81.6	66.2	2.4

difference in the composition of Surgical Subiton RO and Surgical Subiton G. Therefore, the colorless monomer liquid also consists of MMA (98.8%), 1.2% DmpT and approximately 70 ppm hydroquinone (Fig. 178).

For opening the brown glass ampoule, there is no opening aid; the polymer pouch should be opened with a scissors. The polymer powder may be easily poured out of the pouch into the mixing vessel.

Before mixing the cement components, all the powder is put into the bowl, as indicated by the manufacturer. The liquid is then added to the polymer powder, and the clock is started. In a few seconds, a low-viscosity, homogeneous dough

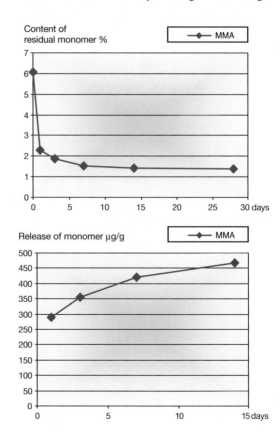

Fig. 180. Content and release of the residual monomer of Surgical Subiton G with time

arises. The viscosity slowly increases, depending on the temperature of components with respect to the temperature of the operating room. For example, the dough may be taken out of the mixing vessel in a non-sticky state after between 2 min 45 s and 3 min if the temperature is 23°C (Fig. 179). The working phase of Surgical Subiton RO is very short (~2 min). After between approximately 4 min 40 s and 5 min, the cement can no longer be handled. By that time, the cement is already very warm. The hardening of the cement occurs 6 min after bringing together the components. Surgical Subiton G, therefore, has to be regarded as a medium-viscosity cement.

The mechanical data are very low (Table 120). In the tested batches, the bending strengths (determined according to ISO 5833 and DIN 53435 protocols) were extremely low. The impact strength determined according to DIN 53435 protocols was 2.4 kJ/m².

The setting time (as determined according to ISO 5833 protocols) is 9 min 50 s. The polymerization temperatures of Surgical Subiton RO and the antibiotic-loaded version are very low. We found values of 60.9°C.

Table 121. ISO 5833 (1992) requirements for the packaging of Surgical Subiton G

Requirements		Com-pliance	Location of information
General	Is the powder packed in a double-layered, sealed container?	+	–
	Is the liquid packed in a double-layered, sealed container?	+	–
Information regarding the powder ingredients	Qualitative	+	FS, PB
	Quantitative	+	FS, PB
Information regarding the liquid ingredients	Qualitative	+	FS, PB
	Quantitative	+	FS, PB
	Warning that the package contains flammable liquid	+	A, AB, FS
	Instructions for storage (≤25°C, darkness)	+	A, FS, PB
	Statement of the sterility of the contents	+	GB, FS
	Warning against reusing the package	–	GB, FS
	Batch number(s)	+	FS, AB
	Expiration date	+	FS, AB
	Name/address of the manufacturer/distributor	+	IB, FS, PB
	Number and date of the standard	+	FS
Information in the package insert	Detailed instructions for handling the components and preparing the cement	+	PB
	A statement drawing attention to the dangers for the patient	+	PB
	Recommendations for using the cement (syringe/dough state)	+	PB
	A statement regarding the influence of the temperature on working times	+	PB
	Graphical representation of the effects of temperature on the length of the phases of cement curing	+	PB

+, complies; –, does not comply; A, ampoule; AB, ampoule blister; FS, carton; GB, shared blister; IB, primary pouch; PB, package insert

The residual monomer content is very high (more than 6% after curing); the same applies to the residual monomer release (Fig. 180). The BPO percentage is comparatively high in the case of this cement, whereas the DmpT percentage is slightly more than 1%. This results in an initiator ratio of four.

It is striking that the qualitative and quantitative compositions of the powder and liquid are only explicitly indicated on the outer carton and in the insert. A notice regarding the prohibition of reuse is missing. There are no indications concerning the batch number and expiration date on the primary vessels. A notice regarding the valid ISO 5833 standard exists (Table 121) but, for this cement, some mechanical tests executed according to this standard were outside the ISO requirements. The key characteristics of Surgical Subiton G are listed in Table 122.

Table 122. The key characteristics of Surgical Subiton G

Medium viscosity
Barium sulfate is the radiopaque medium
The polymer contains a BuMA co-polymer
The polymer is ethylene oxide sterilized
The powder and ampoule are packed together in one blister
Mixing sequence: powder, then monomer
Working time: short
ISO 5833 is not always fulfilled
Molecular weight greater than 350,000 Da
Low bending strength
Low impact strength
Low gentamicin content, low release

BuMA, butyl methacrylate

3.2.4
Comparative Tests of Antibiotic-Loaded Cements

3.2.4.1
Setting Time and Temperature

Having described in detail the antibiotic cements and their packaging, we want to compare them in terms of some important International Standards Organization (ISO) 5833 criteria. Their different abilities to release antibiotic will be discussed in Sect. 3.2.5.7.

The setting temperatures we found are not much different from those of the plain versions. Edwards and Thomasz (1981) noted this for Palacos R (75°C) and Palacos R with Gentamicin (72°C). Hansen and Jensen (1992), however, found temperatures approximately 10°C higher (82.5°C for Palacos R, 81.5°C for Palacos with Gentamicin). The variation found using the ISO method is quite high. No material could be found that did not pass this test.

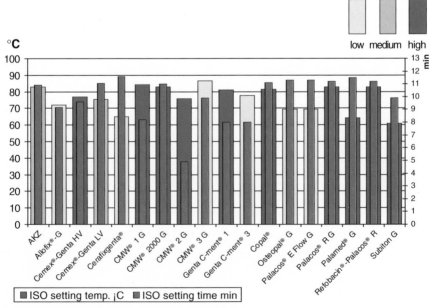

Fig. 181. Setting of antibiotic bone cements, according to ISO 5833

The following cements showed setting temperatures above 80°C: Antibiotic Simplex (Antibiotikahaltiger Knochenzement; AKZ), CMW 1 G, CMW 3 G and CMW 2000 G. However materials with temperatures below 70°C can be found: Cerafix Genta, Osteopal G, Palacos LV/E-Flow, Palamed G and Subiton G.

The antibiotic Cemex cements showed setting temperatures 5–10°C below those of the plain variants. We found the lowest setting temperatures for Subiton G (60°C, as low as for the plain cement; Fig. 181).

In order to decrease the relatively high initial viscosity and to allow for application in mixing systems, pre-cooling of the components is suggested for some cements (Draenert 1988). This practice, common in Germany (Breusch et al. 1999), influences the setting temperatures of Palacos R and Refobacin-Palacos. An exothermic effect (chain growth) initially warms the cold dough after mixing. Because of this consumption of part of the heat of the reaction, the maximum temperature achieved later is reduced by approximately 10°C (Table 123). The dough made under normal conditions (at 23°C) was put into the mold after 1 min, the pre-cooled (4°C) dough was placed in the mold after 3 min. Testing of the pre-cooled material was always was performed with the use of a pre-cooled mixing vessel.

Not only is the setting time prolonged significantly, the peak temperature declines significantly. Hansen and Jensen (1992), however, noted an increase of the polymerization temperature for different cements: the temperatures rose 8.5–15.5°C (from their initial temperatures of 66–82.5°C) after pre-cooling of the components.

A high-viscosity cement with a clearly lower initial viscosity has the advantage that it is feasible to include it in different mixing systems without pre-cooling (Specht and Kühn 1998). If the working time is comparable to that of a high-viscosity cement, this constitutes practical progress. (Kock et al. 1999) have described a new development (Palamed/Palamed G) having these features.

Table 123. Setting times and temperatures, according to ISO 5833 for Palacos R. Comparison of pre-cooled components and those under normal conditions

Palacos R batch		Components at 23°C °C	minutes	Components at 4°C °C	minutes
8409		76.0	10.6	64.0	17.3
		77.0	11.1	64.0	17.7
	average	76.5	10.85	64.0	17.5
8443		76.0	9.9	69.0	17.9
		76.0	10.00	65.5	17.5
	average	76.0	9.95	67.3	17.7
8461		72.0	11.6	65.0	17.0
		75.0	11.3	64.0	16.1
	average	73.5	11.45	64.5	16.55

3.2.4.2
Compressive Strength

The compressive strengths are generally slightly less than those of the plain materials. The antibiotics are never an integrated part of the polymer matrix, thus weakening the cement (though the percentage of the added antibiotic is low).

However, there seem to be exceptions (Fig. 182). For some antibiotic bone cements, the compressive strength is higher than for the plain versions (all Palacos products, Cerafix Genta, CWM 3 G). This was also observed by Ungethüm and Hinterberger (1978), who found a higher compressive strength for Refobacin-Palacos R than for Palacos R.

Lee et al. (1978), however, found a significant decrease in the compressive strength with an increase of added antibiotic. Edwards and Thomasz (1981) had similar results for Palacos R with (89 MPa) and without (100 MPa) antibiotic.

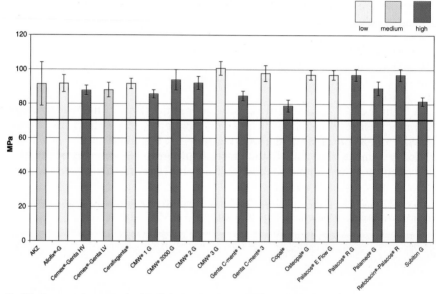

Fig. 182. Compressive strength of antibiotic cements, according to ISO 5833

3.2.4.3
Dynstat Bending Strength

Despite the doubts regarding this test because of the problematic specimens discussed in Sect. 3.2.2.3 – (Dynstat bending strength of plain cements) –, this test (and that for the impact strength) is sometimes performed, as it is easy and quick. It can easily give an idea of whether a material is usable or not. This is why

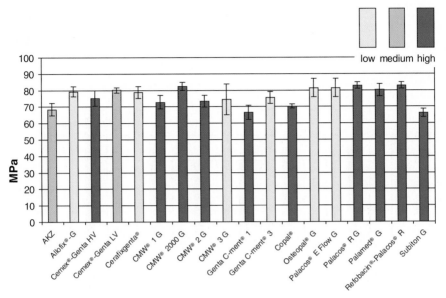

Fig. 183. Dynstat bending strength of antibiotic bone cements, according to German Industrial Standard 53435

it is routinely used as an in-process control by some manufacturers. This makes sense for a valid manufacturing process, because the product quality can readily be assured and traced in this way.

There are no big differences regarding the Dynstat bending strengths of the antibiotic cements. This is not surprising, because the specimens are not stored in water or aqueous solutions.

It can be stated that the bending strengths generally are a bit below those of the plain variants (Fig. 183). The reason is, as already mentioned, that the matrix is weakened by the added antibiotic. This clear trend shows that, despite the use of these small specimens, a reasonable comparative result is given by this method.

3.2.4.4
Dynstat Impact Strength

The tendencies of Sect. 3.2.2.4 (Dynstat impact strength of plain cements), also hold true for the antibiotic cements. The standard deviations of the individual data are relatively high. However, tests with comparable parameters can always indicate the mechanical strengths of the specimens. What this means for the in vivo situation is a different matter.

Again, the cements that were the strongest without antibiotics had the best results. This is another reason for the assumption that this test is appropriate for the judging of bone cements.

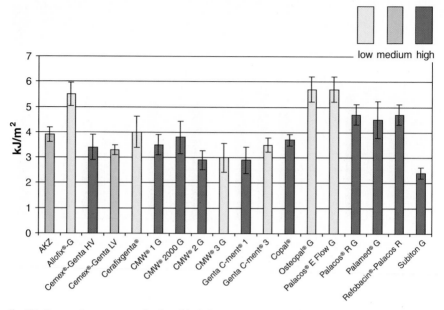

Fig. 184. Dynstat impact strength of antibiotic bone cements, according to German Industrial Standard 53435

The significant differences could be partly due to the different glass transition temperatures (T_gs). We know that co-polymers of methylacrylate (MA) and methyl methacrylate (MMA) have a low T_g and function as plasticizers in the cured cement, thus raising the impact strength. All materials on the chart (with the exception of Allofix G; Fig. 184) having a high impact strength contain co-polymers with MA and MMA in the powder.

3.2.4.5
ISO Bending Strength

All the results are quite similar for the antibiotic cements. The high standard deviations for the Cemex cements and CMW 1 G and CMW 2000 G are notable.

In our opinion, the water storage (50 h) of ISO 5833 generally does not make sense. The results for dry and water-stored samples do not differ sufficiently to justify this time-consuming preparation. The specimens should either be stored in water until saturation (3–4 weeks) before testing or they should simply be tested dry.

Using the ISO method, cements that have a slow water uptake have an advantage (Fig. 185). The differences in water absorption, though small, seem to have an influence on the ISO bending strength.

The results in Table 124 clearly show that water storage results in lower mechanical strength. These results are only available after 2 days. Using dry specimens

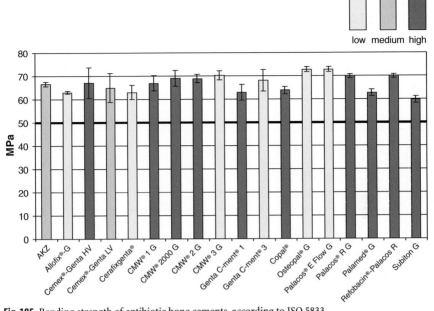

Fig. 185. Bending strength of antibiotic bone cements, according to ISO 5833

tested after 16 h, one can already have the results the next day. Moreover, the effects of the differences in water uptake during the 2-day period makes us think that this method is better in practice.

Table 124. Comparison of the four-point bending strengths and moduli of test samples stored dry for 16 h at 37°C or wet for 50 h at 37°C (Kühn and Ege 1999)

Material	Batch	Four-point bending modulus (dry, 16 h) (MPa)	Four-point bending modulus (wet, 50 h) (MPa)	Four-point bending strength (dry, 16 h) (MPa)	Four-point bending strength (wet, 50 h) (MPa)
AKZ	820287E	2789	2361	67.2	63.0
Refobacin-Palacos R	9022	3044	2681	68.7	62.9
CMW 1 G	Y070A40	2967	2379	64.3	61.6
CMW 3 G	Y069B40	3275	2624	69.1	62.7
Osteopal G	9015	3077	2625	68.9	62.9
Copal	0007	3087	2290	66.5	58.6

3.2.4.6
Modulus of Elasticity

Unlike its plain version, Subiton G is above the lower limit. The modulus of Copal (which is comparatively low; Fig. 186) might be explained by its high content of antibiotics.

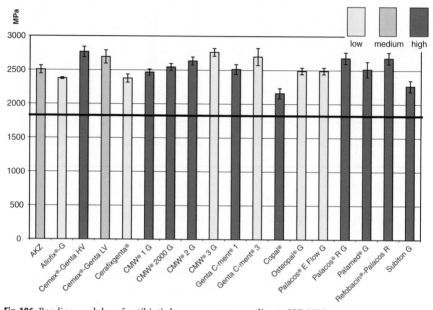

Fig. 186. Bending modulus of antibiotic bone cements, according to ISO 5833

The following scheme holds true for some mechanical tests of bone cements:

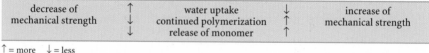

decrease of mechanical strength	↑ ↓ ↓	water uptake continued polymerization release of monomer	↓ ↑ ↑	increase of mechanical strength

↑ = more   ↓ = less

After implantation of the cement dough into the femur and curing, there are two subsequent effects: continuing polymerization, normally resulting in better mechanical strength, and absorption of water, which has a plasticizing effect and decreases the strength. Concomitant with the absorption of water, the release of residual monomer starts. Slow monomer release can result in lower mechanical strength, while rapid diffusion should have a positive influence on the mechanical strength (Hailey et al. 1994, Kühn and Ege 1999).

3.2.5
Further Comparative Studies

For the characterization of bone cements, many physical and chemical properties, in addition to the methods described in the International Standards Organization (ISO) standard, are important for surgeons. For example, the handling behaviors of the cements suggest the time at which the surgeon should insert and fix the prosthesis. If the working phase is too short or the viscosity too high, complications may occur during the operation. The handling behaviors of polymethyl methacrylate (PMMA) bone cements can easily be influenced by the factors described in Sect. 3.2.5.1. Before assuming that a material is defective, it is necessary to know which factors can influence bone-cement properties.

The molecular-weight distribution of the hardened cement (Sect. 3.2.5.2) may significantly influence the fatigue behavior (Sect. 3.2.5.3) of the bone cement. The molecular weight is influenced by the sterilization process. Therefore, the usual sterilization methods for bone cements will be briefly explained.

We will comparatively describe the amount of opacifier used in all examined cements. The differences between the different bone cements on X-rays will be shown.

Because of concerns regarding the toxicities of bone-cement components, the residual monomer release and dimethyl-p-toluidine (DmpT) release of bone cements will be compared (Sect. 3.2.5.6). In addition to fatigue testing, the glass transition temperatures (T_gs; Sect. 3.2.5.6) of all examined bone cements will be described. Finally, the release of gentamicin (Sect. 3.2.5.7) will be described in detail for all the original bone cements we have examined.

3.2.5.1
Working Time

In the following section, we will describe the working phases of all the examined bone cements, because of the importance of the working time for the surgeon. Few of the bone cements examined had a working phase longer than 3 min (Fig. 187). Some cements had a long working phase (as tested by our method; Sect. 2.2.21), but the viscosity during that time was so high that insertion of the dough and subsequent fixation of the prosthesis could not be performed easily.

Some low-viscosity cements have a relatively long working phase; this is not usual for such materials. During the working time, the viscosity varies significantly (from low to high viscosity); therefore, the time available for application is

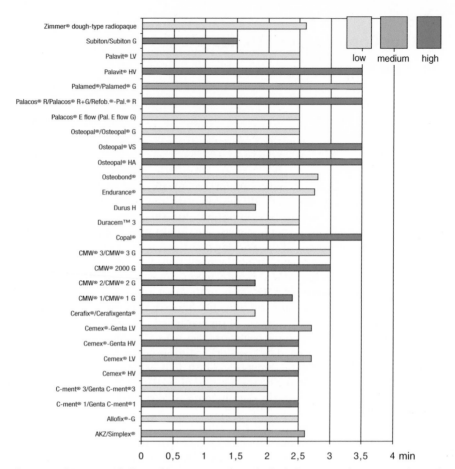

Fig. 187. Working times of all tested bone cements (23°C for both the room and components), tested according to the method described in Sect. 2.2.21

short. Palacos R, Palacos with Gentamicin, Refobacin-Palacos R, Osteopal HA, Osteopal VS, Copal, Palamed and Palamed G have a working phase longer than 3 min.

All the low-viscosity bone cements we investigated initially have a liquid wetting phase. Therefore, homogeneous mixing is easily performed. A relatively long, low-viscosity phase follows, and the nurse and surgeon have to wait for the end of the sticky phase. At the end of the working phase, the viscosities of the low-viscosity bone cements rapidly increase, so the time available for insertion and fixation is usually short. Therefore, it is observed that the dough is often inserted too early or too late when using low-viscosity bone cements. If the dough is inserted too early, the viscosity of the material is too low to prevent the dough from mixing very quickly with blood (because of the higher blood pressure). This becomes apparent when the entire prosthesis (together with the bone

Table 125. Handling times of low-viscosity bone cements (23°C for both the room and components) tested according to the method described in Sect. 2.2.21

Cements	End of sticky phase (min:s)	End of working phase (min:s)
Allofix G	3:45	6:15
C-ment3	4:00	6:00
Cemex LV	3:00	6:00
Cerafix LV	4:30	6:30
CMW 3	4:00	7:00
Duracem 3	3:45	6:15
Endurance	3:15	6:00
Osteobond	4:15	7:00
Osteopal	3:00	5:30
Palavit LV	3:00	5:30
Zimmer dough-type	4:00	6:40

cement) is pushed out by blood flowing back due to hydraulic pressure (Benjamin et al. 1987). The optimal time for application can easily be missed, because the material hardens quickly. In our opinion, such disadvantages mean that low-viscosity bone cements should only be used if the staff is well trained in the handling of such materials.

To demonstrate the problem of the short handling characteristics of low-viscosity bone cements, we have summarized all our results in Table 125. For this purpose, we have listed the time of the end of the sticky phase and that of the end of the working phase for all low-viscosity bone cements examined at 23°C in this study.

Unlike the case for high- and medium-viscosity cements, vacuum mixing (Demarest et al. 1983) of low-viscosity bone cements can only be performed under a low vacuum of approximately 550 mbar. This vacuum is not sufficient to fully eliminate the microporosity (Draenert 1988; Draenert et al. 1999). Vacuum mixing at room temperature at a pressure of 150 mbar results in boiling of the monomer due to its vapor pressure as a function of temperature. Chilling a low-viscosity bone cement before mixing to reduce its viscosity (a practice that is often used for high-viscosity bone cements) does not work because of the extremely late setting time.

For some low-viscosity bone cements, the material can only be used in mixing systems [(Allofix G, C-ment 3, Duracem 3, Genta C-ment 3, Palavit Low Viscosity (LV)]. In our opinion, this procedure may not reduce the disadvantages of the material. Nevertheless, by using low-viscosity bone cements in mixing systems only, one might easily overlook existing problems because of the lack of direct contact with the material. Therefore, the risk of an inappropriate application may increase. In addition to detailed knowledge about the material's properties, the user has to be well trained in the use of the mixing devices. Malchau and Herberts (1998) explained that the unsatisfactory clinical results of bone cements applied by a vacuum-mixing system were due to lack of experience in the use of the mixing device. The authors observed that, with increasing experience, the clinical results improve.

Krause et al. (1982) describe in detail the viscosity of the most important cement types on the market at that time. CMW 1 has the highest viscosity of all examined cements. Therefore it is only suitable for manual mixing. Simplex P is regarded as medium viscous, whereas Zimmer LVC, AKZ and Sulfix 6 are characterized as low viscous. Wixon and Lautenschlager (1998) even regard Palacos R as more viscous than CMW 1. De Wijn et al. (1976) claim that Palacos R is twice as viscous as Simplex P five minutes after start of mixing but has only one third of the viscosity of CMW 1. Ferracane and Greener (1981) also reported on the viscosity of different bone cements.

Because the handling behaviors of bone cements are important to the user, these properties have to be adjusted by the manufacturer for each batch. Therefore, it is important to know what factors can influence the handling properties of the cements (Fig. 188).

relative humidity < 40%	prolongation of working times for 1–3 min consider
	    OR-fully conditioned
	    OR-partially conditioned
	    winter: cold
	    summer: warm

storage in primary container	water-uptake through PE/paper/Tyvek change of mixing properties => better: storage in aluminum pouch
temperature of powder/liquid	at 23 °C: setting e. g. after 6–7 min (ISO) at 2–6 °C: setting e. g. after 12–14 min (ISO)
pre-warmed mixing vessel	high temp.: faster setting low temp.: delayed setting
admixing of antibiotics	inhomogeneous mixture
mixing sequence	strictly follow the package insert, else: une ven wetting of polymer => inhomogeneous mixture
mixing parameters	strictly follow the package insert, e. g. 20 ml liquid + 40 g powder, or 30 ml + 60 g or 5 ml + 10 g, else: change of cement properties
effects of resterilization – heat	destruction of benzoyl peroxide => no curing
– irradiation	fission of polymer chain, reduction of molecular weight => totally different material properties
– gas resterilization	high ethylene oxide residues can only be done using a validated ventilation programm

Fig. 188. Factors influencing the properties of bone cements. OR = operating room

If, for instance, the polymer component is stored at a relative humidity of less than 40%, the working time is prolonged. It is important to know whether the operating room (OR) is fully or partially air-conditioned. In accordance with the manufacturers' instructions, no package should be used unless it is in its original state and there are no doubts regarding the tightness of the seal.

Because of the high dependence of the polymerization on the temperature, the temperatures of the room, the components and the mixing devices have to be taken into account. A significantly lower ambient or component temperature results in slower polymerization and lower viscosity; higher temperatures have the opposite effect.

Mixing vessels may quickly warm due to handling in the OR before mixing. Draenert et al. (1999) describe the time required for the pre-cooled powder to reach the appropriate temperature.

Setting times may vary dramatically with the temperature of the room, mixing vessels or components. Meyer et al. (1973) showed the temperature dependence of the setting time for Simplex P. At an ambient temperature of 4°C, they found a setting time of 60 min; at 37°C, the material was already hardened after 3 min.

Additives mixed into the supplied cement components are very critical. In the industry, production is done with great care, following strict legal requirements to assure consistent quality. With later, manual blending of additives, there is a great risk of getting an inhomogeneous dough. The mechanical strength also drops significantly, especially when adding substances to the liquid (Lautenschlager et al. 1976).

The mixing sequence suggested by the manufacturer should be followed; otherwise, inhomogeneities may result (Draenert et al. 1999). The wetting phase is normally tested and optimized by the manufacturer, thus yielding best mixing results. One should refrain from changing the powder/liquid mixing ratio in order to influence the viscosity; otherwise, the cement properties and mechanical strength can be spoiled.

Resterilization of cement components is strictly forbidden, as all methods have different influences on the material. Heat, for example, degrades the initiator benzoyl peroxide (BPO), thus preventing polymerization. Resterilization by irradiation of powders that were originally gas-sterilized changes the cement properties by degrading the polymer chains. When resterilizing using ethylene oxide (EO) one has to consider that not all EO sterilization methods can be used, and there is a high EO absorption by the powder. The gas has to be desorbed using a valid venting procedure.

3.2.5.2
Molecular Weight

Pure PMMA was the reference (Fig. 1). Figure 189 shows the mean molecular weights, as determined via the relative viscosity. For cements containing both pure PMMA and other polymers in the powder (as is usually the case), there is a minor fault with this method.

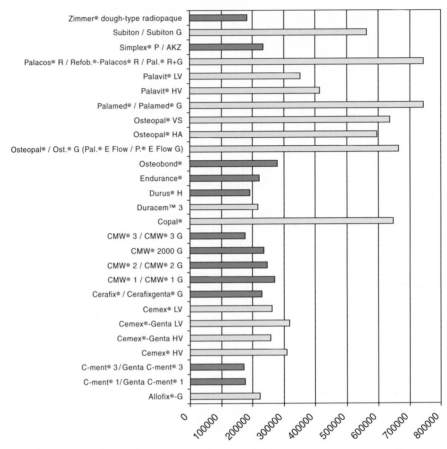

Fig. 189. Molecular weights of bone cements (▢ = EO sterilized, ▮ = Beta/Gamma-sterilized)

For other methods (such as gel-permeation chromatography, GPC), the information about the reference material is often missing. For GPC, it is normally polystyrene. Thus, there is a systematic fault, because only a few cements contain styrene as a co-monomer in the powder.

Looking at the chart, one can easily distinguish two product groups (colored different by us). The dark bars are the cements with irradiated powders.

Normally, ^{60}Co is used as γ-ray source; sometimes ^{137}Cs is used. The advantage is the high penetration depth, which allows the material to be sterilized in the final package. However, it is known that irradiation causes changes in the properties of plastic materials. Especially due to the generation of radicals and ozone, there is both chain fission and cross-linking in the polymer. While degradation is particularly relevant for chains with tertiary carbon atoms, there is a greater tendency of cross-linkage in linear chains (Koppensteiner and Pfeiffer 1993). Appropriate stabilizers may prevent such problems.

γ Irradiation is performed in a few hours. A good dose distribution (which depends on the geometric design of the plant and the dimensions of the goods) must be achieved. The normal dose is 25 kGy.

Bone cement powders always have a lower molecular weight after irradiation (below 300,000 Da). Brauer et al. (1977) and Lautenschlager et al. (1984) found a weight of approximately 242,000 Da for Simplex P. For Osteobond, Wixon and Lautenschlager (1998) found a weight of 260,000 Da. The highly energetic rays clearly reduce the initial molecular weight significantly. Thus, one can deduce that irradiated polymers must have had a much higher molecular weight before the sterilization (~400,000–500,000 Da).

Because of the different polymer structures, the handling properties of cements are quite different before and after irradiation. Actually, they are new products after irradiation. Thus, according to good manufacturing practice, it must be confirmed that the quality is reproducible from batch to batch.

The light-colored bars of Figure 189 are cements sterilized by EO. This method is very complex and is more sensitive. The residual EO also has to be desorbed from the powder using a valid process.

The inactivating effect of EO is based on the high reactivity and oxidizing properties of the molecule. Functional parts of micro-organisms are damaged irreversibly by EO. EO reacts with water to form ethylene glycol and reacts with chloride ions to form ethylene chlorohydrin (Koppensteiner and Pfeiffer 1993). The main parameters to monitor are the application time, the temperatures of the reactants and the reaction chamber, the EO concentration, the pressure and the humidity.

From the literature, it is known that EO sterilization does not affect the molecular weight (Tepic and Soltesz 1996; Lewis and Mladsi 1998). Thus, the molecular weights of Figure 189 are nearly identical to those of the initial polymer components. For Allofix G, the Cemex cements and Duracem 3, polymers with a low molecular weight of 250,000–300,000 Da are used.

The highest molecular weights are found for Copal, Osteopal (with and without gentamicin), Palacos LV/E-Flow (with and without gentamicin), Osteopal HA, Osteopal VS, Palamed, Palamed G, Palacos R (with and without gentamicin), Refobacin-Palacos R, Palavit HV/LV and Subiton (with and without gentamicin). High molecular weights for Palacos R (~800,000 Da) were also noted by Wixon and Lautenschlager (1998) and Lewis and Mladsi (1998). From what was mentioned above, it is clear that, unlike irradiated cements, those sterilized by EO undergo no change in their handling properties.

A clear relationship between the molecular weight and the quasi-static strength could not be found in our study. The following section reports the influence of the molecular weight on the fatigue strengths of low-, medium- and high-viscosity cements.

3.2.5.3
Long-Term Load-Cycling Tests

We show the individual data (test results) plotted as a Wöhler curve for Palacos R in Figure 190. For a better overview, we refrained from presenting such plots in the other figures and only show the regression curves that are relevant for comparison. The ordinate axis is the quasi-static mechanical strength of the water-saturated specimens. The stress levels are plotted against the number of cycles that the individual specimens reached before breaking. The number of cycles (abscissa axis) is plotted in a logarithmic scale. The straight lines generated in this way are fitted using linear regression, with stress as the independent variable.

The extent to which low stress levels are tested determines the length of the Wöhler curve. The slope of the curve depends very much on the average number of cycles reached at the first (highest) stress level. At this point, mistakes are often made. One should consider carefully the mean variation in the number of cycles reached at the first stress level. Of course, the mean data for the lowest level is also very important for the interpretation of the curve, although the regression should represent the mean values of all the measured data.

For all the curves, the specimens that survive the maximum number of cycles (10^7) are the most important criteria in the interpretation of the curve. Thus, a very conservative assessment is preferred. If these specimens are not taken into account, the slope of the curve is higher and the result is worse.

For this study, we intentionally refrained from testing materials using different mixing systems in order to keep the results clear. Normally, vacuum mixing gives

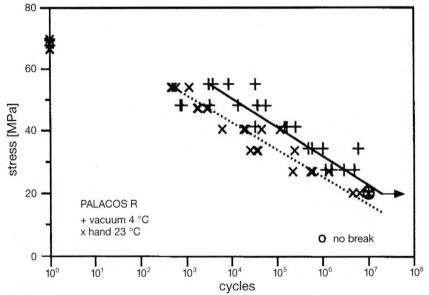

Fig. 190. Comparison of fatigue results for Palacos R, both hand mixed and vacuum mixed (Soltesz and Ege 1993)

significantly better results because of the decrease in the number and size of trapped air bubbles (Lidgren et al. 1984). Using mixing systems may be disadvantageous as a result of poor technique (which, of course, is improved by practice; Malchau and Herberts 1998).

Soltesz and Ege (1993) tested the influence of vacuum mixing on the fatigue strength of Palacos R. The material was mixed manually at 23°C and, for comparison, using a vacuum-cementing system at 200 mbar and component temperatures of 4°C.

It was shown that vacuum mixing leads to a significant increase in fatigue strength, though the quasi-static strengths are practically the same. The reason is considered to be the decrease in the number of pores in the cement dough.

However, an improvement in the fatigue behavior does not seem to be possible for all bone cements via the use of special mixing techniques. The effect seems to be smaller or non-existent if special components in the cement also influence the mechanical strength. Thus, cements with high contents of antibiotics or additional big particles do not show significant improvements as a result of vacuum mixing (Soltesz et al. 1998a, 1998b).

For this study, we compared cements with comparable initial viscosities to minimize the influence of differing miscibilities. It is known, for example, that low-viscosity cements are much less problematic in terms of pores in the dough, as are high-viscosity cements (Soltesz and Ege 1992). One criterion, of course, is a correct and steady way of mixing. We prepared all our test specimens using the same mixing vessels and spatulas. Mixing was done according to the instructions of the manufacturer and was always performed by the same person. The materials used are listed in Table 126.

Comparing the most important high-viscosity cements, CMW 1 and Palacos R, one can see that the quasi-static values differ slightly (Fig. 191). For Palacos, they are higher than for all the samples of CMW 1, as was known after tests performed according to ISO 5833 protocols. This is not significant. However, CMW 1 samples with and without antibiotics have much lower fatigue strengths than do Palacos R with and without antibiotic. Palacos R with antibiotic is even stronger than

Table 126. Bone cements used for fatigue testing

Cement (conventionally mixed)	Viscosity during mixing	Quasi-static starting point (MPa)	Strength after 10^7 cycles	Percentage of quasi-static values after 10^7 cycles
Palacos R	High	67.6	17.8	26.3
CMW 1	High	57.1	12.3	21.5
Refobacin-Palacos R	High	60.4	17.0	28.0
CMW 1 G	High	61.5	14.1	23.0
Palamed	Medium	62.0	17.6	28.0
Simplex P	Medium	60.1	14.2	23.7
Palamed G	Medium	58.6	17.4	30.0
AKZ	Medium	61.0	11.5	18.9
Osteopal	Low	65.6	26.0	40.0
CMW 3	Low	59.7	10.4	17.3
Osteopal G	Low	58.6	20.0	34.0
CMW 3 G	Low	60.0	6.2	10.4

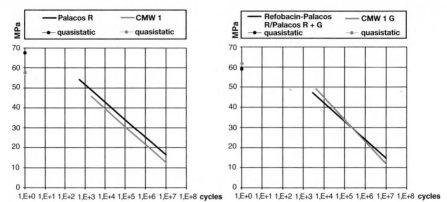

Fig. 191. Wöhler curves for high-viscosity bone cements (without and with antibiotics). Palacos R and CMW 1

plain CMW 1. The differences (given as percentages of the quasi-static values) show this clearly.

Maybe the difference can be explained by the fact that the content of gentamicin is twice as high in CMW 1 G (1.0 g base/40 g) as in Refobacin-Palacos R (0.5 g base/40 g). This is especially important because the plain variant of CMW 1 is weaker than Palacos R. Unlike Refobacin-Palacos R/Palacos R + G, the antibiotic variant of CMW 1 initially has a higher strength but weakens faster.

For the next comparison we used two bone cements (Palamed and Palamed G) which are principally regarded as high viscous. Because of their significantly lower viscosity at the time of mixing, however, they are regarded and compared in this chapter as 'medium viscous'.

For the medium-viscosity cements, we found similar results (Fig. 192). The quasi-static data were also comparable. Simplex P and Antibiotic Simplex (AKZ), however, showed significantly lower fatigue strengths compared with Palamed and Palamed G, respectively.

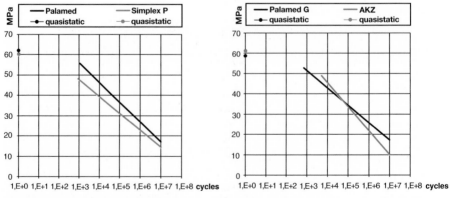

Fig. 192. Wöhler curves for medium-viscosity bone cements during mixing (without and with antibiotics). Palamed and Simplex P

Regarding the two medium-viscosity cements, it is interesting that the fatigue strengths of the plain products are almost identical to those of the cements containing antibiotics. They both have low initial viscosities enabling them to have only a low number of pores. In the subsequent medium-viscosity working phase, the cements seem to behave similarly, though the working phase is clearly longer for Palamed than for Simplex P. Maybe this kind of viscosity behavior, together with the chemical composition, is the reason for the different results during fatigue testing.

Another interesting thing is the influence of a styrene co-polymer on Simplex P and AKZ. Their water uptake seems to be slow, and the specimens are not yet water saturated after the minimum storage time of 4 weeks in water at 37°C. This means that the fatigue strength would be even worse after complete saturation with water. We will discuss this again when we talk about the T_g.

Lewis (1999) tested fatigue strength using "dog bone"-shaped specimens for a maximum of 1.5 million cycles (Fig. 193). For Simplex P, which was manually mixed, he found a fatigue strength much lower than those of Osteopal and Palacos LV. Even more dramatic is the comparison of vacuum-mixed samples: hand-mixed Osteopal/Palacos LV showed a significantly better fatigue strength than vacuum-mixed Simplex P. Though the tests of Lewis (1999) were based on different methods (dry specimens; Weibull 1951; Lewis and Mladsi 1998), his results are comparable to those seen by us.

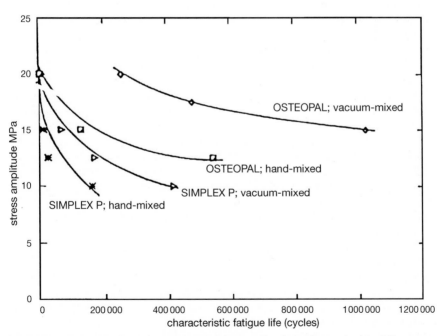

Fig. 193. Comparative fatigue data (Lewis 1999) for Osteopal and Simplex P, mixed in different ways (the plot is created as described in Weibull 1951)

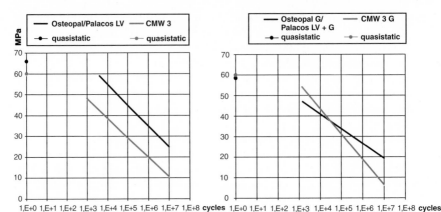

Fig. 194. Wöhler curves for low-viscosity bone cements (without and with antibiotics). Osteopal/Palacos LV/E-Flow and CMW 3

The differences are especially significant for the low-viscosity cements (Fig. 194). Plain CMW 3 already shows a low fatigue strength compared with Osteopal. For the antibiotic variants CMW 3 G and Osteopal G, the differences are even higher. As with the high-viscosity cements, the high initial strength of CMW 3 can drop dramatically. Lewis (1999) also describes very good fatigue behavior for Osteopal.

Based on inhomogeneities in the matrix, crack propagation is often cited as a cause of the failure of cement specimens under cyclic stress. Such inhomogeneities might result from the release of antibiotic from the matrix by diffusion. To determine the influence of a leached antibiotic on strength, Soltesz et al. (1999) tested the fatigue strength of Copal (which has the highest content of antibiotic and the highest release). He compared specimens stored in water (37°C) for 4–8 weeks and for 1 year.

It could be shown that the fatigue strength of Copal is not significantly lower after storage at 37°C for 1 year (Fig. 195). This is also true for the quasi-static and dynamic data.

Significantly, it can be stated that all the tested bone cements exhibited differences in their fatigue strengths that could not be expected based on their quasi-static data. Hopf et al. (1985) also come to this conclusion. Regarding the success of bone cements implanted into the human body, however, the fatigue strength is more important than the quasi-static data. Thus, based on the results of this study, we suggest that fatigue-strength testing be implemented in ISO 5833 as an additional criterion.

The reason for the big differences in the fatigue strengths of the cements is, in addition to the chemical composition, the ability of the monomer to wet the polymer as soon as possible. Thus, the quality of a cement mixture depends on its state 10–15 s after the start of mixing of the components. Furthermore, the way the antibiotics and radiopaque media are implemented in the polymer matrix can lead to significant inhomogeneities.

The molecular weight also has a significant influence on the fatigue strength (Kim et al. 1977; Tepic and Soltesz 1996; Harper et al. 1997; Lewis and Maldsi 1998;

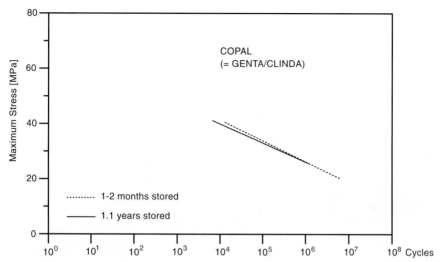

Fig. 195. Comparative fatigue data for Copal stored for different periods in water at 37°C (Soltesz et al. 1999)

Lewis 1999). Regarding the molecular weights, from Sect. 3.2.5.2, one can easily see that the cements with high fatigue strengths have molecular weights above 600,000 Da, while those with low strengths are below the critical limit of 300,000 Da.

The molecular weights of bone cements depend heavily on the way the powder component is sterilized. Palacos R, Refobacin-Palacos R, Palamed, Palamed G, Osteopal and Osteopal G all are EO sterilized, thus avoiding negative influences on the molecular weight. They all have good fatigue strengths. The cements with bad fatigue strengths in our comparison, however, are γ irradiated: CMW 1, CMW 1 G, Simplex P, AKZ, CMW 3 and CMW 3 G.

3.2.5.4
Radiopacity

Without distinct opacity, the surgeon cannot monitor the healing process clearly after a total joint replacement. Therefore, it is very difficult to notice any failure

Table 127. Characteristics of radiopaque media

	Barium sulfate	Zirconium dioxide
Chemical formula	$BaSO_4$	ZrO_2
Comments	Fine white powder	Fine white powder
	Insoluble in water and monomer	Insoluble in water and monomer
Particle diameter (μm)	20–150	1–30
Density (g/cm³)	4.5	1.8
Melting point (°C)	1580	1580
Molecular weight	233.4	123.22

early enough. This is the reason radiopaque media are added to bone cements. Thus, the hardened cement is radiopaque. Either barium sulfate or zirconium dioxide is used as an opacifier for all available bone cements (Table 127).

Adding these substances to the powder normally weakens the cement, because there is no chemical bond to the polymer matrix. Therefore, a compromise must be

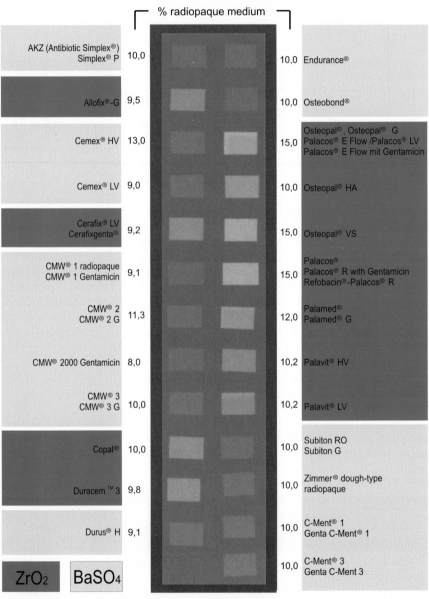

Fig. 196. X-ray opacities of all tested bone cements (40 kV, 2 mAs)

made between sufficient opacity of the cement layer in the body for easy healing control of the cemented prosthesis and the possible loss of mechanical stability.

All bone cements examined contain 8.0–15.0% opacifier in the polymer. In order to compare the bone cements, we made Dynstat samples (Sects. 2.2.13, 2.2.14) of all examined cements. Therefore, we can show the opacity graphically (Fig. 196).

Cements with barium sulfate as the opacifier show the lowest opacity. The lowest barium sulfate content is exhibited by CMW 2000 G (8.0%), whereas Cemex HV contains 13.0% barium sulfate. Most other cements with barium sulfate as the opacifier contain 10.0%. Clear differences in the opacity cannot be observed in these cements.

Compared with bone cements with barium sulfate, bone cements with zirconium dioxide have a significantly higher opacity. Bone cements with more than 15.0% zirconium dioxide in the polymer have the most distinct opacity (Osteopal, Palacos LV, Osteopal VS and Palacos products).

Even bone cements with the lowest contents of zirconium dioxide in the polymer, such as Allofix G (9.5%), have a clearly better opacity than the cements with the highest amount of barium sulfate, such as Cemex HV (13.0%). Comparing the advantages and disadvantages of the different opacifiers in experimental animals (Rudiger et al. 1978) and in more recent studies with cell cultures (Sabokbar et al. 1997; Murray et al. 1999), it can be shown that barium sulfate has more severe osteolytic properties than zirconium dioxide does.

A disadvantage of zirconium dioxide in bone cements is its abrasive property, which can lead to disastrous reactions in the implant bearings in cases of loosening of the implant. Although barium sulfate is almost insoluble, it is known to release toxic barium ions in cases of implant loosening. The precondition for this, however, is the loosening of the implant.

3.2.5.5
Residual Monomer and DmpT in the Polymerized Cement

In the bone cements examined, butyl methacrylate (BuMA) is the only monomer in the liquids aside from methyl methacrylate (MMA). The two monomers do not seem to differ much in terms of their toxicities (Revell 1992). The attention paid to the release of residual monomer from bone cements (Homsy et al. 1972; Kutzner et al. 1974a, 1974b; Scheuermann 1976; Rudigier et al. 1981; Ege and Scheuermann 1987) is based on reports describing allergic reactions (Hollander and Kennedy 1951; Fisher 1956) and the tissue toxicity of MMA (Endler 1953; Hullinger 1962; Willert 1974; Linder 1976). Thus, there was interest in searching for a direct relationship between the properties of MMA and unexplained complications arising from the use of bone cements.

Ever since bone cements have been used in surgery, respiration and circulation effects have been observed during the operation (Ling and James 1971; Schuh et al. 1973; Breed 1974; Kutzner et al. 1974b; Schlag et al. 1976; Wheelwright et al. 1993; Byrick et al. 1994; Turchin et al. 1995; Woo et al. 1995; Draenert et al. 1999), often leading to a patient's death. The explanation, in addition to effects caused by MMA, is still often thought to be emboli induced by the intramedullar increase in pressure. In animal experiments, Rudigier and Grünert (1978) showed that the problems of circulation are a direct consequence of the intramedullar increase in pressure resulting from nervous–reflective processes and not reactions of the body to monomeric MMA (Elmaraghy et al. 1998).

Use of transesophageal, two-dimensional echocardiography (Heinrich et al. 1985; Roewer et al. 1985; Ulrich et al. 1986; Zichner 1987; Wenda et al. 1987a, 1987b, 1988a and b, 1993; Christie et al. 1995) could cause emboli from air or marrow during the implantation of bone cements or the prostheses, respectively. An intramedullar increase of pressure, together with lethal complications, may occur during cementless hip operations (Hofmann et al. 1995, 1999). Today, there are adequate measures against these problems (drill holes for pressure compensation, drains), but the dangers have still not been totally eliminated in endoprosthetic surgery. Draenert et al. (1999) published new results regarding the lowering of the embolic risks.

Based on the composition of the examined bone cements, especially the powder:liquid ratio (mostly 2:1), one can state that the mixed dough contains approximately one third MMA. In the polymerized material, there is approximately 6% residual monomer, as the radical polymerization does not reach a 100% turnover. The reason for this is the rising immobility of the monomer molecules during polymerization. With increasing viscosity, chain propagation slows and finally ends, e.g., by radical recombination. Figure 197 shows the contents of residual monomers of the tested bone cements during the first 28 days.

Allofix G, Cerafix and Cerafix Genta, C-ment 1, C-ment 3 (with and without antibiotic) and Duracem 3 also contain BuMA in the liquid. Because we only tested for MMA, these cements show the lowest MMA contents in the graph.

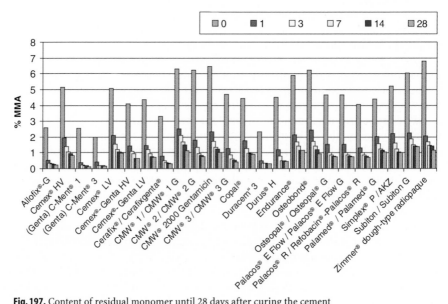

Fig. 197. Content of residual monomer until 28 days after curing the cement

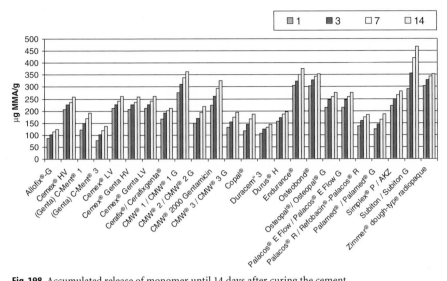

Fig. 198. Accumulated release of monomer until 14 days after curing the cement

The other cements all have 4–7% residual monomer. It can be seen that a powder/liquid ratio differing from 2:1 does not reduce the residual monomer content significantly. This also holds true for the release of monomer. BuMA is less water soluble than MMA, so it may remain in the cured cement for a longer period of time. Moreover, it can be supposed that it is metabolized slower than MMA because of its more hydrophobic structure.

We could not find a relationship between the amount and release of residual monomers and the viscosities of the cements (Fig. 198). The long, low-viscosity phase of the low-viscosity cements and the good mobilities of the monomer molecules do not result in a reduction in the amount of residual monomer. For all cements, there is a decrease of residual monomer with time.

This could be thought to lead to a total release of remaining monomer after a certain time in vivo. However, measurements of the released and remaining monomer have shown that a big part of the initial residual monomer is eliminated by continuing polymerization.

Using animal experiments (dogs and rats) with ^{14}C-marked MMA, Wenzl et al. (1973) showed that, after intravenous application of MMA, more than 90% of the injected radioactivity can be found in the exhaled air; only 5% is found in excrement and urine. Therefore, most of the monomer goes into the blood and is metabolized there quickly (Eggert et al. 1974, 1977, 1980; Cront et al. 1979; Wenda et al. 1985a, 1985b).

Methacrylic acid is first formed by hydrolysis and is then decarboxylated. The reaction with CO_2 is known (Krebs' cycle; Fig. 199; Wenzl et al. 1973).

Significantly, it is found that, of the approximately 6% initial residual monomer, more than three-fourths are consumed by continuing polymerization (Fig. 200; green). Five to six percent (Fig. 200; blue) is released, so only 10–20% of the initial 6% remains in the polymerized cement (Fig. 200; red).

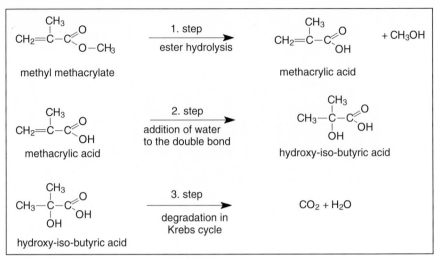

Fig. 199. Biochemical degradation of methyl methacrylate

This is consistent with the results of Ege and Scheuermann (1987), who also described in detail the decrease of residual monomer with time. Even in cements examined during re-operations many years after implantation, a residual monomer content of approximately 0.3–0.5% can be found (Kirschner 1978).

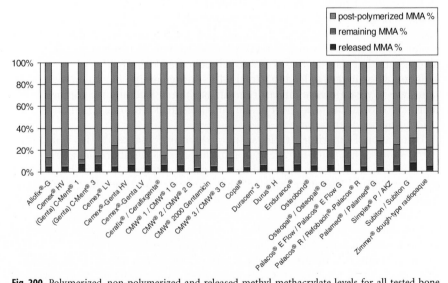

Fig. 200. Polymerized, non-polymerized and released methyl methacrylate levels for all tested bone cements (after 28 days of water storage), expressed as the percentage of the initial residual monomer content

Dimethyl-p-Toluidine

DmpT is regarded as toxic in the literature. Trap et al. (1992) and Taningher et al. (1993) say it harms chromosomes and inhibits the biosynthesis of protein. Bösch et al. (1982), Lintner et al. (1982) and Lintner (1983) report an important influence on the mineralization of bones. DmpT also might be sensitizing to the skin (Tosti et al. 1990; Dutree-Meulenberg et al. 1992; Haddad et al. 1995). A toxic effect of DmpT, however, depends very much on the amount of the substance, and cell damage is reversible in the absence of it. Stea et al. (1998) find a significant ability of cells to recover; 3 days after withdrawing the DmpT, cell growth was at its normal level. Thus, in order to judge possible effects of DmpT when using PMMA bone cements, it is important to know whether, how much and for what period of time it is released in the body.

Theoretically, the ratio of the initiators (BPO:DmpT) in bone is interesting, as are the absolute quantities of the initiators in the cements. All cements on the market have BPO contents of approximately 0.7–2.8% in the polymer. The DmpT content in the monomer is similar. A surplus of BPO may favor a complete turnover of DmpT. A surplus of DmpT, however, results in almost total consumption of the BPO, leaving a high residue of DmpT in the cement.

After setting of the cement, elution in methanol yields approximately 0.1–0.5% residual DmpT (Bösch et al. 1982, 1987; Ege and Scheuermann 1987). Bösch et al. (1987) found 0.2–0.6% DmpT more than 10 years after implantation in cement samples; they found only 0.3% in fresh specimens. Apparently, only a small part

Table 128. Release of dimethyl-p-toluidine (DmpT) from a high-viscosity and two low-viscosity bone cements during curing (Ege and Scheuermann 1987)

Time (min)	DmpT (mg) Palacos R	Palacos E flow	Zimmer bone cement
0–1	0.05	0.05	0.08
1–2	0.08	0.08	0.09
2–4	0.12	0.09	0.15
4–6	0.12	0.11	0.15
6–60	0.12	0.10	0.15

Table 129. Long-term release of dimethyl-p-toluidine (DmpT) from Palacos R at 37°C in Ringer solution (Ege and Scheuermann 1987)

Time (days)	DmpT (μg/cm^2 surface)	DmpT (μg/cm^2 surface/day)
1	0.61	0.61
2–4	0.05	0.016
5–7	0.035	0.011
8–11	0.03	0.0075
12–21	0.067	0.0067
22–42	0.065	0.0025
43–63	0.047	0.0022
64–77	0.03	0.0021

released DmpT ca. 0,1 % Ege and Scheuermann, 1987	reacted DmpT and DmpT remaining in the cement ca. 99,9% (Sato et al. 1975, Boesch et al. 1987)
Total DmpT content of all tested bone cements (0,22 - 0,88 % w/w) = 100 %	

Fig. 201. Amount of dimethyl-*p*-toluidine reacted and remaining unchanged in the cement mantles (Sato et al. 1975; Boesch et al. 1987; Ege and Scheuermann 1987)

of the DmpT is consumed during polymerization (Sato 1975). Of the remaining part, very little is released by elution, leaving the major part in the cement.

The bone cements examined contain approximately 0.22–0.88% DmpT relative to the total amount of cement. Figure 201, Table 128 and Table 129 demonstrate what was found in the literature regarding DmpT in bone cement.

DmpT is not consumed totally during polymerization. Only a small part becomes part of the polymer matrix, while the major part is desalicylated by oxidation to monomethyl-*p*-toluidine. According to Bösch et al. (1987), one can assume that almost all (99.9%) the initial DmpT remains in the cement for years without being released. This means that the risk of cell damage by DmpT when using bone cement can be neglected, especially since it is reversible (Stea et al. 1998).

3.2.5.6
Glass Transition Temperature

In order to determine the T_g, the specialist can use several methods: torsional fatigue testing, shear modulus determination and the dilatometric method (DSC). The DSC method is used most frequently and does not show significant differences between dry and water-saturated materials. The reason for this phenomenon seems to be that only small quantities of granulated material (which dry during heating; 1°C/min) are used (Ege et al., 1998a and b, 1999). The method we use gives results that can be reproduced in every respect, because we use a relatively high amount of material.

Basically, the experiments show that the T_g decreases distinctly by approximately 20°C after water absorption (Fig. 202). Although there is no change in temperature when the samples are stored in dry environment, a continuous decrease in temperature can be observed when stored in water at 37°C. However, when the samples are water-saturated, there are no further changes.

The T_g is directly proportional to the water-absorbing properties of the different examined materials. Because of the comparatively high hydrophobic properties of styrene copolymers (Fig. 205), after 24 h of storage, the examined samples of the Cemex cements, Osteobond and Simplex P have T_gs that are relatively high at first and are – in contrast to the T_gs of all the other materials – still comparatively high (~75°C) after 4 weeks of storage in water. The water absorption of the bone cements with styrene co-polymers is so slow that the T_g adapts

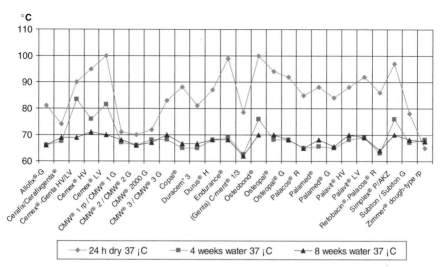

Fig. 202. Glass transition temperatures

itself correspondingly slowly to the temperatures of other cements. After 4 weeks of storage in water, however, these already show nearly the same T_gs as samples stored in water for 8 weeks. For the styrene-containing cements (CMW 2000 G and Endurance), this could not be observed. The reason could be that both cements contain distinctly less styrene than Cemex, Osteobond and Simplex P.

Thus, there were no significant changes after 4 weeks of storage. This observation could be of great importance in determining the fatigue behavior, according to Soltesz (1994), because, in these experiments, it is assumed that the samples are water saturated after storage in water at 37°C for approximately 4 weeks.

Under extreme conditions, the T_g falls approximately 20°C. All other examined bone cements are water-saturated at a temperature of approximately 70°C. This T_g is still distinctly above body temperature, so the risk of sinking of the prosthesis caused by creep is very low.

According to our observations, cements with T_gs of 40–50°C (dry specimens) could lead to disastrous clinical results, because the T_gs of the materials fall below the body temperature after water absorption. This results in considerable creeping of these cements and a higher sinking rate of the prostheses.

3.2.5.7
Release of Active Ingredients

Although there are nearly sterile conditions in modern ORs with air filtration equipment and air-lock systems, infections are still the most frequently occurring early complications after the cementing of artificial joints. It is also known that artificial implants are especially susceptible to infection at their surfaces, because the germs can then escape the natural protection of the body; thus, they can proliferate.

It is known that high concentrations of the active substances are imperative for the antibacterial effect. A single systemic dose of antibiotics after total joint replacement has the disadvantage that, between the location where the active substance is applied and the place where it must be effective, many natural barriers have to be passed. We must also consider that certain antibiotics are toxic for certain tissues or organs and that they have only a low affinity for the area of application. Antibiotics can also be inactivated or excreted too early. Inflamed, infected or necrotic areas are, in general, difficult to reach (Wahlig and Dingeldein 1976, 1980; Wahlig et al. 1984; Wahlig 1986, 1987).

When applying antibiotics locally, bone cements are the carrier matrix. The quantity of active substance released from the matrix clearly has to be above the minimum inhibiting concentration and the minimum bactericide concentration of the respective pathogens. Another advantage of local antibiotic therapy is that the organism is also protected against excessively high quantities of active substances (Elson et al. 1977, Wahlig 1986; Förster et al. 1987).

The release of antibiotics from the bone-cement matrix only depends on the surface, i.e., the release follows the laws of diffusion, which are closely related to water absorption (Wahlig et al. 1972, Marks et al. 1976). According to Wahlig and Buchholz (1972), the release of active substances is directly proportional both to the water-absorbing properties of the cement with respect to time and to the surface of the cement.

Experiments on the release properties show that all the cements at first release a relatively high amount of active substances. This release decreases distinctly within a few days. This retarding release is typical of all the examined cements. Even after 5 years, it could be proved that a very small amount of active substance

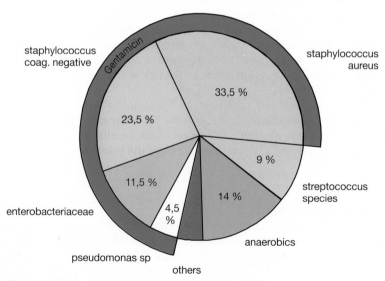

Fig. 203. Antibiotic spectrum of gentamicin (Förster et al. 1988)

is released (Wahlig et al. 1972). Because of this observation, it was feared that long-term release of active substances would favor the formation of resistant bacteria. However, numerous clinical studies soon proved that no resistant bacteria are formed when bone cements containing gentamicin are used, because even a low concentration of active substance still has a certain antibacterial effect (Lorian 1978; Atkinson and Lorian 1984).

The antibiotic used in an endoprosthetic depends decisively on the ability of the chosen active substance to destroy all possible pathogens in endoprosthetic infections. In this respect, mainly gram-positive bacteria – especially *Staphylococcus aureus*, coagulase-negative *Staphylococcus*, *Streptococcus* and aerobic/anaerobic rod bacilli – were found to be relevant. Gram-negative germs, such as *Escherichia coli*, *Enterobacter* and *Pseudomonas aeruginosa* (Förster et al. 1988), could also be examined. This range of germs is well covered by the antibiotic gentamicin (Fig. 203).

In addition to the broad spectrum of efficacy of the chosen antibiotic, its bactericidal properties are also important. Antibiotics with only bacteriostatic effects are not very suitable for this use.

In addition, the active substances have to have good release properties for the carrier matrix. The active substance is only released from the cement matrix by diffusion. In 1984, Wahlig (1987) could already show that the antibiotic gentamicin has the best release properties of 20 different antibiotics tested and out of more than ten different bone cements examined (Fig. 204). In this study, Palacos R was the material that was superior to all other bone cements in terms of the elution of antibiotics.

Further criteria for the choice of suitable antibiotics in bone cements is their heat stability because, during polymerization, higher temperature peaks, which could inactivate or even destroy the antibiotics, may occur. In addition to thermal stability, chemical stability with respect to the monomers used is also important.

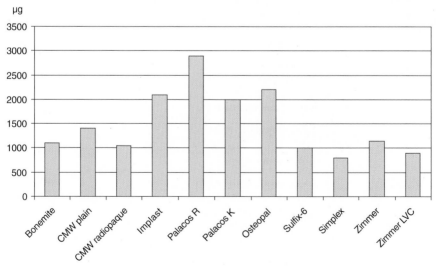

Fig. 204. Release of gentamicin from different bone cements (Wahlig 1987)

Of course, the potential for an allergic reaction to the antibiotic should be as low as possible, as should the influence of the antibiotic on the mechanical properties of the cement. With respect to these factors, gentamicin is the first choice as an antibiotic.

Therefore, it is not surprising that nearly all bone cements with antibiotics contain gentamicin. AKZ, however, is an exception. The antibiotics colistin and erythromycin, which are added to the AKZ polymer powder, do not cover the pathogen spectrum of gentamicin with their effective spectra. Also, these antibiotics act bacteriostatically but not bactericidically. Erythromycin only acts bacteriostatically. Often, there is a primary resistance to Staphylococci and Enterobacteria. The efficacy of erythromycin is generally limited to gram-positive bacteria, which only play a minor role in endoprosthetics (Pneumococci, *Clostridium* spp., Corynebacteria, α-hemolyzing streptococci of group A).

Copal, however, contains both 2.5% clindamicin hydrochloride and a 2.5% gentamicin base. Therefore, we also tested this cement in order to compare its results with the other results. In contrast to Wahlig (1987), we tested the materials of the different manufacturers directly (Fig. 206).

This comparison clearly shows that the products Copal, Osteopal G, Palacos LV G/E-Flow G, Palamed G, Refobacin-Palacos R and Palacos R with Gentamicin, which have MMA/methylacrylate (MA) co-polymers (Palacos-based products), release the active substance best. The comparably good release of Refobacin-Palacos R and Palamed G has already been described (Specht and Kühn 1998; Specht et al 1999). Basically, the chemical composition of these cements leads to comparably quick water absorption (Fig. 205). The use of pure PMMA or chemi-

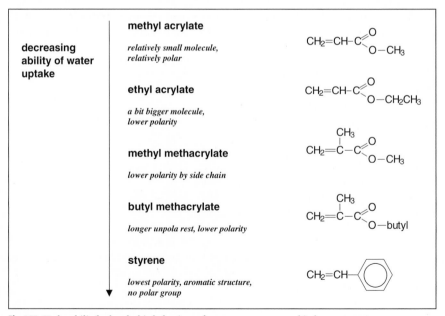

Fig. 205. Hydrophilic/hydrophobic behaviors of some monomers used in bone cements

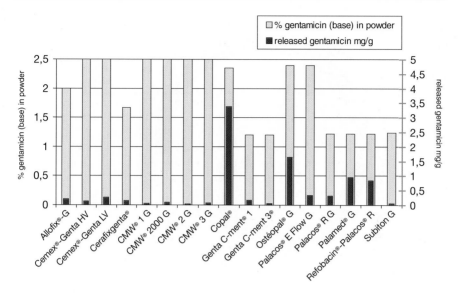

Fig. 206. Accumulated release of gentamicin after 7 days

cally changed co-polymers has a big influence on this property. MMA and ethyl-acrylate – because of their molecular structures – are superior to higher methacrylates (such as BuMA or styrene) in their ability to absorb water quickly (Fig. 205).

The diffusion properties of Palacos-based products are preferable to those of their competitors since, because co-polymers that create more positive preconditions are used. The faster the cement absorbs water, the better the active substance is released from the matrix. The quality of the active substance is as important as the compositions of the different cements. Obviously, it would not sufficient if only the active substance conformed to the pharmacopeia.

The extremely good release of gentamicin from Copal, which is also a cement with a high amount of MMA/MA co-polymer, seems to be additionally favored by the excellent release of the second active substance (Fig. 206). The excellent release properties of Copal are especially important, because this cement was primarily developed to revise infected joints. Therefore, in Copal, the antibiotic clindamicin is used in addition to gentamicin. An effective spectrum is covered by this combination, which responds to nearly 90% of all germs during total-hip replacement (Fig. 207; Kühn and Pfefferle 1998).

Osteopal G and Palacos LV/E-Flow G (two Palacos variants) also release the antibiotic relatively well. Both cements contain approximately 1 g gentamicin base in 40 g polymer powder (2.5%). Refobacin-Palacos R and Palamed G only contain 1.25% gentamicin base in the powder but still release the antibiotic excellently, and Palamed G releases slightly better than Refobacin-Palacos R (Specht and Kühn 1998). Palacos R with gentamicin also follows this tendency. The release it exhibits, however, is lower than the release exhibited by Refobacin-Palacos R.

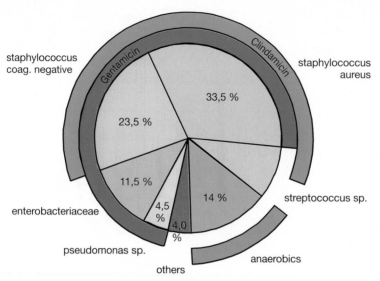

Fig. 207. Antibiotic spectrum of a gentamicin/clindamicin combination (Förster et al. 1988)

The releases of all other examined bone cements – compared with the standard material (Refobacin-Palacos R) – are significantly lower, although the amount of gentamicin per unit in some products is distinctly above those of the Palacos products. All CMW cements (with a 2.5% gentamicin base in the polymer) and the Cemex cements have the highest percentage of gentamicin base. However, their releases are extremely low and are clearly below the releases exhibited by Palacos R with gentamicin and Palacos LV G/E-Flow with gentamicin. The cements CMW 1 G, CMW 2 G, CMW 3 G and Subiton G were found to be the cements with the lowest release rates of all the examined cements.

3.2.5.8
Summarizing Evaluation

In Table 130, we have compiled some important comparative data of the examined cements in order to facilitate quick reference. As the cements passed the requirements of the standard in almost every case, the statement "passed" does not have much significance. Thus, we decided to apply more severe limits for this comparison to make the differences clearer. These were our considerations:

Setting temperature, as determined according to ISO 5833: $\leq 70°C$.

We chose a relatively low temperature, although the found data (as already mentioned in Sect. 3.1.2) do not compare with the actual temperatures reached during a cemented hip operation. One must always consider the influencing factors and the possibility of lowering the temperature, as described in the literature. However, lower maximum temperatures (according to ISO 5833) certainly mean lower temperatures in vivo. Only 14 of the cements showed temperatures at or below our limit of 70°C.

ISO compressive strength	= 70–90 MPa;
ISO elasticity modulus	= 2000–3000 MPa.

In Sect. 3.2.2.2, we explained why we think an upper limit for the compressive strength is important. Brittle materials (high modulus, high compressive strength) have not been very successful in the past. Some cements with promising quasi-static strengths, especially compressive strengths greater than 100 MPa (Sulfix 6 and Sulfix 60) are not marketed any longer. Because almost all cements passed the criteria of the standard, we applied special limits. Regarding the modulus, only three cements did not fulfil our special requirements; 16 cements were within our specifications for the compressive strength.

DIN bending strength (Dynstat):	$\geq$ 80 MPa;
DIN impact strength (Dynstat):	$\geq$ 5 kJ/m^2 (for plain products)
	$\geq$ 4 kJ/m^2 (for antibiotic products).

Dynstat testing is not part of the ISO 5833 protocol. Contrary to the ISO bending strength, which is determined using specimens stored in water at 37°C for approximately 50 h, the Dynstat test is done with dry specimens at least 16 h after preparation. This is why we set higher limits for the Dynstat bending strength. Sixteen cements passed our requirements for the bending strength, and 16 cements passed our requirements for the impact strength.

ISO bending strength:	$\geq$ 70 MPa.

With one exception, all the cements easily reached the bending strength of 50 MPa required in the standard. Thus, we raised our limit to 70 MPa or higher. Ten of the plain cements were still above that limit, but only three of the antibiotic cements were above it. The well-known reason is that the addition of antibiotics lowers the bending strength significantly.

Molecular weight (2.2.10) :	> 350.000 Da.

The importance of the molecular weight for the fatigue strengths of bone cements was described in detail in Sect. 3.2.5.3. For our limit of 350,000 Da, we referred to data from appropriate literature. Only 15 of the cements fulfil this requirement. These are all cements sterilized by EO.

Working phase (Sect. 2.2.21):	$\geq$ 3 min.

A working phase as long as possible is very important for the surgeon. However, only 12 of the examined cements exhibited a working phase at least 3 min long. Some cements, as already described, have working phases so short that application is not easy.

Table 130. Important comparative data for the examined cements

	Setting temperature ≤70°C	Compressive strength = 70–90 MPa	Modulus = 2000–3000 MPa	Bending strength (Dynstat) ≥80 MPa	Impact strength (Dynstat) without (≥5 kJ/m²) and with antibiotic (≥4 kJ/m²)	Bending strength (ISO) ≥70 MPa	Molecular weight ≥350,000 Da	Working time ≥3.0 min at 23°C	Initial content of residual monomer <5%	Release of gentamicin (AB-loaded) >2 mg/g
Antibiotic-free cements										
C-Ment 1		E	E						BuMA	
C-Ment 3			E		E				BuMA	
Cemex Isoplastic (HV)	E		E	E						
Cemex RX (LV)			E	E	E					
Cerafix LV			E		E				BuMA	
CMW 1 radiopaque			E	E						
CMW 2						E				
CMW 3			E			E		E	E	
Duracem 3		E	E	E		E			BuMA	
Durus H						E			E	
Endurance			E			E				
Osteobond			E	E		E				
Osteopal/Palacos LV/E-Flow	E	E	E	E	E	E	E		E	
Osteopal HA	E	E	E		E		E	E	E	
Osteopal VS	E	E	E	E	E	E	E	E	E	
Palacos R		E	E	E	E	E	E	E	E	
Palamed	E		E	E	E		E	E	E	
Palavit HV	E		E		E		E	E		
Palavit LV	E		E		E		E			
Subiton		E					E			
Surgical Simplex P		E	E							
Zimmer dough-type cement	E	E	E							
Antibiotic-loaded cements										
AKZ			E							
Allofix G			E		E				BuMA	
Cemex Genta HV		E	E						E	
Cemex Genta LV		E	E	E					E	
Cerafix Genta	E		E		E				BuMA	
CMW 1 G		E	E							
CMW 2 G			E							
CMW 2000 G			E	E				E		
CMW 3 G			E					E	E	
Copal		E	E				E	E	E	E
Genta C-ment 1		E	E						BuMA	
Genta C-ment 3			E						BuMA	
Osteopal G	E		E	E	E	E	E		E	E
Palacos LV G/E-Flow G	E		E	E	E	E	E		E	E
Palacos R with Gentamicin			E	E	E	E	E	E	E	E
Palamed G	E	E	E	E	E		E	E	E	E
Refobacin-Palacos R			E	E	E		E	E	E	E
Subiton G	E	E	E				E			

BuMA, butyl methacrylate; *E*, fulfils the requirements

Table 131. Criteria for the judgement and registration of bone cements (McDermott 1997) in the USA, as specified by the Food and Drug Administration

Property	Parameter/test method	Standard/method (alternatives)
Chemical composition	Raw materials	NMR (if in the liquid phase), FTIR, HPLC/MS
	Added components	Ash
	Purity	ICP/MS, GC/FTIR/MS, titration
Molecular weight	Relative viscosity (h)	Viscosimetry
	Molecular weight	GPC (polystyrene standard)
Physical properties	Morphology	Light microscopy; SEM
	Porosity	Scanning acoustical microscopy, X-ray
	Aging due to water uptake	ISO 5833 (bending strength)
Handling properties	Doughing time	ISO 5833, ASTM F451
	Setting time	ISO 5833, ASTM F451
	Intrusion/viscosity	ISO 5833, ASTM F451
Polymerization	Maximum temperature	ISO 5833, ASTM F451
	Shrinkage	Density balance, pycnometer (ASTM D2566)
Degree of polymerization	Content of residual monomer	GC, HPLC/GPC, FTIR
	Release of residual monomer	GC, HPLC/GPC
Stability	Monomer stability (enforced)	ISO 5833, ASTM F451
	BPO content	Titration, FTIR
	Doughing/setting time	ISO 5833, ASTM F451
Modulus of elasticity	Four-point bending	ISO 5833
Compression modulus	Compression	ISO 5833
Tensile modulus	Tensile strength	ASTM D638
Fatigue	Tensile/compression fatigue; tensile/tensile fatigue	ASTM D638
	Four-point bending	Method of Dr. Soltèsz, ASTM E399
Fracture toughness	Compact tension/notched bending strength	ASTM E399
Fatigue-crack propagation	Compact tension	ASTM E647
Static strength		ISO 5833
Flexural strength	Four-point bending	ISO 5833
Compressive strength	Uniaxial compression	ISO 5833, ASTM F451
Tensile strength	Uniaxial tension	ASTM D638
Shear strength	Cement–cement shear; ement–implant shear	ASTM D732
Viscoelasticity	DMA/compressive creep	DMA/ASTM D2990
Shelf life	Mechanical properties of the hardened cement	

ASTM, American Society for Testing and Materials; *BPO*, benzoyl peroxide; *DMA*, dynamic mechanical analysis; *FTIR*, Fourier-transform infrared spectroscopy; *GC*, gas chromatography; *GPC*, gel-permeation chromatography; *HPLC*, high-performance liquid chromatography; *ICP*, inductively coupled plasma; *MS*, mass spectrometry; *NMR*, nuclear magnetic resonance; *SEM*, scanning electron microscopy

Content of residual monomer (2.2.7):	≤ 5%.

In our opinion, this value (1 h after curing) should be below 5%. For most of the cements, it is between 4% and 7%; for 16 cements, the monomer content is below 5%. Eight of the cements containing BuMA in their liquid of course have much lower residual monomer contents. They could not be implemented in the comparison.

Release of gentamicin (2.2.8):	> 2 mg/g.

We chose a limit of greater than 2 mg/g. Only six of the cements fulfilled this requirement. In the USA, basic requirements for the registration of bone cements exist (Table 131); these could be a basis for revisions of the standard in the future (McDermott 1997).

In this section, we would like to give an impression of the extent of the efforts that may be necessary for registrations and batch releases in the future. One can see that new products have to pass high hurdles in order to be marketed. Because of the critical uses of bone cements, this is appropriate. However, it has to be determined whether tests can be shortened and simplified while maintaining safety and assuring quality.

References

AMG, Gesetz über den Verkehr mit Arzneimitteln, ECV Editio Cantor Verlag, Aulendorf. 1998

ASTM . Specification F 451–76. Standard specification for acrylic bone cement. Annual Book of ASTM Standards: Medical Devices; Emergency Medical Services. Philadelphia, PA: American Society for Testing and Materials. 1978

Atkinson, B.A., Lorian, V.: Antimicrobial agent susceptibility patterns of bacteria in hospitals from 1971 to 1982. J. Clin. Microbiol. 20, 791–796, 1984

Bargar, W. L., Heiple, K. G., Weber, S., Brown, S. A., Brown, R. H., Kotzar, G.: Contrast bone cement. J. Orthop. Res. 1, 92–120. 1983

Benjamin, J.B., Gie, G.A., Lee, A.J.C., Ling, R.S.M.: Cementing technique and the effect of bleeding. J. Bone Joint Surg, Br. 69, 620–624, 1987

Biehl, G., Harms, J., Hanser, U.: Experimentelle Untersuchungen über die Wärmeentwicklung im Knochen bei der Polymerisation von Knochenzement. Arch.orthop. Unfall-Chir.: 78, 62–69 1974

Bishop, N.E., Ferguson, S., Tepic, S.: Porosity reduction in bone cement at the cement-stem interface. J Bone Joint Surg, Br, 78-B, 349–356, 1996

Bösch, P., Harms, H. Lintner, F.: Nachweis des Katalysatorbestandteiles Dimethylparatoluidin im Knochenzement, auch nach mehrjähriger Implantation. Arch. Toxicol. 51, 157–166, 1982

Bösch, P., Harms, H., Lintner, F.: Zur Toxizität der Knochenzementbestandteile. In: Willert, H.-G., Buchhorn, G.: Aktuelle Probleme in der Chirurgie und Orthopädie, Band 31, Knochenzement, 87–89, 1987.

Brauer, G. M., Termini, D. J., Dickson, G.: Analysis of the ingredients and determination of the residual components of acrylic bone cements. Biomed. Mat. Res. 11, 577–607, 1977

Breed, A. L.: Experimental production of vascular hypotension and bone marrow and fat embolism with Methylmethacrylate Cement. Clin. Orthop. 102, 227–244, 1974

Breusch, S.J., Draenert, K., Draenert, Y., Boerner, M., Pitto, R.P.: Die anatomische Basis des zementierten Femurstieles, Z Orthop. 137, 101–107, 1999

Buchholz, H. W., Engelbrecht, E.: Über die Depotwirkung einiger Antibiotika beim Vermischen mit dem Kunstharz Palacos. Chirurg 41, 511–515, 1970

Buchholz, H. W., Elson, R. A., Engelbrecht, E., Lodenkämper, H., Röttger, J., Siegel, A.: Management of Deep Infection of Total Hip Replacement. J. Bone and Joint Surg. 63 B, 342–353, 1981

Burke, D. W., Gates E. I., Harris, W. H.: Centrifugation as a method of improving tensile and fatigue properties of acrylic bone cement. J. Bone Joint Surg. 66, 1265–1273, 1984

Byrick, R.J., Mullen, J.B., Mazer, C.D., Guest, C.B. Transpulmonary systemic fat embolism: studies in mongrel dogs after cemented arthroplasty. Am J Respir Crit Care Med, 150, 1416–1422, 1994.

Charnley, J.: Anchorage of the femoral head prosthesis of the shaft of the femur. J. Bone Joint Surg. 42 Br: 28–30, 1960

Charnley, J.: Acrylic cement in orthopaedic surgery. Baltimore: Williams and Wilkins, 1970.

Christie, J., Robinson, C. M., Pell, A. Ch., McBirnie, J., Burnett, R.: Transcardiac echocardiography during invasive intramedullary procedures. J Bone Joint Surg. Br: 77 B, 450–455, 1995

Connelly, T. J., Lauenschlager, E. P., Wixson, R. L.: The role of porosity in shrinkage of acrylic cements. Transactions of the 13th Meeting of Society, 12, 114, 1987

Cront, D. M. G., Corkill, J. A., James, M. L., Ling, R. S. M.: Methylmethacrylate metabolism in man. Clinical Orthop. and Rel. Res. 141, 90–95, 1979

Davies, J. P., Jasty, M., O'Connor, D. O., Burke, D. W., Harrigan, T. P., Harris, W. H.: The effect of centrifuging bone cement. J. Bone Joint Surg. 71B, 39–42, 1989

Davies, J. P., O'Connor, D. O., Burke, D. W., Harris, W. H.: Comparison of the diametral shrinkage of centrifuged and uncentrifuged Simplex P, Proc. 16th Annu. Mtg. Soc. Biomater. Charleston, SC; 23, 1990

Debrunner, H. U.: Untersuchungen zur Porosität von Knochenezementen. Arch. Orthop. Unfall-Chir. 86, 261–278 , 1976

Demarest, V. A., Lautenschlager, E. P., Wixson, R. L.: Vacuum mixing of methylmethacrylate bone cement. Trans. Soc. Biomat. 6, 37, 1983

De Wijn, J. R., Sloof, Th. J. J. H., Driessens, F. C. M.: Characteriziation of bone cements. Arch. Orthop. Unfall-Chir. 72, 174–184, 1972

De Wijn, J. R., Driessens, F. C., Slooff, T. J.: Dimensional behavior of curing bone cement masses. J. Biomed. Mat. Res. 9, 99–103, 1975a

De Wijn, J. R., Slooff, T. J., Driessens, F. C.: Characterization of bone cements. Acta Orthop. Scand. 46, 38–51, 1975b

DIN 53435: Prüfung von Kunststoffen, Biegeversuch und Schlagbiegeversuch an Dynstat-Probekörpern. Normenausschuß Kunststoffe (FNK) im DIN e.V., Normenausschuß Materialprüfung (NMP) im DIN, 1983

Draenert, K.,: Zur Praxis der Zementverankerung. Forschung und Fortbildung in der Chir. des Bewegungsapp. 2, München: Art and Science, 1988

Draenert, K., Draenert, Y., Garde, U., Ulrich, Ch.: Manual of cementing technique. Springer Verlag, Heidelberg, 1999

Dutree-Meulenberg, R. O., Kozel, M. M., van Joost, T.: Burning mouth syndrome: A possible etiologic role for local contact hypersensitivity. J Am Acad Dermatol, 26, 935–940, 1992

Edwards, R. O.: Thomas, F. G. V.; Evalution of acrylic bone cements and their performance standards. J Biomat Mat Res 15, 543–551, 1981.

Ege, W.: Knochenzement. In: Planck, H., Kunststoffe und Elastomere in der Medizin, Kohlhammer GmbH, Stuttgart, 112–121, 1993

Ege, W.: Material properties of PMMA bone cements. In: Buchhorn, G.H. and Willert, H.-G. (Herausg.), Technical Principles, Design and Saftety of Jont Implants. Hogrefe & Huber Verlag, Göttingen, 49–53, 1994.

Ege, W.: Twenty five years experience in the development of bone cement. In: Bone Cement and Cement Techniques. Eds. G. H. I. M. Walenkamp, Marbella, 1999, in press

Ege, W., Scheuermann, H.; Freisetzung von Restmonomer und N,N-dimethyl-p-toluidin aus Knochenzementen während der Aushärtung und bei Langzeitlagerungen – Eine in-vitro-Untersuchung. In: Willert, H.-G., Buchhorn, G (Hrsg.), Aktuelle Probleme in der Chirurgie und Orthopädie, Band 31, Kochenzement, 79–82, 1987

Ege, W., Kühn, K.-D., Maurer, H., Tuchscherer, Chr.: Physical and chemical properties of bone cements. In: Biomaterials in Surgery, ed. by G.H.I.M. Walenkamp, Thieme-Verlag, Stuttgart, 39–42, 1998a

Ege, W., Kühn, K.-D., Maurer, H., Tuchscherer, Chr.: Glass transition temperature of various bone cements. Abstracts: North Sea Biomaterials, The Hague, NL, 177, 1998b

Ege, W., Kühn, K.-D., Maurer, H., Tuchscherer, Chr.: Glass transition temperature of various bone cements. J. Mater. Sci.: Mater. Med., in press, 2000

Eggert, A., Huland, H., Runke, J., Seidel, H.: Der Übertritt von Methylmethacrylat-Monomer in die Blutbahn des Menschen nach Hüftgelenksersatzoperationen. Chirurg 45, 236–242, 1974

Eggert, A., Seidel, H., Wittmann, D. H.: Beitrag zur Pharmakokinetik von Methylmethacrylat Monomer aus Knochenzementen. Der Chirurg 48, 316–318, 1977

Eggert, A., Eckert, W., Seidel, H.: Zur Ausscheidung von Knochenzementmonomer in der Atemluft. Arch. Orthop. Traumat. Surg. 97, 221–224, 1980

EG-GMP-Richtlinien, in: EG-GMP-Leitfaden einer guten Herstellpraxis für Arzneimittel, ECV Editio Cantor Verlag, Aulendorf, 5. Auflage. 1998.

Elmaraghy, A, Humeniuk, B, Anderson, G.I., Schemitsch, E.H., Richards, R.R.: The role of methylmethacrylate monomer in the formulation and haemodynamic outcome of pulmonary fat emboli. J.Bone Jont Surg, Br, 80-B, 156–161, 1998.

Elson, r. A., Jephcott, A. E., McGechie, D. B., Verettas, D.: Antibiotic-loaded acrylic cement: J. Bone Joint Surg. 59 B, 200–205, 1977

Endler, F.: Die allgemeinen Materialeigenschaften der Methylmethacrylat-Endoprothesen für das Hüftgelenk und ihre Bedeutung für die Spätprognose einer Hüftarthroplastik. Arch. Orthop. Unf. Chir. 46, 35, 1953

Eriksson, R.A., Albrektsson, T.: The effect of heat on generation. An experimental study in the rabbit using bone growth chamber. J Oral Maxillofac Surg, 42, 707–711, 1984

Eyerer, P., Jin, R.: Title Influence of mixing technique on some properties of PMMA bone cement. J. Biomed. Mat. Res., 20, 1057–1094, 1986

Feith, R.: Side-effects of acrylic cement implanted into bone. A histological, (micro)angiographic, fluorescense-microscopic and autoradiographic study in rabbit femur. Acta Orthop. Scand. Suppl., 161, 1975

Ferracane J. L., Greener, E. H.: Rheology of acrylic bone cements. Biomat. Med. Dev. Artif. Organs, 9:213–224, 1981

Fisher, A. A.: Allergic sensitization of skin and oral mucosa to acrylic resin denture materials. J. prosth. Dent. 6, 593, 1956

Foerster,G. v., Buchholz, H. W., Lodenkämper, H, Lodenkämper U.: Antibiotika und Knochenzement – die lokaltherapeutische Bedeutung. In: Willert, H.-G., Buchhorn, G (Hrsg.), Aktuelle Probleme in der Chirurgie und Orthopädie, Band 31, Kochenzement, 227–233, 1987

Foerster, G. v., Buchholz, H. W., Heinert, K.: Die infizierte Hüftendoprothese – Spätinfektion nach der 6. postoperativen Woche. In: Cotta, H, Braun, A (Hrgs.), 124–135, 1988

Haas, S. S., Brauer, G. M., Dickson, G. A.: Characterization of polymethyl-methacrylate bone cement. J. Bone Joint Surg (Am), 57 A, 380–391, 1975

Haboush, E. J.: A new operation for arthroplasty of the hip based on biomechanics, photoelasticity, fast setting dental acrylic and other considerations. Bull. Hosp. It. Dis N.Y.14, 242, 1953.

Haddad, F. S., Lvell, N. J., Dowd, P. M., Cobb, A. G., Bentley, G.; Cement hypersensitivity: A cause of aseptic loosening. J. Bone Joint Surg, 77B, 329–330, 1995

Hailey, J. L., Turner, I. G., Miles, A. W., Price, G.: The effect of post-curing chemical changes on the mechanical properties of acrylic bone cement. J. Mater. Sci.: Mater. Med. 5, 617–621, 1994

Hansen, D., Jensen, J. S.: Prechilling and vacuum mixing not suitable for all bone cements. Handling characteristics and exotherms of bone cements. J. Arthroplasty 5, 287–290, 1990

Hansen, D., Jensen, J. S.: Mixing does not improve mechanical properties of all bone cements. Manual and centrifugation-vacuum mixing compared of 10 cement brands. Acta Orthop. Scand. 63:13–18 1992

Harper, E.J., Braden, M., Bonfield, W., Dingeldein, E., Wahlig, H.: Influence of sterilization upon a range of properties of experimental bone cements. J. Mat. Sci.; Materials in Medicine, 8, 849–853, 1997

Havelin, L. I., Espehaug, B., Vollset, S. E., Engesaeter, L. B.: Early aseptic loosening of uncemented femoral component in primary total hip replacement: a series based on the Norwegian Arthroplasty Register, J. Bone Joint Surg. 77B, 11–71, 1995a

Havelin, L. I., Espehaug, B., Vollset, S. E., Engesaeter, L. B.: The effect of cement type on early revision of Charnley total hip prosteses. J. Bone Joint Surg. 77A, 1543–1550, 1995b

Heinrich, H., Kremer, P., Winter, H., Wörsdorfer, O., Ahnefeld, F. W.: Transoesophageale zweidimensionale Echokardiographie bei Hüftendoprothesen. Anaestheses 34, 118–123, 1985

Henrichsen, E., Jansen, K., Krogh-Poulson, W.: Experimental investigation of the tissue reaction to acrylic plastics. Acta orthop. Scand 22 , 141–146, 1953

Hofmann, S., Hopf, R., Huemer, G., Kratowill, C., Koller-Strametz, J., Schlag, G., Salzer, M.: Modified surgical technique for reductionof bone narrow spilling in cement-free hip endoprosthesis. Orthopäde., 24(2), 130–137, 1995

Hofmann, S., Hopf, R., Mayr, G., Schlag, G., Salzer, M.: In vivo femoral intramedullary pressure during uncemented hip arthroplasty. Clin-Orthop. 360, 136–146, 1999

Hollander, L., Kennedy R. M.: Dermatitis caused by autopolymerizing acrylic restoration material. Dent. Dig. 57, 213, 1951

Homsy, C. A., Tullos, H. S., Anderson, S. M., Differante, N. M., King, J. W.: Some physiological aspects of prothesis stabilization with acrylic polymers. Clin. Orthop. 83, 317–328, 1972

Hopf, Th., Zell, J., Sellier, Th., Hanser, U.: Methodik der Dauerschwingfestigkeitsprüfung von PMMA-Knochenzementen. Med.-orthop.-Techn 105, 20–25, 1985

Hullinger, L., Untersuchungen über die Wirkung von Kunstharzen in Gewebekulturen. Arch. Orthop. Unf. Chir. 54, 581, 1962

Huiskes, R.: Some fundamental aspects of human joint replacement. Analyses of stresses and heat conduction in bone-prosthesis structures. Acta Orthop. Sand., 185 (Suppl), 1980

ISO. International standard 5833/1: Implants for Surgery-Acrylic Resin Cements. Orthopaedic Application. 1979

ISO. International standard 5833/2: Implants for Surgery-Acrylic Resin Cements. Orthopaedic Application. 1992

Jasty, M., Jensen, N. F., Harris, W. E.: Porosity measurements in centrifuged and uncentrifuged commercial bone cement preparations. Poster presentation: 2nd World Congress of Biomaterials, Washington, 1984

Jasty, M., Davies, J. P., O'Connor, D. O., Burke, D. W., Harrigan, T. P., Harris, W. H.: Porosity of various preparations of acrylc bone cements, Clin. Orthop. Rel. Res. 259, 122–129, 1990

Jasty, M., Maloney, W. J., Bragdon, C. R., O'Connor, D. O., Zalenski, E. B., Harris, W. H.:
The initiation of failure of cemented femoral components of hip arthroplasties. J. Bone Joint Surg. 73 B, 551–558, 1991

Judet, J., Judet, R.: The use of an artificial femoral head for arthroplasty of the hip joint. J. Bone Surg. 32 Br, 166, 1956.

Keller , J.C., Lautenschlager E.P.: Experimantal attempts to reduce acrylic porosity. Biomat Med Dev Art Org., 11, 221–236, 1983.

Kiaer, S.: Preliminary report on arthroplasty by use of acrylic head. Cliniquièm congrès international de Chirurgie orthopèdique, Stockholm, 1951

Kim, S.L., Skibo, M., Manson, J.A., Hertzberg, R.W.: Fatigue crack propagation in polymethyl-methacrylate: effect of molecular weight and internal plasticization. Polymer Engineering and Science, 17 (3), 194–203, 1977

Kindt-Larsen, T., Smith, D. B., Jensen, J.S.: Innovations in acrylic bone cement and application equipment. J.Appl. Biomat. 6, 75 – 83, 1995

Kirschner, P.: Experimentelle Untersuchungen mechanischer und chemischer Eigenschaften von Knochenzementen nach Langzeitimplantation im menschlichen Körper.

Habilitationsschrift, Mainz, 1978

Kleinschmitt, O.: Plexiglas zur Deckung von Schädellücken. Chirurg. 13, 273, 1941

Kock, H.J., Specht, R., Kühn, K.-D., Ege, W.: Rationale for Palamed®/Palamed® G – a new bone cement. In: Bone Cement and Cement techniques, Marbella, Ed. G.H.I.M. Walenkamp., in press, 1999.

Könning, H, Ackermann, T, Seifert, C, Wirth, C.J.: Peroperative Kostenanalyse zementierter versus nicht-zementierter Hüfttotalendoprothesen zum klinischen und ökonomischen Management. Z. Orthop. 135, 479–485, 1997.

Koppensteiner, G., Pfeiffer, M.: Sterilisationsverfahren und deren kunststoffgerechte Anwendung. In: Planck, H.: Kunststoffe und Elastomere in der Medizin. Kohlhammer-Verlag, Stuttgart Berlin Köln, 1993

Krause, W., Krug, W. Miller, J.: Cement bone interface effect of cement technique and surface preparation. Orth. Transactions 4, 204, 1980

Krause, W. R., Miller, J., Ng, P: The viscosity of acrylic bone cements. J. Biomed. Mater. Res. 16:219–243, 1982

Kühn, K.-D.: Distribution of vesicular-arbuscular mycorrhizal fungi on a fallow agriculture site. II. Wet habitat. Angew. Botanik 65, 187–203, 1991.

Kühn, K.-D. and Pfefferle, H.J.: A gentamicin/clindamicin containing bone cement. Abstracts: North Sea Biomaterials, The Hague, NL, 168, 1998

Kühn, K.-D., Specht, R., Ege, W., Kock, H.J: Mechanical properties of bone cements. In: Bone Cement and Cement techniques, Marbella, Ed. G.H.I.M. Walenkamp, in press, 1999.

Kühn, K.-D. and Ege, W.: Influence of a change of storage conditions in ISO 5833 on the mechanical results. Abstracts: North Sea Biomaterials, Bordeaux-Arcachon, F, 1999

Kummer, F. J.: Bone cements: effects of pressurization on structure and mechanical properties. Trans Orthop Res Soc, 21, 245–149, 1974

Kusy, R. P.: Characterization of self-curing acrylic bone cement. J. Biomed. Mater. Res. 12, 271–305, 1978

Kutzner, F., Dittmann E. Ch., Ohnsorge, J.; Atemeffekte durch Knochenzement auf Methylmethacrylatbasis. Z. Orthop. 112, 1053–1062, 1974a

Kutzner, F., Dittmann, E. Ch., Ohnsorge, J.: Restmonomerabgabe von abhärtendem Knochenzement. Arch. Orthop. Unf. Chir. 79, 247–253, 1974b

Labitzke, R, Paulus, H.: Intraoperative Temperaturmessungen in der Hüftchirurgie während der Polymerisation des Knochenzementes Palacos. Arch. Orthop. Unfall-Chir. 79, 341–346, 1974

Lautenschlager, E. P., Jacobs, J.J., Marshall, G.W., Meyer, P.R. Jr.: Mechanical properties of bone cements containing large doses of antibiotic powders. J Biomed Mat Res 10, 929–938, 1976

Lautenschlager, E. P., Strupp, S. I., Keller, J. C.: Structure and properties of acrylic bone cement. In: Duchaynep Hasting G. W. ed.: Functional behavior of orthopaedic biomaterials, vol II. Applications, CRC Series in structure-property relationships of biomaterials. Boca Raton. FL: CRC Press, 1984

Lee, A. C. J., Ling, R. S. M., Wrighton, J. D.: Some properties of polymethylmethacrylate with reference to its use in orthopaedic surgery. Clin. Orthop. 95, 281, 1973

Lee, A. J. C., Ling R. S., Vangal, S. S.: Some clinically relvant variables affecting the mechanical behaviour of bone cement. Arch. Orthop. Traumat Surg, 92, 1–18, 1978

Lehmann, R. A., Jenny, M.: Tierexperimentelle und histologische Ergebnisse bei der Frakturleimung mit dem Polyurethanpolymer Ostamer® Schweiz. Med. Wochenschr. 91, 908-914, 1961

Lewis, G.: Properties of acrylic bone cements: state-of-the-art-review. J Biomed Mater Res (Appl Biomater) 38, 155–182, 1997

Lewis, G.: Relative influence of molecular weight and mixing method on the fatique performance of acrylic bone cement: Simplex®P versus Osteopal®. In: Bone cement: Practice & Progress, Kings College Hospital, London, 1999.

Lewis, G., Austin, G. E.: Mechanical properties of vacuum-mixed acrylic bone cement. J. Appl. Biomater. 5, 307–314, 1994

Lewis, G., Mladsi, S.: Effect of sterilization method on properties of Palacos® R acrylic bone cement. Biomaterial 19, 117–124, 1998

Lidgren, L., Drar, H., Moller, J.: Strength of polymethylmethacrylate increased by vacuum mixing. Acta Orthop. Scand. 55, 36–541, 1984

Linden, U.: Porosity in manually mixed bone cement. Clin Orthop, 231:110–112, 1988

Linder, L. G., Harthon, L., Kullberg, L.: Monomer leakage from polymerizing acrylic bone cement. An in vitro study on the influence of speed and duration of mixing, cement volume and surface area. Clin. Orthop. 119, 242–249, 1976

Linder, L: Reaction of bone of the acute chemical trauma of bone cement. J. Bone Joint Surg., 59 A, 82–87, 1977

Lindner, L.: Tissue reaction to Methylmethacrylate Monomer. Acta orthop. Scand 47, 3–10, 1976

Lindwer, J., van den Hooff, A.: The infuence of acylic bone cement on the femur of the dog. Acta Orthop Scand, 46, 657–671, 1975

Ling, R. S. M., James, H. L.: Blood pressure and bone cement. Brit. Med. J 1971 II, 404, 1971

Lintner, F., Bösch, P., Brand, G.: Histologische Untersuchungen über Umbauvorgänge an der Zement-Knochengrenze bei Endoprothesen nach 3–10jähriger Implantation. Path. Res. Prac. Res. 173, 376, 1982.

Lintner, F.: Die Ossifikationsstörung an der Knochenzement-Knochengrenze. Acta. Chir. Austr. Suppl. 48, 1983.

Lorian, V.: Effects ofsubinhibitory concentrations of antibiotics. 10. Int. Congr. of Chemotherapy, Zürich, Proceedings: Current Chemotherapy, Am. Soc. for Microbiol. Washington, D.C.,1 72–74, 1978

Marks, K. E., Nelson, C. L., Lautenschlager, E. P.: Antibiotic impregnated bone cement. J. Bone Joint Surg. 58 A, 358–364, 1976

Malchau, H., Herberts, P.: Prognosis of Total Hip Replacement. Surgical and Cementing Technique in THR: A Revision-Risk Study of 134.056 Primary Operations. Scientific Exhibition, 63rd Annual Meeting of the American Academy of Orthopaedic Surgeons, Atlanta, USA. 1996

Malchau, H., Herberts, P.: Prognosis of Total Hip Replacement. Scientific Exhibition. Presented at the 65th Annual Meeting of the American Academy of Orthopaedic Surgeons, New Orleans, USA. 1998

McDermott, B.: Darft – Preclinical testing of PMMA bone cement, FDA-guidance, 1997

MPG (Medizinproduktegesetz): Gesetz über Medizinprodukte vom 2. August 1994 sowie Erstes Gesetz zur Änderung des Medizinproduktegesetzes (1. MPG-ÄndG) vom 11. August 1998

Meyer, P. R. jr., Lautenschlager, E. P., Moore B. K.: On the setting properties of acrylic bone cement. J. Bone Joint Surg. 55 A, 139–156, 1973

Miller, J., Krause W. R.: The effect of viscosity on intrusion and handling of bone cement. Orthop. Trans. 5, 352–353, 1981

Mjöberg, B., Franzen, H., Selvik, G.: Early detection of prostethic-hip loosening. Comparison of low- and high-viscosity bone cement. Acta Orthop Scand 61 (3), 273–274, 1990

Mjöberg, B.: Loosening of the cemented hip prosthesis. The importance of heat injury. Acta Orthop. Sand. Suppl, 221, 1986

Müller, K.: A practice orientated study of the complex „Processing and handling – Application-Resultant Properties of autopolymerizing PMMA bone cements". Werkstofftech 10, 30–36 (1979)

Murray, D., Sabokbar, A., Fujikawa, Y., Athanasol, N.: Radio-opaque agents and osteolysis. In: Bone Cement and Cement techniques, Marbella, Ed. G.H.I.M. Walenkamp., in press, 1999.

Oest, L., Müller, K., Hupfauer, K.: Die Knochenzemente. Ferdinand Enke Verlag Stuttgart, 1975

Rau, H.: Plastische Deckung deformierter Schädeldefekte. Arch Chir, 304, 926–929, 1963.

Reckling, F. W., Dillon, W. L.: The bone-cement interface temperature during total joint replacement. J Bone Joint Surg, 59 A, 80–82, 1977

Revell, P., George, M. Braden, M., Freeman, B., Weightman, B.: Experimental studies of the biological response to a new bone cement, I. Toxicity of n-butylmethacrylate monomer compared with methylmethacrylate monomer. Jour. Mat. Sci: Mat.in Med., 3, 84–87, 1992.

Rimnac, C. M., Wright, T. M., McGill, D. L.: The effect of centrifugation on the fracture properties of acrylic bone cements. J. Bone Joint Surg. 68A, 281–287, 1986

Roewer, N., Beck, H., Kochs, E. Kremer, P., Schröder, E. Schöntag, H., Jungbluth, K. H., Schulte am Esch, J.: Nachweis venöser Embolien während intraoperativer Überwachung mittels transoesophagealer zweidimensionaler Echokardiographie. Anästh. Intensivther. Notfallmed. 20, 200–205, 1985

Rudigier, J., Grünert, A.: Tierexperimentelle Untersuchungen zur Pathogenese intraoperativer Kreislauf- und Atmungsreaktionen bei der Implantation sogenannter Knochenzemente in die Markhöhle eines Röhrenknochens. Arch. Orthop. traumat. Surg. 91, 85–95, 1978

Rudigier, J., Scheuermann, H., Kotterbach, B., Ritter, G.: Restmonomerabnahme und –freisetzung aus Knochenzementen. Unfallchirurgie 7, 132–137, 1981

Sabokbar, A, Fujikawa, Y, Murray, D.W., Athanasou, N.A.: Radio-opaque agents in bone cement increase bone resorption. J. Bone Jount Surg., Br, 79-B, 129–134, 1997

Saha, S., Pal, S.: Mechanical properties of bone cement: a review. J. Biomed. Mater. Res 18, 435–462, 1984

Sato, T., Keta, S., Otsu, T.: A study an initiation of vinyl polymerization with diacylperoxide-tertiary amine systems by spin trapping technique. Macrmol. Ch., 176, 561, 1975.

Scheuermann, H.: Bestimmung des Monomergehaltes von Knochenzementen und Bestimmung der Monomerfreisetzung an wässrigen, physiologischen Medien während der Verarbeitungsphase und im ausgehärteten Zustand. Ingenieurarbeit Fachhochschule Fresenius, Wiesbaden, 1976

Scheuermann, H., Ege, W.: Aufbau und Zusammensetzung handelsüblicher Knochenzemente. In: Willert, H.-G., Buchhorn, G.: Aktuelle Pürobleme in der Chirurgie und Orthopädie, Band 31, Knochenzement, 17–20, 1987.

Schlag, G.-, Schliep, H.-J., Dingeldein, E., Grieben, A., Ringsdorf, W. Sind intraoperative Kreislaufkomplikationen bei Alloarthroplastiken des Hüftgelenks durch Methylmethacrylat bedingt? Anaesthesist 25, 60–67, 1976

Schreurs, D. W., Spierings, P. T. J., Huiskes, R., Slooff, T.J. J. H.: Effect of preparation techniques on the porosity of acrylic cements. Acta Orthop. Scand. 59, 403–409, 1988

Schuh, F. T., Schuh, S. M., Viguera, M. G., Terry, R.N.: Circulatory changes following implantation of Methylmethacrylate Bone Cement. Anaesthesiology 39, 455–457, 1973

Soltész, U.: The influence of loading conditions on the lifetimes in fatigue testing of bone cements. J. Mater. Sci.: Mater. Med. 5, 654–656, 1994

Soltész, U. und Ege, W.: Fatigue behavior of different acrylic bone cements. Fourth World Biomaterial Congress, Berlin, 90, 1992.

Soltész, U. und Ege, W.: Influence of mixing conditions on the fatigue behaviour of an acrylic bone cements. 10. Europ. Conf. of Biomaterials., Davos, 138, 1993.

Soltész, U., Schäfer, R., Kühn, K.-D.: Effekt of vacuum mixing on the fatigue behaviour of particle containing bone cements. Abstracts: North Sea Biomaterials, The Hague, NL, 69, 1998a.

Soltész, U., Schäfer, R., Kühn, K.-D.: Einfluß von Anmischbedingungen und Beimengungen auf das Ermüdungsverhalten von Knochenzementen. 1. Tagung des DVM-Arbeitskreises "Biowerkstoffe", 89–94, 1998b

Soltész, U., Schäfer, R., Kühn, K.-D.: Fatigue behaviour after aging of a bone cement with high content of antibiotics. Abstracts: North Sea Biomaterials, Bordeaux-Arcachon, 1999.

Specht, R and Kühn, K.-D.: Palamed® and Palamed® G: new bone cements. Abstracts: North Sea Biomaterials, The Hague, NL, 169, 1998.

Specht, R., Kühn, K.-D, Kock, H.J: Mechanical testing of Palamed. In: Bone Cement and Cement techniques, Marbella, Ed. G.H.I.M. Walenkamp, 1999.

Stea, S., Granchi, D., Zolezzi, C., Ciapetti, G., Visentin, M., Cavedagna, D., Pizzoferrato, A.: High-performance liquid chromatography assay of N,N-dimethyl-ptoluidine release from bone cements: evidence for toxicity. Biomaterials 18, 243–246, 1997.

Taningher, M., Pasquini, R., Bonatti, S.: Genotoxicity analysis of N,N-dimethyl-p-toluidine. Environ Mol Mutagen, 21, 349–356, 1993

Thanner, J., Freij-Larsson, C., Karrholm, J., Malchan, H., Wesslen, B.: Evaluation of Boneloc chemical and mechanical properties. Acta Orthop. Scand. 66, 207–214, 1995

Tepic, S., Soltész, U.: Influence of gamma sterilization on the fatigue strength of bone cement, Proc. 42nd ORS, Atlanta, GA; 445, 1996

Toksvig-Larsen, S., Franzen, H., Ryd, L.: Cement interface temperature in hip arthroplasty. Acta Orthop. Scand. 62, 102–105, 1991

Tosti, A., Bardazzi, F., Piancastelli, E., Basile, G. P.: Contac stomatitis due to N,N-dimethyl-paratoluidine. Contac Dermatitis, 22, 113–115, 1990

Trap, B., Wolff, P., Steen Jensen, J.: Acrylic bone cements: residuals and extractability of methacrylate monomers and aromatic amines. J Apll Biomater, 3:51–57, 1992

Turchin, D. C., Anderson, G. I., Schemitsch, E. H., Byrick, R. J. Mullen, B. M., Richards, R. R.: Pulmonary and systemic fat embolization following medullary canal pressurization. Trans Orthop Res Soc, 20, 252, 1995

Ulrich. Ch., Burri, B., Wörsdorfer, O., Heinrich, H.: Intraoperative Transoesophageal Two-dimensional Echocardiography in Total Hip Replacement. Arch. Orthop. traumat. Surg. 105, 274–278, 1986

Ungethüm, M., Hinternberger, J.: Die Normung von Implantatwerkstoffen am Beispiel Knochenzemente. Z. Orthop. 116, 303–311, 1978

Vieweg, R. Esser, F.: Polymethylmethacrylate. C. Hauser Verlag, München, 1975.

Wahlig, H.: Die Geschichte der Biomaterialien als Wirkstoffträger. MPS, Berichte aus der Pharma-Forschung 6, Mainz, 1986.

Wahlig, H.: Über die Freisetzungskinetik von Antibiotika aus Knochenzementen – Ergebnisse vergleichender Untersuchungen in vitro und in vivo. In: Willert, H.-G., Buchhorn, G (Hrsg.), Aktuelle Probleme in der Chirurgie und Orthopädie, Band 31, Kochenzement, 221–226 (1987)

Wahlig, H., Buchholz, H. W.: Experimentelle und klinische Untersuchungen zur Freisetzung von Gentamycin aus einem Knochenzement. Chirurg. 43: 441–445 (1972)

Wahlig, H., Hameister, W., Grieben A.: Über die Freisetzung von Gentamycin aus Polymethylmethacrylat. Langenbecks Arch. Chir. 331, 169–212, 1972

Wahlig, H., Dingeldein, E.: Gentamicin in Alloarthroplastic. Clinical and Experiment results. Chemotherapie 1, 189–193, 1976

Wahlig, H., Dingeldein, E.: Antibiotics and Bone Cements. Experimental and Clinical Long-Term Oberservations. Acta Orthop. Scand. 51, 49–56, 1980

Wahlig, H., Dingeldein, E., Buchholz, H. W., Buchholz, M., Bachmannn, F.: Pharmakokinetic Study of Gentamicin based cement in total hip replacements. J. Bone and Joint Surg., 66 B, 175–179, 1984

Wang, J.-S., Franzèn, H., Jonsson, E., Lidgren, L.: Porosity of bone cement reduced by mixing and collecting under vacuum. Acta Orthop. Scand. 64, 143–146, 1993

Wang, J. S., Franzèn H., Toksvig-Larsen, T.: A comparison of seven bone cement mixing systems. Acta Orthop. Scand. 65 (suppl. 260), 62, 1994

Wang, J.-S., Franzèn, H., Toksvig-Larsen, S., Lidgren, L.: Does vacuum mixing of bone cement affect heat generation? Analyses of four cements brands. J. Appl. Biomater. 6, 105–108, 1995

Weibull, W.A.: Statistical distribution function of wide applicability. J. Appl. Mech., 18, 293, 1951

Weber, S. C., Bargar, W. L.: A comparison of the mechanical properties of Simplex, Zimmer, and Zimmer low viscosity bone cement. Biomater. Med. Devices Artif. Org. 11, 3–12, 1983

Wenda, K, Rudigier, J., Scheuermann, H., Weitzel, E.: How to avoid circulatory reactions in total hip replacements with bone cement. 11th Annual Meeting of the Society for Biomaterials, San Diego, Transactions, Vol. VIII: 125, 1985a

Wenda, K., Rudigier, J., Scheuermann, H., Biegler, M: Pharmakokinetic of methylmethacrylat monomer during total hip replacement in man. 2nd International Conference on polymers in medicine, Capri, 1985b

Wenda, K., Grieben, A., Rudigier, J., Scheuermann, H.: Pharmakologische Effekte und Kinetik von Methylmethacrylat-Monomer. In: Willert, H.-G., Buchhorn, G., Aktuelle Probleme in der Chirurgie und Orthopädie, Band 31, Knochenzement, 83–86, 1987a

Wenda, K., Issendorf, W. D. v., Rudigier, J., Ahlers, J.: Blood pressure decrease after bone cement – effect of monomer or intramedullary pressure? 13th Annual Meeting of the Society for Biomaterials, New York, Transactions, Vol. X: 220, 1987b

Wenda, K., Ritter, G., Rudigier, J., Degreif, J.: Der intramedulläre Druck während Marknagelosteosynthesen. Chirurgisches Forum 88 f. experim. u. klin. Forschung. In: Schriefers, K. H., et al. (Hrsg.), Springer-Verlag, Berlin, Heidelberg, 153–158, 1988a

Wenda, K., Scheuermann, H., Weitzel, E., J. Rudigier: Pharmacokinetics of Methylmethacrylate monomer during total hip replacement in man. Arch.orthop. traumat. Surg. 107, 316–321, 1988b.

Wenda, K., Degreif, J., Runkel, M., Ritter, G.: Pathogenesis and prophylaxis of circulatory reactions during total hip replacement. Arch Orthop Trauma Surg, 112, 260–265, 1993

Wenzl, H., Garbe, A, Nowak H.: Experimentelle Untersuchungen zur Pharmakokinetik von Methylmethacrylat. In: Erlacher, PH., Zemann, L, Spitzy, K. H. (Hrsg.),1–16, 1973

Wheelwright, E.F., Byrick, R.J., Wigglesworth, D. F. et al.: Hypotension during cemented arthroplasty: Relationship to cardiac output and fat embolism. J Bone Joint Surg (Br), 75 B, 175–203, 1993

Willert, H. G.: Die quantitative Bestimmung der Abgabe von monomerem Methylmethacrylat verschiedener Knochenzemente an das umliegende Gewebe während der Polymerisation. Batelle Information 18, 48, 1974

Willert, H.-G, Buchhorn, G.: (Hrsg.): Knochenzement: Werkstoff, klinische Erfahrungen, Weiterentwicklungen. Aktuelle Probleme in Cirurgie und Orthopädie, Bd. 31: Huber Verlag, Bern, Stuttgart, Toronto, 1987

Wiltse, L.L., Hall, R.H., Stenehjem, J.C.: Experimental studies regarding the possible use of self curing acrylic in orthopaedic surgery. J Bone Joint Surg, 39-B, 961–972, 1957.

Wixson, R. L., Lautenschlager, E. P., Novak, M.: Vacuum mixing of methylmethacrylate bone cement. 31st Annual Orthop. Res. Soc. (ORS). Meeting in Las Vegas, 1985

Wixson, R. L., Lautenschlager, E. P., Novak, M. A.: Vacuum mixing of acrylic bone cement. J. Arthroplasty 1, 141–149, 1987

Wixson, R. L., Lautenschlager, E. P.: 9. Methyl Methacrylate. In: The adult hip, Ed. Callaghan, J.J., Rosenberg, A.G., Rubash, H.E. Lippincott-Raven Publisher, Philadelphia, 135–157, 1998

Woo, R., Minster, R.J. jr., Fitzgerald, R., Mason, L:D: Lucas, D.R., Smith, F.E.: Pulmonary fat embolism in revision hip arthroplasty. Clin Orthop 319, 41–53, 1995

Worringer, E., Thomaslke, G.: Über die plastische Deckung von Schädelknochendefekten mit autopolymerisierender Kunstharzmasse. Eine neue Schnellmethode. Arch. Psychiatr Nervenkr 191, 100–113, 1953

Zichner, L.: Embolien aus dem Knochenmarkkanal nach Einsetzen von intramedullären Femur kopfendoprothesen mit Polymethylmethacrylat. In: Willert, H.-G., Buchhorn, G (Hrsg.), Aktuelle Probleme in der Chirurgie und Orthopädie, Band 31, Kochenzement, 201–205, 1987

Subject Index